PATIENT
HEAL THYSELF

DESTINY IMAGE BOOKS BY JORDAN RUBIN

Essential Oils

Planet Heal Thyself

Maker's Diet Meals

The Maker's Diet

The Joseph Blessing

Re-size America

The Maker's Diet Revolution

PATIENT
HEAL THYSELF

A Remarkable Health Program Combining
ANCIENT WISDOM
with Groundbreaking Clinical Research

JORDAN RUBIN

DESTINY IMAGE® PUBLISHERS, INC.
P.O. Box 310, Shippensburg, PA 17257-0310
"Promoting Inspired Lives."

This book and all other Destiny Image and Destiny Image Fiction books are available at Christian bookstores and distributors worldwide.

For more information on foreign distributors, call 717-532-3040.
Reach us on the Internet: www.destinyimage.com.

ISBN 13 TP: 978-0-7684-4352-3
ISBN 13 eBook: 978-0-7684-4353-0
ISBN 13 HC: 978-0-7684-4355-4
ISBN 13 LP: 978-0-7684-4354-7

For Worldwide Distribution, Printed in the U.S.A.
1 2 3 4 5 6 7 8 / 22 21 20 19 18

IMPORTANT NOTICE

This book is not intended to provide medical advice or to take the place of medical advice and treatment from your personal physician. Readers are advised to consult their own doctors or other qualified health professionals regarding treatment of their medical problems. Neither the publisher nor the author takes any responsibility for any possible consequences from any treatment, action, or application of medicine, supplement, herb, or preparation to any person reading or following the information in this book. If readers are taking prescription medications, they should consult with their physicians before beginning any nutrition or supplementation program.

DEDICATION

To all people afflicted with illnesses that leave them fearful and hopeless and who suffer needlessly and don't experience the abundant life we were all meant to enjoy. This book and my prayers go out to each and every one of you.

CONTENTS

Part III: Health and Healing

FOREWORD

by

Dr. Josh Axe, DC, CNS, DNM

Best-selling author of *Eat Dirt: Why Leaky Gut May Be the Root Cause of Your Health Problems and 5 Surprising Steps to Cure It*

I'm indebted to Jordan Rubin in many ways, but what I will never forget is how I was inspired by the principles of his "Maker's Diet" when my mother was facing a life-threatening disease—breast cancer—more than a decade ago.

I was twenty-four years old, in school training to become a physician and working as a nutritionist outside of Orlando, Florida, when I received a phone call from home. My mother, Winona, was on the line, and she sounded upset.

"What's wrong, Mom?" I asked.

"The cancer has come back," she said through sniffles.

Back when I was in seventh grade and growing up in Dayton, Ohio, Mom had first learned she had breast cancer when she was just forty-one years old. The prognosis was so serious that she underwent a total mastectomy of her left breast and started four tough cycles of chemotherapy that greatly weakened her. Seeing my mother suffer so greatly led me to say to myself, *I never want to see Mom or anyone else go through chemotherapy again.*

My mother proved to be a fighter and eventually recovered, but the cancer left its calling card. A gym teacher at a local public school, Mom felt lousy every single day, which left her depressed.

Hearing her distressed voice again shook me back to the present. "My oncologist told me they found a tumor on my lungs that was 2.5 centimeters," my mother said. "He wants to do surgery and start radiation and chemotherapy right away."

I expressed my sorrow and did my best to encourage my mother. From my studies in the medical field, I knew we had to stop feeding the cancer cells and get to the root cause of the disease. "Your body can heal itself from cancer, but you'll have to follow a detailed plan that I lay out for you."

I decided to fly home to Dayton immediately. When we sat down in the living room, I asked her about any symptoms she had been experiencing and other health problems. Mom replied that she had been dealing with multiple food sensitivities and had been diagnosed with hypothyroidism, but it was her last health symptom that shocked me.

"I've been having an average of one bowel movement a week for the last ten years," she said.

"Why didn't you say something earlier?" I asked.

"Because I thought it was normal."

"One or two bowel movements a week is definitely *not* normal, but we can do something about that."

Mom needed to clean up her diet. I explained that we were going to start all over in her pantry and refrigerator—out with the old processed foods and anything in a box and in with new organic foods, especially organic fruits and vegetables as well as wild-caught salmon and pasture-raised chicken.

This is where Jordan Rubin was a big help. I knew Jordan through mutual friends, and when I reached out to him, he suggested that I have my mom start taking a probiotic supplement with soil-based organisms (SBOs). Known as "good bacteria," or probiotics, SBOs increase the absorption of nutrients and improve bowel function.

Mom—who knew her days could be numbered—followed my diet and lifestyle advice to the letter. The SBOs helped her constipation problems tremendously. She began having one bowel movement every day and lost twenty-two pounds. A big smile returned to her face.

When my mom went in for another biopsy, not only was her blood work normal, but her cancer markers dropped dramatically. Because her largest tumor had shrunk by 52 percent, her doctors told her that they were postponing surgery. Mom completed a radiant health comeback, and I'm deeply appreciative of the role that Jordan played in helping her defeat a significant disease that nearly took her life. I must also mention that Jordan's discovery of SBOs inspired me to write my best-selling book, *Eat Dirt*.

Jordan is no stranger to comeback stories like my mother's because he is a living example of someone who was at death's door yet persevered to make a health comeback that ranks as one of the most dramatic natural healing stories ever told.

Although Jordan came from a family that stressed a healthy diet, his own deteriorating dietary habits while a student at Florida State University may have contributed to the onset of his nearly terminal case of Crohn's disease. Once the diagnosis had been made, initial medical treatments, which consisted of massive doses of intravenous and oral antibiotics and anti-inflammatory drugs, only exacerbated his condition.

Faced with his own battle to stay alive, Jordan searched the world for answers. He learned about the amazing dietary secrets employed by our ancestors that allowed them to live long, disease-free lives. Most of all, his consumption of beneficial microbes found in pristine soils helped him return to excellent health.

But even greater than his own healing journey are the secrets of health and longevity that Jordan has gathered together for the benefit of all humanity. Throughout *Patient Heal Thyself*, Jordan shares the concepts of ancient healing that have been lost through time and modernity but are absolutely essential to becoming—and staying—healthy.

In Jordan's prescription for health, you'll find nutritional treasures that are far more powerful than simply your run-of-the-mill vitamins and minerals. Primitive dietary essentials such as health-giving phytochemicals found in herbs and whole foods, the ever-important essential fats, and, of course, the role of SBOs are all part of the healthy diet. Jordan calls his eating program the Maker's Diet, which will be explained in detail in this profound work.

I truly believe the information in the chapters ahead will form the foundation for your journey to super health or recovery from disease. That's why I encourage you to enjoy *Patient Heal Thyself* and to pay close attention.

Your health and the health of your loved ones may depend on it.

INTRODUCTION

by

Jordan Rubin

Everyone flocks to see today's heroes play music to thousands of adoring fans, dunk a basketball with thunderous power, or glide their way to Olympic gold in the downhill skiing event.

We see these modern-day heroes at their best, at their shining moments, standing on the crest of the mountain looking down at the rest of us. But think for a moment. These heroes each put in thousands of hours of sweat, toil, and failures with no screaming fans to encourage them. They made sacrifices far beyond what any of us have made. They swam hundreds of laps in cold pools in the wee hours of the morning while we were still asleep. They played music in dingy clubs to a handful of people who weren't even paying attention to them. They practiced day in and day out, even when their friends were out having fun.

The common denominator in the lives of these superstars was an insatiable drive and determination to succeed. The truth is that the chance of any one of us becoming a rock star, an all-star basketball player, or an Olympic gold medalist is smaller than winning the lottery.

I believe that the process of overcoming an incurable illness is much the same as training for and winning the Olympics. The individuals who have the courage to take charge of their own health have the unending determination to make the near impossible sacrifices it takes to be one of the select few who beat illness and choose life. They are today's true heroes.

My own healing journey from death's door to a return to super health was not an easy one. I made a lot of mistakes along the way. But I know in the end that my journey produced lasting changes in my life, and I hope that by sharing what I have learned with you, you can take charge of your own health and realize your body's phenomenal potential.

In the midst of life's trials and tribulations, we often ask why God would allow us to go through such ordeals. But I now know more than ever, God would never allow anyone to suffer like I did without a divine plan.

The fact is, I went through a real-life "hell" and nearly died. I truly believe, though, that this was part of God's plan so that I might become your teacher and show you, as well as others, how to regain your birthright of great health.

In the pages that follow, you will learn the health secrets that allowed our ancestors to live long, disease-free lives. You will learn how to regain your health if you've lost it or how to maintain the excellent health that you currently enjoy and even slow premature aging.

But let me warn you. Some of the recommendations in this book may surprise you. In fact, many of my instructions fly in the face of what "they" are telling you. The "they" are the traditional medical establishment and many governmental agencies. If a politically correct approach to health and nutrition is what you're looking for, you've come to the wrong place. If you're looking for an optimal health plan for you and your family that is validated by history, science, and our Creator, however, then buckle up. You're in for a wild ride!

If I had to boil my message down to one sentence, it would be this: *No matter what health challenges plague you today, there is hope for an answer.* It's time to get armed with powerful truths from our Creator. It's time to provide your body with the nutritional tools it needs to regenerate from head to toe. The time is now.

Patient, heal thyself!

PART I

PATIENT HEAL THYSELF

1

THE JOURNEY

There I was, standing on the field at Doak Campbell Stadium at Florida State University, doing the tomahawk chop with my fellow cheerleaders and 80,000 screaming fans as our Seminoles marched their way to their first-ever NCAA national championship.

The year was 1993. Life couldn't have been better. I was an eighteen-year-old freshman on an academic and athletic scholarship, with more friends than I could spend time with and a member of a great fraternity. In my spare time, I was a soloist in a traveling singing group and a quarterback for my intramural football team. I lived with seven of my friends in a house just outside of campus. Life was great.

Then, it happened.

The summer after my freshman year, I was working as a counselor at a day camp in Central Florida to earn extra money. I remember the afternoon I first started getting sick. I was riding on a bus with the kids at camp. I was feeling sleepy, which was unusual for me because I usually had an energy level that rivaled the Energizer Bunny. I just kept going and going and going. At one point, though, while riding on the bus, I actually fell asleep.

"Jordan, Jordan! Wake up!"

One of the kids was shaking me to wake me up, which was embarrassing. Unfortunately, falling asleep at inopportune times such as this became a regular occurrence for me. I also became frequently tired during the day and lacked energy.

Shortly after my noticeable loss of energy, I remember getting terrible stomach cramps that had me running to the bathroom several times a day with diarrhea. Before long, frequent trips to the toilet were routine for me. Even though I was feeling lousy, I didn't want to admit it to myself. Getting sick didn't really fit into my schedule, if you know what I mean.

In fact, I even decided to attend a week-long overnight camp, in spite of my need to be close to a toilet. What was I thinking? Camping out in the summer heat of Florida is tough enough on a healthy person. My nausea was making me feel even worse, and the usual camp "chow" wasn't helping. I found myself gulping iced tea and beating a well-worn path to the outdoor bathrooms.

The next fact I want to tell you is quite startling. In seven days, I lost twenty pounds. That's *twenty* pounds in one week. For some people, losing twenty pounds in a week would be a dream come true. But for me, it was a nightmare. I remember trying to tackle a friend of mine during a camp football game and getting trampled. I realized how much weaker I had become. At this point, I had to face reality to a certain extent. Something was really wrong with me.

Like a seasick passenger on a long bumpy boat ride, my upset stomach was constant. I became completely dehydrated, and my mouth felt like I had a large ball of cotton stuffed in it. My gums were riddled with canker sores and ulcers.

I had become so sick and fatigued that I couldn't even make it through one week of overnight camp. I had to have someone drive me four hours south to my family's home in Palm Beach Gardens. When I got there, I was in denial. I hugged my mom and dad and did my best to hide my illness from my parents, which was sort of dumb because my father is a naturopathic doctor.

Actually, I *had* to hide my illness. If my parents had any idea how sick I really was, they would have made me go to the hospital. Or worse, they would not have let me go back to school, and the new semester was starting in only ten days. This was my sophomore year, and I was sure that if I could hang on until school started, everything would be fine. I just needed to get back into the swing of things.

Without telling my parents, I visited a family doctor in our community. I detailed my symptoms—nausea, constant diarrhea, weight loss, cotton-mouth, and fatigue. That was just the beginning of my list.

The doctor put me through a series of tests looking for viruses, including the HIV virus that causes AIDS, but none were detected. He ordered a stool culture that came back negative and prescribed a course of antibiotics for me to take. Neither the doctor nor I ever asked why I had developed severe digestive problems.

Looking back, I sure wish I or someone else had. I mean, I don't want to sound like a bad sport or an ungrateful patient, but when something goes wrong, it's often a good idea to find out *why*. In any event, I took the antibiotics with me on my return to school. Unfortunately, my condition only worsened, and I began experiencing even more severe gastrointestinal problems.

I did everything I could to ignore what was happening to my body. I kept busy by trying to go to class, but I had to discontinue all of my extracurricular activities. I was forced to quit the cheerleading squad and the fraternity I was joining. I also had to quit studying to pass my American College of Sports Medicine exam in preparation for becoming a fitness professional.

I weighed about 145 pounds at that time, down from my normal 175 to 180 pounds. As the days went by, my health worsened. I was falling apart. I was running fevers of 104 degrees every night. I barely slept because I was getting up to run to the bathroom all night.

To make matters worse, my gastrointestinal problems had become systemic, affecting my joints. My hip constantly popped out of its socket whenever I did anything. I would suffer minor dislocations even getting in and out of cars. I remember the situation became so severe that my hip popped out once as I was walking to class. I was forced to turn around and go back to my house rental.

Before I left for school, my father had given me a cache of dietary supplements to take with me back to college. As a naturopath, my father was taught to work with the whole person and to use safe and natural, nontoxic healing methods.

While exploring this collection one afternoon, I saw that he had given me probiotics, digestive enzymes, and other herbal and nutritional dietary products. I didn't know much about nutritional supplements. I did, however, believe that these products would help me get well. Perhaps I made myself believe that.

Thus began my "magical mystery tour" of alternative medicine. Besides these first nutritional supplements, I also tried different diets. After I discovered that the cotton feeling in my mouth was oral thrush, which was linked with candida infection, I tried several anti-candida diets. My father also put me on the Specific Carbohydrate Diet, which was purported to have been used successfully to treat people with Crohn's disease, ulcerative colitis, irritable bowel syndrome (IBS), celiac disease, cystic fibrosis, and chronic diarrhea.

The premise of the Specific Carbohydrate Diet is that damage done to intestinal walls by bacterial/fungal overgrowth is part of a vicious cycle that wreaks havoc with the body's health and immunity. The diet attempts to eliminate the type of carbohydrates—grains, sugar, dairy, corn, and potatoes—that tend to nourish "bad" bacteria and fungal species. The Specific Carbohydrate Diet often helps to lower their populations and restores the body's balance or inner ecology.

I stopped eating sugar, molasses, sucrose, high fructose corn syrup, or any other processed sugars. I tried to avoid corn, wheat, barley, oats, rye, rice, and other grains. I also sought to avoid starchy foods such as potatoes, yams, and parsnips. I forgot about drinking milk and eating cheese. Pasta was also a food of my past. That was just the beginning of the dietary restrictions.

The Specific Carbohydrate Diet may have helped some. Trouble was, I didn't have the self-discipline necessary to stay on a diet as rigorous as this one. Well, let me amend that statement. I could stay on the diet for periods of time—until my roommate who worked at a sorority house brought home leftovers from the kitchen. Suddenly, after eating a plate of spaghetti, I wasn't on the Specific Carbohydrate Diet anymore, though I promised myself I would get back on it as soon as I was through pigging out.

You see, I was hungry all the time. I had a ravenous appetite, but I only wanted to eat foods that tasted good to me, which, of course, happened to be unhealthy. Yet no matter how much I ate, I continued to lose weight.

When you are as sick as I was, toilet locations become an obsession. No matter where I went, I had to know where a toilet was located. Even if I felt well enough to go out with friends, I wouldn't go unless I knew where a decent bathroom was. Long car rides were definitely out. My daily plans were dominated by the question, "Where's the bathroom?" That may sound funny to most people, but not to the millions of people who suffered as I did.

I finally broke down and called my parents and told them how sick I really was. They were very concerned and made plans for me to fly home the next day. When I arrived, I walked in the front door with a temperature of 105 degrees. I was burning up!

My dad took one look at me, packed the bathtub with ice cubes, and dunked me in ice-cold water. I remember freezing in the ice water and overhearing my father crying out to my mother, "My God, I don't want my son to die."

I was confused. I didn't know what was happening. All I could think about was that I didn't want to die. I wanted to return to school. I wanted my old life back.

The very next morning, my father and mother took me to the emergency room—the first time I had ever been in a hospital since I was born in a hot tub. (That's another story.) I was hoping it would be a quick visit, that I'd get some "cure all" medication and be on my way back to school.

My "quick visit" lasted two weeks. During this period, I would lie in a hospital bed with an IV pole attached to each arm, receiving intravenous antibiotics and nutrients, and watch TV.

The doctors prescribed antibiotics and antiparasitic drugs that had to be given intravenously for maximum effect, but my body was so overridden by infection that it had become terribly inflamed. To combat this, I was prescribed two heavy-duty and highly toxic steroid medications—hydrocortisone and prednisone.

I was also given every kind of test imaginable. I got more X-rays in those two weeks than most people get in a lifetime. Both my upper and lower gastrointestinal tracts were scanned—and believe me, these weren't the usual short bursts of radiation you get with dental X-rays. I felt like radiologists were conducting an in-depth tour of my gut.

I was told that I had Crohn's disease, a condition primarily involving the small bowel and proximal colon that causes the intestinal wall to thicken and cause narrowing of the bowel channel, blocking the intestinal tract. The result was abnormal membrane function, including nutrient malabsorption.

I had an even worse variation of the disease. The doctors noted I had duodenitis, an inflammation of the duodenum, which is at the beginning of the small intestine. In addition, there was widespread inflammation throughout my large and small intestine. Although less than 1 percent of Crohn's disease patients specifically experience duodenitis, it appeared that I was one of the chosen few with both duodenal and total colonic inflammation.

At this point, the doctor ordered total parenteral nutrition (TPN). This is where nutrients were delivered intravenously and directly into the bloodstream. I was rampant with infection, inflammation, and pain.

Crohn's disease was a much worse diagnosis than I had imagined. I was not in a good state of mind at this point—especially when the doctor told me the disease was incurable. Patients with Crohn's disease experience frequent and progressive symptoms of abdominal pain, diarrhea, and extreme weight loss as seen in other wasting conditions such as cancer and AIDS. Many patients experience premature death.

How's that for making you feel hopeful about your diagnosis! One thing was for sure, I was going to have to take medication if I wanted to stay alive. Yet the side effects of the medications that keep me alive were almost as bad as the disease itself.

∞

I was among the 1.3 million Americans who suffered from an inflammatory bowel disease, which includes Crohn's disease and ulcerative colitis, according to the Centers for Disease Control and Prevention. Today, the incidence of Crohn's disease is 201 persons per 100,000 adults, a figure slightly less than ulcerative colitis.

Although I can speak with experience and knowledge about bowel disease today, back in 1994 I was just a nineteen-year-old suffering from a chronic disease that I was told would require a lifetime of medication. I was confused about how my entire life got so turned upside down in a matter of months. I didn't know anyone with Crohn's disease and didn't know where to go for help in those pre-Internet days. I was too embarrassed to even tell my friends what my symptoms were. When they asked what was going on, I just told them I was sick. I refused to go into detail.

I left the hospital and returned home still desperately hoping to improve enough to return to school in a few weeks. I thought that there must be some kind of magic bullet that would get me well. But this new existence via medications was not a good one. True, I was no longer being given intravenous drugs, but this was only because the doctor had prednisone and other medications administered orally.

What a dangerous drug prednisone is. I hallucinated the first day I took it. I began crying. I was emotionally wrought. I also was taking asacol (Mesalamine), an anti-inflammatory used to treat ulcerative colitis, and two more antimicrobials—metronidazole (Flagyl) and fluconazole (Diflucan)—for what had become a chronic case of thrush. To ensure I improved, the doctors also put me on ciprofloxacin (Cipro), which we now know is also prescribed for anthrax. Because a side effect of prednisone was heartburn, I had to be put on ranitidine (Zantac).

The worst part of this ordeal was that I wasn't getting better. I was still using the toilet a dozen to thirty times a day. Most of my stools were bloody.

The nighttime was worse. You don't know what sleep deprivation is until you experience chronic nocturnal diarrhea. The trips to the bathroom went on all night—every forty-five minutes to an hour. If I got more than an hour of sleep during the entire night, it was a miracle. The cramps were often so intense that I wanted to pull my hair out or bang my head against the wall. I existed in a state of fatigue and exhaustion.

Not surprisingly, I almost completely lacked iron. In fact, at one point, I went more than an entire year with an almost unheard-of serum iron level of 0—zero, nada. My serum levels of the blood protein albumin were so low that they indicated my body was suffering from a severe wasting disease known as cachexia. This was quite serious on both accounts. Iron is an essential component of hemoglobin, the oxygen-carrying protein in the blood. Iron is normally obtained through food in our diet and by the recycling of iron from old red blood cells. Iron-deficiency anemia means the tissues are receiving inadequate oxygen.

As for my albumin levels, this test helped to determine that not enough protein was being absorbed by my body. Albumin is the protein of the highest concentration in plasma. Albumin transports many small molecules in the blood such as bilirubin, calcium, progesterone, and drugs. This protein is also of prime importance in maintaining the oncotic pressure of the blood, which keeps fluid from leaking out into the tissues. Low albumin levels also often indicate malnutrition. I was definitely malnourished.

But while the consumption of large amounts of dairy may have played a role in the onset of my condition, I believe one of the exacerbating influences was my high-carbohydrate, low-fat diet. Put simply, bad bacteria in the gut love the types of sugary, high-carbohydrate and refined foods in the modern diet.

∞

When I started eating large amounts of sugary foods in college, it was the bad bacteria that got the head start in repopulating the barren property within my gut after my friendly bacteria were decimated by the large doses of antibiotics I had taken.

The growth of yeast, fungi, parasites, and disease-causing bacteria within my gut seriously damaged my gut lining, promoted the absorption of internally produced toxins, and impaired the absorption of nutrients. With this bacterial imbalance (dysbiosis) also came the breakdown of my body's immune barrier.

The gastrointestinal tract is critical to the body's immune function because the gut is where most of the body's antibody-producing cells reside. To put it bluntly, my dysbiosis led to a host of debilitating illnesses. During my illness, I had all of the following conditions:

- chronic candidiasis, of which I was given the absolute worst rating given for candida from the diagnostic laboratories that tested me

- infestation by *Entamoeba histolytica,* also known as amebic dysentery
- cryptosporidiosis, caused by a protozoa infection in the gastrointestinal tract
- incipient diabetes with extremely poor circulation (my whole lower leg was purple)
- jaundice plus other liver and gallbladder problems
- insomnia (the most I ever slept continuously was an hour and fifteen minutes)
- hair loss, which was awful to suffer from (I was nineteen…need I say more?)
- endocarditis (a heart infection)
- eye inflammation
- prostate and bladder infections
- chronic electrolyte imbalance due to dehydration
- elevated C-reactive protein, which was indicative of chronic inflammation and bacterial infection, as well as increased susceptibility to heart attack and stroke risk
- anemia, which meant that too few red blood cells were present in the bloodstream and insufficient oxygen reached muscle tissues and organs
- chronic fatigue, a mysterious, debilitating ailment known for unceasing fatigue, headaches, weakness, muscle and joint aches, and the inability to concentrate
- arthritis, which inflames the joints and causes stiffness and pain
- leukocytosis, which is caused by an abnormal increase in white blood cells
- malabsorption syndrome, meaning I could not assimilate the nutrients in the food I ate

Because of my dad's naturopathic background, I had it in me to try natural methods that I hoped would turn on my body's healing response. Not long after I was discharged from the hospital, my father and I made the decision to try to find natural pathways to do just that.

I tried everything. And I do mean *everything*. Getting well became an obsession for both my dad and me. Together we began a search around the world that took me to seventy health practitioners from seven different countries, including medical doctors, chiropractors, immunologists, acupuncturists, homeopaths, herbalists, nutritionists, and dieticians.

I mentioned earlier my experience with the Specific Carbohydrate Diet. At this point, I still believed that this restrictive diet could help me if I had stayed on it perfectly with no deviations, so I decided to try it one more time. I became a strict devotee and even consulted daily on the phone with Elaine Gottschall, who devised the diet and wrote about it in her book *Breaking the Vicious Cycle*.

She had worked with a physician, Elson Haas, to heal her daughter of ulcerative colitis, a disease similar to Crohn's disease. I stayed on the Specific Carbohydrate Diet with fanatical adherence for three to six months on three different occasions. Unfortunately, the diet didn't work for me.

I moved on and tried just about every other diet that has ever been written about. I consulted with some of the foremost practitioners and diet experts throughout the world. I visited Dr. Robert Atkins, the physician and cardiologist behind the Atkins Diet. I met with eicosanoid guru Barry Sears, Ph.D., author of *The Zone*. I contacted Jeffrey Bland, Ph.D., a highly regarded functional medicine expert.

I didn't have any luck with any of these extremely knowledgeable and highly educated health professionals. They truly wanted to help, and I knew they were sincere. Their diets had many solid underpinnings, but something was missing because none of them were able to help.

So I kept searching.

I estimate that over the course of about two years, my father spent $150,000 on natural health treatments. (That amount would be $250,000 today.) I took dozens of probiotic formulas, as well as enzyme, fiber, anti-candida, and antiparasitic formulas. At one point, I was taking upwards of six bottles a day of expensive probiotics. I remember using two bottles of powdered acidophilus, two bottles of bifidus, and two bottles of *Lactobacillus bulgaricus* every day, which was costing my parents hundreds of dollars daily.

When someone told me my liver was the problem, I tried liver detoxification, using live cell therapy with injectable sheep cells taken from sheep embryos. The "health expert" who provided the products told me that in the United Kingdom he had cured some 250 Crohn's disease patients. All I remember is that the needles were huge and I didn't get better.

Then I read that cabbage juice was good for the gut and was rich in organic sulfur compounds, so I ingested large amounts of cabbage juice. I used plenty of other detoxification formulas. I did retention enemas and colonics and more liver detoxification. I tried glandulars from every conceivable organ. I used injectable vitamins and minerals. For this regimen, I was instructed to inject myself *seven times a day.* I used a needle reserved for insulin injections. I became so emaciated that when I injected myself in the shoulders and the sides of my hip, I could feel the needle hitting my bone.

I used injectable thymus gland extract. I consumed wheat grass juice. I tried Chinese herbs, Peruvian herbs, Japanese kampo, olive leaf extract, and shark cartilage. I tried macrobiotics. I used nitrogenated soy. I visited alternative clinics in Mexico and Germany, often in a wheelchair and often returning worse than when I began. One doctor who treated me characterized my appearance as that of a "Nazi concentration camp survivor."

As my search grew more frantic and desperate, I grasped for straws. I took something called adrenal cortical extract, or ACE, an extract of bovine adrenal gland that is thought to possess the powers of hydrocortisone and was once used extensively in medicine. Only belatedly did I learn that many such batches were contaminated with *Mycobacterium abscessus,* a rapidly growing bacterium distantly related to the tuberculosis organism.

My dad, through reading health magazines and calling colleagues, found all kinds of clinics and therapies for me to try. The number of machines that were hooked up to my body could fill a science fiction novel! I tried various forms of electro-dermal screening (EDS), a form of computerized information gathering based on physics.

For that, a blunt, noninvasive electric probe was placed at specific points on my hands, face, or feet, corresponding to acupuncture points at the beginning or end of the energy meridians. Minute electrical discharges from these points served as information signals about the condition of the body's organs and systems. According to the doctor who probed me with his EDS machine, my illness was due to electromagnetic fields in my house. The next thing I knew, I had to sleep in a steel cage that was put around my room. At night, I began to shut off the TV and clocks—all electrical devices. I don't need to tell you whether this worked. I think you know the answer.

This was all weird science, and it could only have come from the outer reaches of the alternative health field. Another so-called alternative health practitioner told me I was sensitive to the movements of a certain satellite that orbited the Earth every ten years. He said that I was one of the rare, unlucky people that the satellite influenced—and that I would have to wait a considerable period of time before the satellite left the Earth's orbit.

You might say I'm still waiting.

∞

Taking various medications and supplements was my life. Unless I was visiting a doctor, which I did several times a week, I stayed home. I passed the time by watching cooking shows and fantasizing about foods that I could eat someday. I felt a special bond with Chef Emeril, who was in his heyday on the Food Network.

I also read just about every piece of literature and book about health that I could get my hands on. I consumed three hundred books on health and nutrition during my illness, but I was still puzzled over what products to use and which products could help me.

I didn't just read health books. I often sought out the doctor who wrote the book and consulted with him or her in person or on the phone. All the doctors and health practitioners I spoke with said they could cure me in a short period of time. They had never failed to cure their patients, they added. All of them made promises, but very few of them had any clinical validation to verify their claims. My willingness to believe them and put all my faith in them, however, demonstrates what people who are desperately ill go through.

Because I was so weak, traveling from clinic to clinic was an ordeal, especially by airplane. I oftentimes got bladder as well as eye infections. I remember one time, as I sat in my seat waiting for an airplane to take off, I said to myself, "If this plane went down, it wouldn't be that bad." I was not suicidal, but I just couldn't handle the pain anymore. I reasoned that if I died, at least I could join my Creator.

I hit rock bottom on a trip to Germany, where I traveled to take yet another herbal IV treatment. At that time, the U.S. Food and Drug Administration (FDA) did not permit this supplement to be imported, so I had to go to Germany to take it. The timing for a European trip couldn't have been worse because I was weaning myself from other medications. I had gotten off prednisone, but when I did that, I experienced a complete adrenal shock. I couldn't catch my breath.

My mother accompanied me to the German clinic. Upon landing, we missed a train by a few minutes because my mom and I couldn't manage to drag our luggage through the station on time. Because we missed the train, we were stuck in the station for *six more hours*! All the time I was dragging my jet-lagged body back and forth to a bathroom.

Once at the clinic, the German doctor made an interesting diagnosis. He concluded that my problem rested with my immune system. He declared that certain parts of my immune system were overactive and certain parts were underactive, and I needed to stay at the clinic for six weeks to receive treatment. My mother, a schoolteacher, returned to the United States and left me in Germany while I underwent the six-week treatment protocol.

What an awful experience! For instance, after my six-hour IV treatments, no one would come to help me back to my room. There I sat, all alone, shaking with cold chills, feeling like I was about to have a seizure. No one ever came by to check up on me. After a while, I would do my best to fall asleep.

I certainly slept more while I was in Germany because I was put on high doses of opium. In Germany, doctors prescribe a tincture of opium to slow down peristalsis and keep patients from having to go to the bathroom so much. When I failed to improve, the doctor, who was egoistical, decided that I wasn't getting well because I had mental problems.

I reached rock bottom. Think about my circumstances: I was nineteen years old. I had dropped out of college. I was far away from family and friends. My mother had left me in a German health clinic where nobody spoke English. My feeble attempts at speaking German got me nowhere.

Not only did I feel like I was in a prison, I was imprisoned in my own body. I was miserable and constantly in pain. I contemplated dark and dreary thoughts, wondering if I would ever enjoy normalcy again, if I would ever wake up without pain and be healthy like I once had been.

Finally, my parents and I decided it was time for me to come home. To catch my airplane flight, I had to leave at 5 a.m., but nobody in the clinic was awake that early. I was too frail and thin to carry my own luggage, but I tried anyway. I couldn't find switches to turn on lights in the halls and tripped down some stairs in the dark. I finally managed to get my suitcases to the lobby, but when the taxicab showed up I couldn't open the front door to the clinic. I found a back entrance, managed to wheel my bags out, but tripped down another set of steps and fell flat on my face.

The taxi driver, upon arriving at the airport, fetched a wheelchair for me. After wheeling me to the ticket counter, the agent had to summon someone who spoke English, but he couldn't find any record of my ticket.

Now what do I do? I had no money. My credit card was declined for some reason. I was completely sick. I had a urinary tract infection (UTI) in addition to my massive bowl problems. I was on opium. And now I couldn't go home.

I was literally at the end of my rope.

All I could do was whisper a quick prayer: "Lord, I cannot do a single thing. Please help me get out of this situation. I feel completely hopeless."

In a couple of minutes, the agent told me that my ticket had been found. I got on the plane. I took a ten-hour flight to the United States, missed a connecting flight, waited around for the next one, and finally made it to Miami. Getting home was a thirty-hour ordeal.

I cannot describe how relieved I was to be back in my old house. I remember lying on the couch listening to *The Annette Funicello Story* on television. Notice that I said *listening* because I had compresses over my eyes for double conjunctivitis. When I had to go to the bathroom, I had to walk quickly even though my eyes were closed. Bowel movements were painful and urination burned. But in spite of my illness and pain, I was thrilled to be home again with my family—at least as thrilled as could be expected from someone who lacked hope of recovering from a terminal illness. I say *terminal* because I really thought I was going to die.

Shortly after my return home from Germany, I was hospitalized a second time. I was completely dehydrated and had a resting heart rate of between 160 to 180 beats per minute. I couldn't keep water down. My weight dropped to 104 pounds, the lowest ever. The nurses tried to get IVs into me so I could be rehydrated, but they couldn't get any blood to return because my veins were dry and tapped out. One time, it took the nurses and doctors two and a half hours to get an IV into my body.

I remember hearing one of the nurses crying in the hallway. She told another nurse, "That poor boy isn't going to make it through the night."

Feeling more hopeless than words can describe, I only knew to pray. I didn't blame God. Even while feeling grim and believing I was going to die, I always held a glimmer of hope that God would choose to cure me. If not, I was prepared to meet my Maker. I was disappointed that I had never fallen in love or married. But I had had a great, great life. I trusted God's plan for my future and put myself in the only capable hands I knew of—my heavenly Father's. I thanked my Creator for every moment He'd given me and expressed my gratitude. That night, I lay in bed, alone in my room, fully prepared to die.

When I woke in the morning, I was surprised that I was still there. I looked up and saw my Grandmother Rose, who'd placed her hand on my forehead and spoke soothing thoughts. Soon, several nurses entered. They tried to hook me up to an IV and were elated when they were able to get a blood return. Overnight, they calculated that I gained ten pounds of water weight. That's how dehydrated I was!

I felt a new resolve in my body. I wanted so badly to live. A glimmer of sunshine entered my life, giving me newfound hope—real hope.

That feeling of hope was short-lived, however, when doctors got hold of my body. Once again, I became a human drugstore. The doctors prescribed the same medications I had been given the first time I was hospitalized—the usual antibiotics, antifungals, and antiparasitics, along with the steroids hydrocortisone and prednisone. When the time came to leave the hospital and they switched me from IV to oral medications, I had hallucinations. As baseball sage Yogi Berra once said, "It was déjà vu all over again."

Back at home, I managed to break through the hallucinations to say something to my mom. I had an unusual demand that completely startled her.

"I want you to take a picture of me," I said.

She stammered and then refused. She couldn't fathom why anyone would want a picture to commemorate such a pathetic condition. But even with everything I had been through and all those doctors who failed to help me, I still had faith in my God's ability to deliver me from my despair. I wanted to document the moment that I was at my absolute lowest.

I remember my mom asking, "Why in the world do you want me to take a picture of you?"

I answered with my best attempt at a smile, "Because no one will believe me when I get well. No one will believe that I was this sick. I'm getting out of bed, and I need you to take my picture." There were no selfies in those days.

I nearly fell to the floor climbing out of bed. My legs were sticks, and my torso was skin and bones. I needed help standing up, and even then staying upright on my two feet was a struggle. The picture you see on the cover of this book is the photograph my mother took. I weighed 114 pounds, and that was after gaining ten pounds of water weight in the hospital.

I had a beard because I was too weak to shave and couldn't afford to cut myself with my unsteady hand. My skin-and-bones body looked like someone who had been in a concentration camp or held as a prisoner of war. My skin looked dead.

One doctor told me my only hope was to go to Mount Sinai Hospital in New York City, where surgeons would expertly remove all of my large colon and part of my small intestine. Or I could undergo another kind of surgery, experimental at the time, called a J-pouch procedure. This surgery was a way to try and preserve bowel function once I had my colon removed.

As I was considering what to do, I read the doctors' transcripts of my medical records. My primary physician called my condition the worst case of Crohn's disease he had ever seen and doubted I would live to return home.

It was crazy. The medications were only making me worse. At least their effects could probably be reversed, but surgery to remove my large colon? That was permanent. Not only that, I learned that nearly 75 percent of people with Crohn's who have surgery must undergo a second surgery.

After talking things through with my family, I decided to go to Mount Sinai and get whatever surgery I needed. That's what I would have to do to stay alive.

◌◌

It was early 1996, and I hadn't left for New York City yet. I still held out hope that I could avoid ostomy surgery.

One day, my father came into my bedroom and told me that he had just spoken to an eccentric nutritionist named Bud Keith on the phone. The nutritionist told my father that he believed I was ill because I was not eating the diet of my ancestors, based upon biblical principles.

When my father told me about all of this, I was naturally curious. My father investigated the nutritionist's program and thought it was worth a shot. I would do anything to avoid surgery, so I decided to try out his ideas, which fit into my belief system.

In an effort to start over, I took myself off all nutritional products and read the Bible to see what people ate thousands of years ago. I also learned that the longest living cultures in the world had one thing in common—they consumed living foods that abounded with beneficial microorganisms.

A few weeks later, I got on a plane, still bound to my wheelchair, and headed for San Diego to live closer to Bud Keith, who would teach me how to eat from the Bible. After integrating his program along with some of my own findings about nutrition and health from the Bible, I saw some improvement.

While I was gone, my father had promised that he wouldn't send me nutritional supplements to try; he did anyway. One day, I received a package from him containing a plastic bag containing black powder. He said it was a probiotic, but I had already tried over thirty different probiotics. Now was I supposed to eat this stuff that looked like dirt?

Forget it, I thought.

My dad called on the phone and urged me to give the probiotic a try.

"It may look like dirt, but it isn't," he said. "It contains healthy organisms from the soil."

An article that accompanied the package explained that this nutritional pack contained nutrients missing from today's pesticide-sterilized, barren soils. They weren't trace minerals but organisms known as soil-based organisms or SBOs. These were living organisms that had been wiped out by the pesticide treatment of America's farmlands, pasteurization of foods, and modern man's disdain for all microorganisms—even those life-supportive bugs our bodies need for great health.

I decided to include these SBOs in my daily diet, which also included raw goat's milk in the form of fermented kefir; different organically grown free-range or grass-fed meats; natural sprouted or sourdough breads made from whole grains that were yeast-free; organic fruits and vegetables like raw sauerkraut, carrots, and other vegetable juices. These were all "live" foods with their beneficial enzymes and microorganisms intact.

Improvement didn't come immediately. In fact, I had somewhat of a Herxheimer reaction, which is an allergic response resulting from the death of large numbers of pathological organisms. This is also known as a "die-off."

The collective effects of organism die-off often temporarily worsen one's symptoms. Holistic physicians who practice environmental medicine believe this die-off reaction indicates that the patient is having an excellent backlash effect to good treatment.

Since the time of Hippocrates, it has been understood that symptoms of most diseases, other than degenerative disorders where irreversible organic damage has been sustained, represent the efforts of the body to eliminate toxins. In 1848, Thomas Sydenham, the so-called English Hippocrates, wrote, "[a] disease, however much its cause may be adverse to the human body, is nothing more than an effort of Nature who strains with might and main to restore the health of the patient by the elimination of the morbific matter."

One month after adding the "black powder" to my diet, I noticed an elimination of black, tar-like stuff during a bowel movement. I also had newfound energy, and I went to the bathroom less frequently.

At this point, my father purchased a used motor home for me while I was living in San Diego. He thought that staying close to the ocean and breathing the salt air would be good for me. While driving around beach communities like Ocean Beach and Pacific Beach in my motor home, I felt like a bum trying to find places to park at night—an unusual experience for an upper-middle-class kid like me.

You may ask how on Earth I was able to drive a motor home in my condition. My answer is simply: Only the Lord knows. It helped that friends from my hometown of Palm Beach Gardens flew out to San Diego to stay with me in my motor home and take care of me.

During my forty days and nights of parking my motor home close to the beach, I prayed, listened to music, and planned everything around buying, preparing, and eating my food. My weight jumped from 122 to 151 pounds, which meant I gained 29 pounds in forty days! The photograph of me on the beach that you see on the book cover was taken during this period. I was not completely well yet, but I had made miraculous strides toward full recovery. I continued to gain weight and strength, and by my twenty-first birthday, I weighed 170 pounds—practically my original weight before I got sick. I doubt if anyone in the world was happier than me.

The terrain of my body and my intestinal tract were rebuilt, and it appeared that somehow the SBOs were taking care of my underlying condition. All in all, in three months I gained over fifty pounds.

I am convinced that the combination of the biblical diet and the SBOs restored my health. I still went through periods of detoxification every few months or so, but I continued to persevere. In December 1996, I returned home to Florida at my normal weight. I was ready to start my life again. I was finally healthy!

I had done what hundreds of thousands of disease sufferers desperately want to do—make a full recovery to good health. My first idea was to go back to the many doctors who had treated me and tell them about the biblical or Maker's Diet and the SBOs. I mailed my "before" and "after" pictures to the doctors I had consulted with. I thought everyone would be so eager to learn what had healed me. I even thought the doctors would want to include the Maker's Diet and SBOs in their treatment programs.

While some health professionals were genuinely excited to hear about my recovery, including Elaine Gottschall, author of *Breaking the Vicious Cycle,* very few of them wanted to try my Maker's Diet and SBOs with their patients. I felt like I had something to help other sufferers of digestive disorders, especially other Crohn's disease sufferers, but no one in the traditional medical world wanted to hear about it.

Dr. Morton Walker, a medical journalist who had given me information for some of the clinics I visited, offered to write an article outlining my story for the *Townsend Letter for Doctors and Patients,* a prestigious health publication that focuses on alternative medicines and treatments. The article about my recovery generated over two thousand phone calls from doctors as well as individuals suffering from bowel disease.

Literally overnight, I had to find a way to distribute the SBOs that had helped me get well. I started a whole-food nutrition company to help ill and hurting people like myself who were seeking to regain their health.

I believe I went through my ordeal for a reason. I consulted seventy doctors and took five hundred health products for a reason. Because I have personally experienced and survived my walk through the valley of disease but have remained healthy as a horse for the last twenty years, I believe I can speak to you as an authority.

People say Crohn's disease is incurable, but from my experience, no disease is incurable. Some people may be too far gone and may not ever get completely well, but every single disease and every single state of health can be improved through whole-food nutrition and whole-food supplements that bring us back to a diet and a lifestyle that has been proven to work for thousands of years.

My goal after getting well was to create a vehicle whereby I could reach people who were suffering from digestive and immune system disorders. I began to design products based on the theory of anthropological nutrition or, simply, the nutrition of our history.

But now that I was better, I also wanted to know everything there was to know about how I got better. I wanted to design a program so that everyone who suffers from illness can take their health into their own hands.

You'll learn about my health program in the coming pages of *Patient Heal Thyself,* but first, we need to take a gut check.

2

I'VE GOT A GUT FEELING

Why do we say that a performing artist, when his or her songs are full of feeling, sang from the gut?

Why do performers get "butterflies in their stomach" before going on stage?

Why does indigestion produce nightmares?

Why are antidepressants used for gastrointestinal ailments?

I like interesting questions like these. I also like word games and definitions, so here's another one: Where does the word *gut* come from?

Let's start with the *Merriam-Webster's Collegiate Dictionary*, which tells us that the etymology of the word *gut* dates back to the Middle English word *guttas*, which has its roots in the 12th century Old English word *geotan*, meaning "to pour."

Your gut, the dictionary says, is "the basic visceral or emotional part of a person," "the alimentary canal or part of it (as the intestine or stomach)," and "the inner essential parts." As we go along, keep these definitions in mind.

It turns out that both our gut and our brain originate early in fetal development when a clump of tissue called the neural crest appears and divides. While one section turns into the central nervous system, another piece migrates to become the enteric nervous system (ENS). Only later are the two nervous systems connected via a cable known as the vagus nerve, the longest of all the cranial nerves whose name is derived from the

Latin word for *wandering*. In keeping with its etymological origins, the vagus nerve meanders from the brain stem through organs in the neck and thorax before ending up in the abdomen. This is how the brain-gut connection happens.

So profoundly influential is the state of the gut upon people's health that I have coined the term *gastro-neuroimmunology* to try and capture the essence of the link between our two brains and our immune function.

I came up with the term because a healthy gut allows us to enjoy neurological and psychological as well as immunological health. This is not to discount the highly important mass of gray between our ears—the human brain. This is simply to say that the body has two brains—the brain between our ears and the second brain, our gut.

Everyone talks about their gut feelings, especially gut-wrenching feelings. No wonder we tell people to trust their gut. But are we living too much in our head? Should we think with our gut?

Maybe we should. Did you know that one-half of all our nerve cells are located within the gut? Did you know that our capacity for feeling and emotional expression depends primarily on the gut and, to a lesser extent, the brain?

Furthermore, did you know that your gastrointestinal health is a major key to your overall and total health?

Do you have a gut feeling where I'm headed with all of this?

I hope so because we take our gastrointestinal tract or gut for granted. We really shouldn't.

Sandra Blakeslee, writing in the *New York Times*, had this to say about the link between our gut and the brain:

> Have you ever wondered why people get butterflies in the stomach before going on stage? Or why an impending job interview can cause an attack of intestinal cramps? Or why antidepressants targeted for the brain cause nausea or abdominal upset in millions of people who take such drugs?

The reason for these common experiences is because each of us literally has two brains—the familiar one encased in our skulls and a lesser-known but vitally important one found in the human gut. Like Siamese twins, the two brains are interconnected; when one gets upset, the other does, too.

The gut's brain, known as the enteric nervous system (ENS), is located in sheaths of tissue lining the esophagus, stomach, small intestine, and colon. (Enteric is derived from the word *entera*, simply meaning we also have a nervous system in our entera or intestinal tract.)

Considered a single entity, the ENS is packed with neurons, neurotransmitters, and proteins that zap messages between neurons and support cells like those found in the brain. The ENS contains complex circuitry that enables it to act independently, learn, remember, and, as the saying goes, produce gut feelings.

In his book *The Second Brain,* Dr. Michael Gershon, a professor of anatomy and cell biology at Columbia-Presbyterian Medical Center in New York City, dubbed the entire gastrointestinal system, the body's second nervous system.

"The brain is not the only place in the body that's full of neurotransmitters," wrote Dr. Gershon. "A hundred million neurotransmitters line the length of the gut, approximately the same number that is found in the brain.… The brain in the bowel has got to work right or no one will have the luxury to think at all."

Scientists have long been fascinated with the gut. The field of neurogastroenterology—now there's a tongue twister—finds its start with the 19th century English investigators William M. Bayliss and Ernest H. Starling, who took anesthetized dogs and applied pressure to the intestinal lumen, which is the cavity of the tubular gastrointestinal organ. This pressure caused contraction and anal relaxation, followed by a propulsive wave. It is this propulsive wave or peristaltic reflex that scientists call the "law of the intestine."

Peristalsis moves—rather, propels—food through the digestive tract. In experimental studies, even when all nerves connecting the bowel to the brain and spinal cord were severed, "the law of the intestine" prevailed and digestion continued. Thus, the scientists surmised the ENS to be independent from the central nervous system.

After the initial work of Bayliss and Starling and experiments some eighteen years later by German scientist Paul Trendelenburg, which confirmed their findings, science moved on, however. After researchers discovered other chemical neurotransmitters such as epinephrine and acetylcholine, they lost interest in the law of the intestine.

Exacerbating the situation, the publisher of Trendelenburg's results (reported in 1917) was John N. Langley, who went on to author *The Autonomic Nervous System* in 1921. Langley was also editor and publisher of the *Journal of Physiology* and had over the years alienated many of his colleagues. Many of the theories he popularized were ultimately trivialized in a case of wholesale scientific revenge. In a move involving an ultimate scientific insult, scientists at the Physiological Society, which took over the journal after Langley's death, reclassified the enteric nerves as simply part of the parasympathetic nervous system.

It wasn't until the period between 1965 and 1967 that Dr. Gershon proposed, in a series of papers in *Science and the Journal of Physiology*, that there existed a third neurotransmitter, namely serotonin (5-hydroxytryptamine, 5-HT), that was both produced in and targeted to the ENS. Now we know this neurotransmitter is also found in the central nervous system.

Details of how the ENS mirrors the central nervous system have been emerging in recent years. Nearly every substance that helps run and control the brain has turned up in the gut. In fact, many major neurotransmitters generally associated with the brain, such as serotonin, dopamine, glutamate, norepinephrine, and nitric oxide, are found in plentiful amounts in the gut.

Some two dozen small brain proteins, called neuropeptides, are also found in relatively high amounts in the gut, which makes them major cells of the immune system. For instance, enkephalins, one class of the body's natural opiates, are plentiful in the gut. And in a finding that confounds many researchers, the gut is a rich source of benzodiazepines—the family of psychoactive chemicals that includes such ever-popular drugs as Valium and Xanax, Blakeslee reported.

We all think that the brain in our skull is the "Big Cheese" or majordomo of the body—literally chief of the house. Trouble is, when you start counting nerve cells, there are several hundred million of them in the gut alone—and about as many as in the spinal cord. When you add in the esophagus, stomach, and large intestine, you suddenly have more nerve cells in the gut than in the entire remainder of the peripheral nervous system.

Talk to people and most will tell you the brain determines whether you are happy or sad. But contrary to what most think, this may be backward. Perhaps the gut is more responsible than we ever imagined for our mental well-being and how we feel.

No wonder Karl Lashley, generally considered the founder of neuropsychology, noted, "I am coming more and more to the conviction that the rudiments of every human behavioral mechanism will be found represented even in primitive activities of the nervous system." He wrote this in 1951.

As more light is shed on the circuitry between the two brains, researchers are beginning to understand why people act and feel the way they do. The brain and gut are so much alike that during our sleeping hours both have natural ninety-minute cycles. For the brain, this slow wave sleep is interrupted by periods of rapid eye movement sleep—the time when dreams occur. For the gut, the ninety-minute cycles also involve slow waves of muscle contractions, but as with REM intervals, these are punctuated by short bursts of rapid muscle movement.

Could it be that both brains influence each other? The answer is probably "yes." We know that REM sleep is a sleep phase characterized by arousal, altered activity of the autonomic nervous system, and altered colon (large intestine) function.

We also know that patients with bowel problems tend to have abnormal REM sleep. Poor sleep has been reported by many—perhaps a majority of—patients with IBS and non-ulcerative dyspepsia—also known as "sour stomach." These poor folks complain of awakening tired and unrefreshed in the morning. Even if they awake from what they describe as a "sound sleep," they report a general feeling of tiredness and fatigue.

Abnormal REM sleep is reduced by low-dose treatment with the antidepressant amitriptyline, which has also been shown to be effective in treating IBS and non-ulcerative dyspepsia. The sleep disturbance is likely to play an important role in the chronicity of symptoms by setting up a vicious cycle of pain, fatigue, and emotional distress, which alters the body's arousal systems during sleep. In turn, poor sleep quality increases sensitivity to bowel and somatic (skin and muscle) stimuli, leading to more pain and distress. This finding supports traditional folk wisdom that indigestion produces nightmares.

On a personal note, I believe that sleep is the single most important ingredient for digestive health. I believe that getting enough sleep at the right time (sleep before midnight is the most valuable) will do wonders for your digestion.

Many drugs designed to affect the brain also affect the gut. For example, the gut is loaded with the neurotransmitter serotonin. In fact, more serotonin is produced there than anywhere else in the body. Serotonin is linked with initiation of peristalsis.

About 25 percent of people taking fluoxetine (Prozac) and other types of similar-acting antidepressants experience gastrointestinal problems such as nausea, diarrhea, and constipation. The problem with these drugs is that they prevent uptake of serotonin by cells that should be using it. While this enables the depressed person to have more serotonin in the brain, less serotonin is available for use by the cells of the gastrointestinal tract.

"Serotonin is calming to the digestive tract, initiating peristaltic and secretory reflexes," noted nutritionist June Butlin, M.Sc, Ph.D. "Long-term use or the wrong dosage may cause fluctuations between nausea, vomiting, constipation, and diarrhea, and can cause depression, anxiety, insomnia, and fluctuations in appetite."

In a study reported in a *New York Times* article, Dr. Gershon and his colleagues explained Prozac's side effects on the gut when they mounted a section of guinea pig colon on a stand and put a small pellet in the "mouth" end. The isolated colon whipped the pellet down to the anal end of the column, just as it would inside an animal.

When the researchers put a small amount of Prozac into the colon, the pellet "went into high gear," Dr. Gershon explained to the *New York Times*. "The drug doubled the speed at which the pellet passed through the colon, which would explain why some people get diarrhea," the newspaper article said.

"No wonder, in small doses, Prozac is used to treat chronic constipation. If a little is beneficial for constipation, a lot is not. When the Gershon team greatly increased the amount of Prozac in the guinea pig colon, the pellet stopped moving at all. Hence, a little cures constipation; a lot causes it. Prozac stimulates sensory nerves, thus can also cause nausea."

The gut has opiate receptors much like the brain. "Not surprisingly, drugs like morphine and heroin that are thought to act on the central nervous system also attach to the gut's opiate receptors, producing constipation," explained pain management specialist Michael Loes, M.D., M.D.(H.), author of *The Healing Response*. "Both brains," he said, "can be addicted to opiates."

Many Alzheimer's and Parkinson's disease patients are constipated. A sickness we think of as primarily affecting the brain or central nervous system also impacts the gut.

Our gut also *helps* us in some amazing ways by producing chemicals called benzodiazepines, the same chemicals used to alleviate pain and found in antianxiety drugs like Valium. Perhaps our gut is truly our body's anxiety and pain reliever, which explains why when we're anxious we tend to overeat. Perhaps our body is trying to produce extra benzodiazepines.

While we are not sure whether the gut synthesizes benzodiazepine from chemicals in our foods, bacterial actions, or both, we know that in times of extreme pain, the gut goes into overdrive to deliver benzodiazepine to the brain. The result is to render the patient unconscious or at least reduce the pain, said Dr. Anthony Basile, a neurochemist with the Neuroscience Laboratory at the National Institutes of Health in Bethesda, Maryland.

So take care of your gut. It's taking care of you.

Dr. Gershon has said that "the gut may be more intellectual than the heart and may have a greater capacity for feeling." He also believes that our society's many gastrointestinal problems originate from imbalances within the gut's brain.

"Throughout the world's healing and mystical traditions, the belly is seen as an important center of energy and consciousness," added Fernando Pages Ruiz, a contributing editor to *Yoga Journal.* "You've probably noticed that many of India's great spiritual adepts sport prodigious bellies. These tremendous tummies are thought to be full of prana. Hence, Indian artists often depict their deities with a paunch. In China, the gentle art of tai chi emphasizes the lower abdomen as a reservoir for energy."

In his online article, Pages Ruiz quotes tai chi teacher Kenneth Cohen, author of *The Way of Qigong,* and says that, according to Cohen, "It's possible to strengthen the abdominals by learning how to compact qi (prana) into the belly."

"From the Chinese viewpoint," he quotes Cohen, "the belly is considered the *dan tian* or 'field of the elixir,' where you plant the seeds of long life and wisdom."

Lastly, in biblical times, the seat of emotion, which we call the heart, is actually referring to the bowels. That thought in itself conjures up an image of a young Romeo sending a love note to his girlfriend with the inscription, "Baby, you really move me."

The trouble with these modern times is that many influences today are counterproductive to gastrointestinal health. As a result, we are experiencing health problems that could be overcome if we knew they were centered in the gut. No wonder so many of us have poor health.

We've neglected the health of our gut for far too long, and that has to change.

3

BEYOND PROBIOTICS

U p to this point, I've been talking about how the center of health is the gut—the body's gastrointestinal tract. When it comes to good nutrition and taking nutritional supplements, I've always said, "You are not what you eat but what you assimilate."

But the gut is more than the second brain; it is also the seat of the body's defenses and the center of immune function. In addition to the lymphoid tissue concentrated within the lymph nodes and the spleen and immune cells circulating in our bloodstream, lymphoid tissue and immune cells are also found at other sites, most notably the gastrointestinal tract, respiratory tract, and urogenital tract. Such lymphoid tissue is termed *MALT*, or mucosal-associated lymphoid tissue. In the gastrointestinal tract, however, it's called the GALT, or gut-associated lymphoid tissue.

Our gut produces about 75 percent of our body's total immune system cells. So when we want to boost immunity, we must also look at improving gastrointestinal health.

Studies show that over 40 percent of patients visit their doctors for gastrointestinal problems, with complaints ranging from IBS and abdominal bloating to diarrhea and constipation. Often there are no answers to these problems because of a lack of diagnosed anatomical or chemical defects. Doctors routinely tell patients that their gut problems are imaginary, emotional, or all in their heads, attributing their problems to malfunction in the brain.

Needless to say, the quality of life for these patients will remain poor until their problems are understood and a method to enhance the body's healing response is found. It would help matters if today's doctors had an understanding of the ENS and the importance of the gut to overall well-being and its ability provide cures for many conditions well beyond those found in the gastrointestinal tract. This is important because the gut is the center of our own happiness and well-being.

A lot of diseases, we now realize, result from living too far removed from our microscopic allies, the beneficial bacteria in our environment. This is why SBOs can be so beneficial and a topic that I want to address fully in this chapter.

Dr. Morton Walker, who wrote about my health comeback in the *Townsend Letter for Doctors and Patients*, reported on the discovery of soil-based organisms in this manner:

> There are relatively few areas of the world today whose natural ecology has been untainted by modern man. While hiking through a remote area on another continent in the 1970s, an American scientist discovered some mounds on the ground that he recognized as soil-based organisms of an unusual nature.

> He brought a small quantity of the SBOs to the United States for use in experimentation. Because these bacteria are not regularly found on the North American continent, the scientist had to create a new culture for research purposes. Over the next three years, his research team performed studies on the unknown soil-based organisms.

> These researchers: (1) identified exactly what the various strains were; (2) determined toxicity or pathogenicity of the bacteria for humans or animals; (3) ascertained if the SBOs were beneficial for animals or humans and found they were useful to both. Tests on rodents and other animals proved that nothing toxic came from the bacteria. Botany studies conducted indicated the SBOs were beneficial to plants and soil.

> Next, at U.S. and Mexican institutions, human beings—including the biochemist himself—underwent clinical tests with the bacteria by applying them topically to open wounds. Then the organisms

were ingested. No toxicity reactions or side effects were observed; in fact, the SBOs offered no adverse responses in the test subjects even with greater amounts consumed. Over time, the scientist and his co-workers perfected a process for selectively breeding superior strains of the microorganisms until they produced cultures that furnished good, positive body reactions such as more normal bowel movements, improved sleep patterns, fewer colds and flu, and greater amounts of energy. During the breeding experiments, the scientist brought his SBOs to university laboratories in California for experiments. He collaborated with professors and utilized the universities' computer data banks.

Dr. Walker reported that neither the scientist nor his collaborators ever made any changes to the bacteria by mutation or other means. These SBOs, he said, appeared to be as old as the Earth.

∞

I mentioned that once my story became public through the *Townsend Letter,* demand for these homeostatic soil organisms was incredible. I became the "hub" for anyone in the world with a gastrointestinal problem who couldn't get better, and soon I began receiving thousands of letters and phone calls in those pre-Internet days. Eventually, I created a formula containing these organisms and produced an SBO probiotic supplement for the marketplace.

Among the most critical areas for the nutritional products industry are sourcing raw materials and their handling, all the way from soil to store shelf. You probably don't know this, but most herbs today are fumigated and irradiated in order to kill all microorganisms. Not very natural, if you ask me. I wanted to use all-organic ingredients, if possible, which was rare, even in the natural products industry. I also found that vegetables and herbs were better absorbed when they are predigested through lactic acid fermentation, and that these herbs are more potent when grown in certain areas of the world.

I worked with a team that came up with a unique fermentation process that encouraged the production of populations of beneficial microorganisms that made our whole foods and herbs much more available to the body, even disease-weakened ones.

I'm very pleased with what were able to do, and my nutritional formulations were well-received in the marketplace.

Asthma

Allergies

IBS

Rheumatoid arthritis

Lupus

Crohn's disease

Chronic fatigue syndrome

Immune disorders

All are reaching epidemic proportions.

To protect yourself from these disorders and insure long-term super health—as well as to aid your body's healing quest in the case of these and other related disorders—may I respectfully suggest that you eat some dirt?

Do not be surprised by what I say. Dirt—or to be more specific, the Earth's soil—is one of your body's best friends.

Dirt or topsoil is so essential to health that if you or a loved one is suffering from any of the above conditions, this may be due to a lost connection with our planet.

Back in the era of primitive man, we got dirty and were exposed to all sorts of microscopic bugs. Our food was dirty, our clothes were dirty, and our bodies were dirtier. But was this all bad? Not really, and it's a shame that "dirt" has such a negative concept as in, "Don't touch! That's dirty."

Growing up, we were meant to make mud pies, to play in the sand box, and get dirty. Those things, it turns out, are necessary to our long-term health as almost anything. Our immune systems need this kind of exposure to know how to react to real or not-so-real threats to our health.

You see, without early exposures to all sorts of organisms in the soil, when our immune systems are exposed to various intruders later in life, our bodies may overreact. Hence, we develop autoimmune diseases, some types of asthma, and debilitating allergies. But that's just one of the consequences of our lost connection to Earth. Our immune systems may never truly reach their full zenith of defensive powers against disease-causing organisms or chemical toxins without reestablishing this lost connection to our planet's crust.

So while modern civilization proceeds full speed ahead with hand-held technology and interconnectivity, we must not allow ourselves to become apart from Nature. I believe it's in our best interest to maintain contact with the good Earth. It's a shame that most of us don't.

Therefore, my main premise is that most of us will benefit by returning to our bodies these missing microorganisms. Prestigious health experts at our most respected medical and scientific institutions worldwide have come to these same conclusions.

In fact, society's growing separation from dirt and germs may well be the cause of the growing incidence of a wide range of maladies, says epidemiologist David Strachan, who first advanced the over-cleanliness theory when he was at Britain's London School of Hygiene and Tropical Medicine.

While conducting research, Dr. Strachan noticed that children belonging to large families were much less likely to develop asthma, hay fever, or eczema. Dr. Strachan theorized that older children coming home dirty with all sorts of resident soil microorganisms were actually protecting their younger brothers and sisters.

When Dr. Strachan says we need dirt, I think he's on to something.

∽

Throughout the world, scientists are carrying spoons and sandwich bags no matter where they go, in search of ever-exotic sources of such soil organisms. They are seeking out new and unique soil organisms in bat caves, hot springs, undersea volcanoes, and even from mummies. Each exotic locale may yield a completely new resource for SBOs. Consider these discoveries:

- While vacationing in Norway, an employee at Sandoz Pharmaceutical took home a mold found in soil that later led to development of the anti-rejection transplant drug cyclosporin.
- A scientist scouring the soil of an Indonesian temple discovered microbes that can turn starch into sugar.
- In Japan, a scientist picked up a clump of soil from a golf course and used it to cure parasitic infections plaguing livestock.

- Most current antibiotics come from microbes in the soil, including streptomycin, the first treatment for tuberculosis, and vancomycin, currently the drug of last resort for the toughest infections.

And consider this—unknown organisms make up 99.9 percent of all the microbes in the soil. One gram of soil—the weight of a packet of sugar—can contain as many as 10,000 species *unknown* to science, notes Jo Handelsman, a professor of plant pathology at the University of Wisconsin.

"Now, for the first time, she [Handelsman] and her colleagues, along with several other research groups working independently, are learning to extract the DNA of these mysterious creatures and clone it," said an article in *Business Week*. "They are finding that the microbes differ so profoundly from known bacteria that they could represent entirely new kingdoms of life—as different from other bacteria as animals are from plants. That means that the proteins produced by these creatures could have properties unlike any other such substances known." Already, Handelsman says, several new antibiotics have been identified from such soil microbes.

But here's the clincher: From the same article in *Business Week,* there was a great explanation as to why anyone with Crohn's or any other disease might well benefit from SBOs, and it all starts with the human intestines—an environment that most people consider pretty familiar.

The gut is home to perhaps 10,000 kinds of microbes, and one of the surprises in the decoding of the human genome is that the gut contains more than 200 genes that come from bacteria. These microbes not only keep us alive, but in some small part, we are made of them. The *Business Week* article went on to say this:

> [Researchers are] now looking at how these largely unknown microbes might play a role in Crohn's disease, an inflammation of the small intestine. [They have] found that the makeup of the mixed "community" of microbes in the intestines changes in people with the disease. A similar thing might happen with tuberculosis…leading [researchers] to wonder whether some diseases might be caused not by a single dangerous microbe but by a change in the microbial community—an ecological imbalance inside the human body.

So there you have it. Our soil is home to countless numbers of microorganisms, and our gut is populated with far more microbes than we have ever known. Inside and out, we are at one with the Earth. At least we should be. After all, the Bible says that man was made from the dust of the Earth. That is a bit of wisdom that we can't even yet begin to understand or comprehend.

The idea that dirt is good for our health is paradoxically due to our exposure to both protective and infectious microorganisms found in soil. According to a key report in the *New Scientist,* researchers have discovered the microorganisms found in dirt influence maturation of the immune system so that it is either functional or dysfunctional. The organisms to which we are exposed "condition" our immune system so that it intuitively knows when to produce and activate T-helper (Th) cells.

Let me talk a little bit more about T-helper cells. Among the cells of the immature immune system are so-called non-differentiated T-helper cells (Th cells), which are primarily produced by the thymus gland. These Th cells control the initiation or suppression of the body's immune reactions and regulate many other immune cells. Among the Th cells are two types that develop as we mature: Th1 and Th2 helper cells.

The quality of an individual's immune system can be evaluated through the balance of cytokines that it is producing. This increasingly popular classification method is referred to as the Th1/Th2 balance.

Interleukins and interferons are called "cytokines" that can be grouped into those secreted by Th1 type cells and those secreted by Th2 type cells. Th1 cells promote specialized cell-mediated immunity, while Th2 cells induce humoral immunity. (This refers to immunity to infection created by proteins termed *antibodies,* or specialized proteins secreted by "B" cells or B lymphocytes.)

Th1 cells are the quintessential cop who does his job of defending your body efficiently—with little wasted effort. The body's Th1 cells produce only as many germ-zapping antibodies as necessary to stop an invader. The message here is economy of action.

But on the other hand, Th2 cells are the armed forces of the body, and when they go out to do battle, it's like sending in the U.S. Army, Navy, Marines, and Air Force. The Th2 cells are "total response" defenders.

These two different methods by which the body fights infections exist side by side. While cellular immunity (Th1) directs natural killer T cells and macrophages to attack abnormal cells and microorganisms at sites of infection inside the cells, humoral immunity (Th2) results in the production of antibodies used to neutralize foreign invaders and substances outside of the cells. Imagine the skies over Syria some time and you get a sense for the possible mayhem created by Th2 cells when they are in overdrive and overproducing germ-zapping antibodies.

In many cases, an infection is fought with both arms of the immune system. At other times, predominantly one is needed to control an infection. Therefore, a healthy immune system needs to be balanced and dynamic between Th1 and Th2 activity, switching back and forth between the two as needed. This allows for a quick eradication of a threat and then a return to balance before responding to the next threat.

The inability to respond adequately with a Th1 response can result in chronic infection, chronic fatigue syndrome, and even cancer. On the flip side, an overactive yet paradoxically ineffective Th2 response can contribute to allergies and various syndromes and play a role in autoimmune disease.

∞

Children who are exposed to an adequate number of viruses and bacteria and other microorganisms from playing in the dirt, making mud pies, and putting fingers in their mouths will develop mature Th cells that mature in the proper proportion into desirable Th1 cells. But without adequate internal exposure to soil microbes, immune cells will have a tendency toward overreactions and become more likely to mature into Th2 cells.

Too many children, today and in the last twenty or thirty years, have been denied this much-needed exposure to soil microorganisms. There are all sorts of reasons: safety in the neighborhood, urban and suburban development, and the rise of electronic gaming, but the result is that we live in too clean an environment. The immune systems of children and adults are no longer being built up properly.

Perhaps the pendulum needs to swing away from elimination of microorganisms from our environment. This, coupled with the fact that most kids aren't allowed to "explore" or live in urbanized neighborhoods and have lost contact with our bacterially rich Earth.

Moreover, we oversterilize everything. We have disinfectant dishwashing soap and disinfectant body lotions and skin bars with disinfectants like triclosan—and even disinfectant produce washes when, in fact, we need the beneficial organisms in our food supply.

An even bigger issue is how agricultural soil has been sterilized with pesticides and herbicides, destroying beneficial and harmful bacteria alike, even harming plants' natural immune systems. Our food used to have loads of bacterial organisms that became part of the plant we consumed. Now that our soil is sterile, our foods are sterile. Pesticides and herbicides have done pretty much to the soil what overuse of medical antibiotics has done to the human gut—eliminate not only the bad guys but also the good guys. And that's not good.

Oh, sure, we are exposed to some of these microorganisms every now and then, but leading researchers say that on a daily basis, most people are no longer exposed to large enough quantities of microorganisms from dust, soil, air, water, and foods to achieve optimal health.

With an overly sterile environment, our relationship to Earth has been severed. We live in air-conditioned offices and homes and pass from one to the other walking upon concrete or asphalt pavement after traveling in cars on polluted highways. Our foods are irradiated to further kill the microorganisms. We use antibacterial preservatives. The idea of consuming fermented foods like sauerkraut and kefir is almost foreign to Americans. With our modern, high-tech processing methods, food manufacturers remove and destroy many of our food's most important life-giving nutrients.

From the first settlers in the 17th century up until the 1950s, the American agricultural system raised fruits and vegetables in soil exceedingly rich in bacteria and other organisms. After World War II, however, these SBOs were displaced as a result of chemical farming and pesticide usage by Big Agriculture.

In their quest to reduce unwanted disease-causing pathogens, agribusiness conglomerates have sterilized the soil and water through chlorination, thereby eliminating the beneficial bacteria as well as the harmful ones. It's normal for large cattle-raising companies to give antibiotics, hormones, and other drugs to their livestock.

Even if we don't take antibiotics, we almost certainly consume them when we eat meat and dairy products. Cattle, pigs, and poultry are routinely given big helpings of antibiotics to prevent infections from spreading in their stressful, crowded quarters. In Europe, giving antibiotics to cattle is outlawed, as is the importation of American beef; this is, in part, due to all the antibiotics fed to U.S. cattle. Researchers estimate that by consuming just one glass of commercial milk, we are unknowingly ingesting the residues of up to one hundred different antibiotics.

This constant exposure to low-dose antibiotics is leading to an increase in antibiotic-resistant bacteria.

∞

A healthy intestine in both children and adults contains billions of bacteria—including up to 10,000 different species. Optimally, the body's beneficial or benign bacteria should outnumber the cells of the body by approximately a hundredfold! This is no longer the case, however.

These friendly bacteria are our first line of immune defense. They displace and fight off unfriendly bacteria and internal fungi that can set the stage for both adult and childhood illness. They even increase the body's levels of interferon, a mighty immune-boosting chemical. Good bacteria are as essential to good health as clean water and organic food.

But here's the problem that adults—and children especially—face as they grow up in a toxic world. Stress, medications, and poor diet reduce friendly bacteria even further, leaving us even more vulnerable to disease. Antibiotics can be the biggest culprits in destroying our friendly bacteria. At high dosages, they wipe out all bacteria inside your child's body—the good along with the bad.

Once that happens, the race is on as to which microorganisms—the good guys or the bad guys—set up shop in that empty real estate inside you or your child's gut.

This is why we must be extra careful to replenish and stabilize friendly bacteria in the gastrointestinal tract. By making a conscious effort to consume SBOs, you can position a massive army of health defenders in your intestines that are on guard to protect your health as well as maintain a balanced immune system, reacting only as needed and never overreacting or underreacting.

The way SBOs stimulate the immune system's Th cells will also influence other immune cells, especially B lymphocytes that are manufactured in the bone marrow and produce nonspecific or unprogramed antibodies. These unprogramed antibodies have the ability to take a fresh, new look at newly introduced bodily invaders. They have not been preprogramed to overreact and are freely available to travel where and when needed.

The beauty of it all is that this huge reservoir of extra antibodies is always on hand for the immune system to utilize as long as the individual is taking SBOs in a supplement form regularly. Without them, this reservoir of extra antibodies is unavailable. Thus, by ingesting SBOs on a regular basis, the effectiveness of one's immune system becomes vastly enhanced.

What the SBOs do is to help accomplish the educational process that was earlier disturbed when the link between beneficial soil organisms and the human body was broken. By this, I mean they help to educate the body's Th cells in a way that didn't happen during childhood. The process might be more aptly called building immune "tolerance" or "maturation."

Through constant exposure to the lost SBOs, the body's Th cells become reeducated and "tolerant" and mount only necessary, but not excessive, immune responses. In a sense, this formula gives the immune system the workout it missed when the patient was young and living in our modern, highly sanitized world. But that is only part of what SBOs do. Like any other great advance in healing, the science is there to back up the positive clinical outcomes that complementary physicians are seeing with their patients.

In the natural environment, SBOs help plants to digest inorganic substances, protect root systems from parasites, yeast, and fungi, and provide growth factors and different hormones. They do the same for human health and the gastrointestinal tract. We are, after all, part of Nature.

William C. Bryce, M.D., Ph.D., of Huntington Beach, California, notes: "Just as SBOs destroy molds, yeasts, fungi, and viruses in the soil of the organic garden, they perform the same function with pathological organisms present in the gut, which greatly enhances the body's immune system."

⚭

Scientists and doctors are prone to use fancy words that leave the average person wondering what the heck they're jabbering about. This imbalance, when pathogenic microorganisms outnumber beneficial bacterial species, is referred to as *dysbiosis*. Put simply, dysbiosis is one of those fancy words for a condition that occurs when the population of organisms residing within the gastrointestinal tract becomes imbalanced, often resulting in acute or chronic sickness.

Normally, populations of pathogenic organisms are kept in balance by competition from good bacteria because of symbiosis, which is the mutually interdependent relationship among the hundreds of intestinal microbial species. According to Dr. Michael Gershon, author of *The Second Brain*, "One reason that the bacteria in the lumen of the colon do not break out and infect the body is that they are at war with one another. No one kind of germ gains ascendancy and takes uncontested possession of colonic turf. The constant competition between otherwise nasty germs helps to keep the bacterial population under control."

The problem is that after antibiotics have wiped out all or much of the entire gastrointestinal landscape, the bad bacteria have the upper hand because they love the types of foods that we typically consume in our diet, especially the carbohydrates found in bread, pasta, milk, candy, baked goods, and soft drinks.

So when the balance of good and bad bacteria is disturbed by antibiotics, it's the bad bacteria that get the head start in repopulating the barren property within your gastrointestinal tract. Another point to consider is this: the kind of food people who are sick or have been sick love to eat is what we call comfort food—you know, milkshakes, breads, pastas, cookies, and fries. These are the very kinds of food that promote the growth of disease-causing bacteria.

Dysbiosis results in abnormal fermentation in the small intestine. In the large intestine, some fermentation is desirable because it produces butyrate and other short-chain fatty acids that nourish the cells of the intestinal wall. In the small intestine, however, growth of yeast, fungi, and/ or fermenting pathogenic bacteria can result in damage to the gut lining, absorption of toxic by-products, and impaired absorption of nutrients.

Repeated use of broad-spectrum antibiotics, oral contraceptives, and steroid medications can set up conditions for opportunistic overgrowth of organisms that are not affected by the drugs or that are able to recolonize rapidly once treatment has ended. This is particularly true of yeast and fungal organisms. Their metabolic products appearing in urine are the strongest physical evidence of intestinal overgrowth of these organisms.

At the end of the day, *dysbiosis* is a fancy word for the imbalance of microorganisms in your gastrointestinal tract. But what you need to keep in mind is that persistent dysbiosis can have serious health consequences that lead to a weakened immune system. As the body loses its ability to cope with the offending infections and pathogens, a host of chronic conditions appear that, on the surface, seem to have little to do with gastrointestinal disturbances.

This means that gastrointestinal health has far-reaching implications for general health, much more so than is commonly recognized. Indeed, doctors may have to do quite a bit of medical sleuthing to track down patients' complaints to finally attribute them to dysbiosis or an imbalance of their gastrointestinal bacteria. But once patients take appropriate pathways to enhance the healing response, they often respond far more favorably than anticipated.

When the friendly bacteria are decimated by antibiotics, other harmful bacteria, yeast, and fungi already living in the body, which were held in strict check by the friendly bacteria, begin to multiply profusely. The overgrowth of one especially potent yeast-like fungus, *Candida albicans*, leads to a potentially serious condition called candidiasis. Depending on its locale of action, candidiasis can inflame the tongue, mouth, or rectum. It can also cause vaginitis and may be instrumental in triggering a range of mental and emotional symptoms, including irritability, anxiety, and even depression. Many allergies that manifest themselves as digestive disorders, such as bloating, heartburn, constipation, and diarrhea, also have been causally linked to candida yeast overgrowth.

Knowing how to use antibiotics in a safe and effective manner is critically important to doctors, pharmacists, and consumers alike. A good place to start is with our children. The American Academy of Pediatrics has observed that 95 percent of children in the United States will be treated with antibiotics for a middle ear infection by the age of five. Some children will shake off the effects of antibiotics just fine, but others won't. Their systems might become ravaged by the antibiotics, and their populations of beneficial bacteria could be decimated.

∞

Not surprisingly, dysbiosis and its prevention or treatment are among the most topical and challenging problems doctors face today. In dysbiosis, when protective friendly bacterial species are reduced in population, even organisms traditionally thought to have little ability to cause disease, including usually benign bacteria, yeasts, and some parasites, can induce illness by altering our nutritional status or immune response.

The consequences of intestinal dysbiosis extend beyond the immediately obvious gastrointestinal distress. Studies have implicated intestinal bacterial imbalances as a basis for conditions ranging from recurrent infections and immune breakdown to chronic fatigue.

In today's world, when we're looking to maximize our health, dysbiosis may leave us predisposed to a host of common ailments including diarrhea, constipation, IBS, colon cancer, allergies, vaginitis, increased susceptibility to infection, food cravings, lack of mental clarity, hypoglycemia symptoms, and many more conditions that doctors rarely connect to the bacterial populations of the gastrointestinal tract.

Equally important, however, are the effects on tissues far from the intestinal site, such as the brain, joints, and muscles, as well as on the immune system. Effects can be as diverse as headaches, learning disorders, insomnia, immune dysfunction, behavioral disorders, chronic fatigue, joint pain, and nutritional deficiencies.

More familiar to many patients are conditions such as IBS, Crohn's disease, fibromyalgia, leaky gut syndrome, wasting disease, diverticulitis, hemorrhoids, and breast and colon cancer—all of which may have their genesis in an upset in the gastrointestinal tract's bacterial population.

Abnormal bacterial populations that lead to dysfunctional gut fermentation have adverse effects on nutrient assimilation and production, especially the B vitamins, and the absorption of calcium, magnesium, and zinc. These nutritional deficits explain how abnormal bacterial gut populations may cause many other significant adverse effects on health.

∞

Today, we know that digestive diseases and other conditions related to unhealthy imbalances of intestinal flora not only have an enormous impact on our health but are also extremely costly to the nation.

Digestive, liver, and pancreatic diseases, which often are caused in part by or result in dysbiosis, result in more than 100 million outpatient visits and 13 million hospitalizations at a cost of $141.8 billion, according to a report commissioned by the National Institutes of Health. The cost in human life is 230,000 deaths annually.

The costliest digestive diseases, in both direct and indirect costs, are:

- digestive cancers ($24.1 billion)
- liver disease ($13.1 billion)
- gastroesophageal reflux disease (GERD) ($12.6 billion)
- gallstones ($6.2 billion)
- abdominal wall hernia ($6.1 billion)
- diverticular disease ($4.0 billion)
- pancreatitis ($3.7 billion)
- vital hepatitis ($3.3 billion)
- peptic ulcer disease ($3.1 billion)
- appendicitis ($2.6 billion)

Digestive diseases have an enormous impact on the health care system in the United States. New technologies and new drugs have revolutionized the understanding and treatment of peptic ulcer disease and gastrointestinal esophageal reflux disease (GERD). While successful outcomes of future research will continue to reduce the economic and health care costs related to diagnosing and treating digestive diseases, the fact is that no matter what new medicines we come up with, the bottom line remains this: Your body desperately requires healthy intestinal flora, while many environmental and dietary conditions threaten this balance. We should be handing out SBOs to everyone.

So where did it all start? As the practice of soil and water sterilization increased over the years, the beneficial bacteria in Americans' bodies decreased correspondingly. Normally we should have a balance of 85 percent "good" bacteria to 15 percent "bad" bacteria in the intestinal tract, but today, most of us show the reverse ratio. Therefore, it's no coincidence that the incidences of chronic and degenerative diseases have multiplied dramatically since World War II.

Sophisticated lifestyles among Western industrialized countries contribute greatly to critical gastrointestinal disruption among the populations. Antibiotic usage, excessive stress, heavy consumption of excess sugar and alcohol, the regular drinking of carbonated beverages, and frequent consumption of over-the-counter drugs alter the acid/alkaline balance of the intestinal tract, creating the perfect environment for pathogenic microbial activity.

Nutritional researchers are convinced that as much as 90 percent of known systemic diseases may be caused or exacerbated by gastrointestinal imbalances. My case of Crohn's disease was a severe example of what can occur from gut bacterial imbalances.

The water we drink isn't helping things. Once, drinking water teemed with mycobacteria, a type of germ. Now, I'll be the first to tell you that some of these pathogens were deadly, and the fact that today our water supplies are disinfected has made our tap water much safer and greatly reduced morbidity and mortality as compared to a century ago.

On the other hand, though, I want to point out that populations in countries with low rates of asthma still drink water with billions of mycobacteria per liter. The chlorination process used to disinfect water also disinfects the human body, eliminating both good and bad microorganisms.

In order to restore health, many people need to restore their connection to the soil. While obviously not everyone can go out and start making mud pies, do a little gardening, or hike in the mountains, there is another way of doing so, and that's by consuming nutritional supplements with SBOs. I believe SBOs can prove to be the healing link between our soil and our bodies.

By reintroducing SBOs to the human body, persons in pain—and who are suffering from immune disorders including food allergies, IBS, rheumatoid arthritis, lupus, and Crohn's disease, and many other conditions—finally have the missing link their bodies require to enhance the healing response.

Years ago, I met a board-certified gastroenterologist named Joseph Brasco, M.D., while attending a nutritional seminar. I was there both to speak and because I was researching more about the principles of the ancestral diet. Dr. Brasco attended because he was investigating new options for his patients with gastrointestinal disorders. When it came time for my talk, Dr. Brasco sat in the front row. He had read about me in the *Townsend Letter* and was intrigued by my story.

We went to lunch afterward, where he picked my brain. "I'm intrigued by what you shared today," he told me. "What you said makes great sense—your inclusion of kefir and other fermented foods, and the use of soil-based organisms in nutritional supplements. I've already been prescribing these supplements to patients. In my own practice, however, I'm taking things one step further. You see, my idea is that we can take the healing of patients through diet and universalize it not just to an individual but to a whole group of people—all our patients."

Eventually our partnership resulted in writing a book together entitled *Restoring Your Digestive Health*. To this day, Dr. Brasco remains a fan of SBOs when it comes to his patients' health problems and for maintaining their health. He is also keen on the inclusion of fermented foods in our diet and the role they can play in the healing process. Indeed, SBOs and fermented foods naturally fit well together.

Keep in mind Dr. Brasco is a board-certified gastroenterologist and comes from a traditional background in medical training and education. Here's what he says about the value of SBOs in his own practice and why he thinks they are so essential to our health and well-being:

> Eating vegetables directly out of the soil as part of food was good for primitive man. The organisms living in that soil caused primal man to thrive. Today is so different, however. Given the paranoia that modern men and women in Western society feel against ingesting soil of any kind, these ancient soil-based organisms no longer are part of our food supply. Yes, times do change!

It used to be that a pioneering farmer working his fields, the so-called sod-buster who became hungry, simply dug into the ground, pulled up some carrots, brushed off the dirt, and chomped away on vegetables containing the residual dirt and all. The farmer kept his gastrointestinal tract functioning well by ingesting these extracurricular homeostatic soil organisms. But that's not the way it is anymore. So fastidious are residents of Western industrialized nations that too much cleanliness has become somewhat detrimental to one's gastrointestinal tract. We have to eat dirt once in a while. We really do.

But, in fact, the reestablishment of the SBO–body link yields far more benefits than simply aiding in cases of autoimmune disease. Overall, bodily functions and immunity are greatly improved. Cholesterol levels are naturally reduced, energy levels are increased, and resistance to disease-causing organisms is enhanced.

With soil organisms, I was able to enhance my own body's healing response. Upon ingesting them, the soil organisms maintained a healthy balance of intestinal flora by producing organic compounds such as lactic acid, hydrogen peroxide, and acetic acid, which increased the acidity of the intestine and inhibited the reproduction of massive amounts of harmful microorganisms. These soil organisms also produced substances called bacteriocins, which act as natural antibiotics to kill almost any kind of pathological bacteria and to fend off threats they themselves face from pathogenic microorganisms.

Two of the soil organisms that intrigued me in my research were *Bacillus subtilis* and *Bacillus lichenformis*. In studies conducted in Germany at the University of Berlin's Max Volmer Institute, both were shown to inactivate human immunodeficiency, herpes simplex (HSV-1 and HSV-2), simian immunodeficiency, feline calicivirus, murine encephalomyocarditis, and other lipid envelope viruses—along with mycoplasmas, fungi, and bacteria. They did so by producing a potent chemical called surfactin, a detergent-like substance that dissolves the lipid membranes of lipid envelope viruses, thereby rendering them completely inactivated.

The soil organisms provided even more important health benefits. They established colonies in the entire digestive system, starting in the esophagus and ending in the colon, by attaching themselves to the walls of these organs. Burrowing behind the putrefaction, which lines the intestinal walls, they ate and destroyed unfriendly microorganisms. The decay was then dislodged and flushed out of the body in the normal evacuation process.

This aided in detoxification of the intestinal tract, increased the body's ability to absorb nutrients, and, again, made the immune system super-strong by removing mucoid plaque that covered the GALT, especially aiding the body's ability to fight off infectious viruses and bacteria.

What science is determining is that SBOs are extremely aggressive against all pathological molds, yeasts, fungi, and viruses and they help the body to efficiently eliminate such pathogens. Moreover, protozoa, worms, and other parasites are eliminated as well by the aggressive action of the SBOs, both within the intestines and throughout the other organs and tissues. *C. albicans,* other yeasts, and molds are obliterated.

Here's a list of the health benefits we receive from ingestion of the soil organisms:

SBOs pool new RNA/DNA in the cells.

SBOs are rich sources of DNA and RNA, the naturally coded instructions for the cells to reactivate their own repair. Working in a symbiotic relationship with bodily tissues, SBOs create a pool of extra DNA/RNA raw materials that are immediately available when needed, accelerating healing of wounds and other tissue disturbances including burns, surgical incisions, and infections.

SBOs quench free radicals by creating SOD, a powerful antioxidant.

SBOs produce the free radical-quencher superoxide dismutase (SOD), a wonderful antioxidant. Unless extinguished at once, free radicals attack any physiological molecule, causing cancers and other tissue damage. SOD, working enzymatically, is a first-line defense against free radicals before they can cause organ damage.

SBOs stimulate alpha-interferon production.

SBOs stimulate the production of a key immune system regulator known as the polypeptide alpha-interferon (a molecular protein). The scientific community has long known about the virus-fighting ability of alpha-interferon and sought to enhance the body's production to aid the healing response when faced with certain health maladies. Research documents over fifty immune-regulating effects.

Alpha-interferon has been synthesized and used for a variety of illnesses, notably cancer, but the recombinantly derived version is extremely costly, inefficient, and has many adverse side effects. Researchers at the State Academy of Medicine in Apodaca, Mexico, report that the SBO formula, when consumed at the recommended dosage, stimulates the body's endogenous alpha-interferon production.

"The product itself does not contain any alpha interferon but comprises a singularly efficient set of nutrients that seem to increase specifically and most effectively the body's natural alpha interferon production," the researchers said. Working on human patients with various immune dysfunctions, the research team demonstrated the human body requires only small daily quantities of alpha-interferon to maintain a lively and effective immune response.

Scientists note that even small increases in the body's production of this therapeutic substance, produced by the immune system in reaction to soil organisms, can become an effective neutralizer of the toxic effects of pathogenic viruses that cause herpes, hepatitis B, hepatitis C, influenza, and other potentially life-threatening illnesses.

SBOs stimulate the production of human lactoferrin.

Present in the homeostatic soil organisms themselves is a certain substance that stimulates the formation of human lactoferrin, a member of the family of iron-carrying proteins. Lactoferrin is found in the specific granules of neutrophils, where it exerts antimicrobial activity by withholding iron from ingested pathogenic bacteria and fungi. For this reason, SBOs exhibit characteristics akin to fungicides, virucides, bactericides, and parasiticides. Iron carried by lactoferrin is extremely bioavailable—greater than 95 percent—yet it will not be delivered to noxious microbes.

∽

So wide-ranging is the impact of our gut on human health that each of the following conditions may be caused by intestinal toxemia and can be aided by soil organisms:

- **Allergies.** William Lintz, M.D., reported in *Gastrointestinal Allergy, The Review of Gastroenterology* that he successfully treated 474 patients suffering allergies by elimination of pathogenic bacteria and their toxins.
- **Asthma.** Dr. Allan Eustis, an instructor at Tulane University of Medicine in the early 20th century, noted that eliminating intestinal toxemia relieved 121 cases of bronchial asthma.
- **Arthritis.** Dr. Anthony Bassler treated some 344 arthritic patients by relieving intestinal toxemia.
- **Cardiac arrhythmias.** Dr. D.J. Beary, a professor of physiology at Queens College, Cork, England, noted this: "There seems to be little doubt that substances that have a deleterious action on the heart musculature and nerves are formed both in the small and large intestine, even under apparently normal circumstances."
- **Ear, nose, and throat problems.** J.A. Stucky, M.D., noted, "In several hundreds of cases of diseases of the nasal accessory sinuses, middle and internal ear…I have found unmistakable and marked evidence of toxemia of intestinal origin as evidenced by excessive indications in the urine, and when the condition causing this was removed there was marked amelioration or entire relief of the disease."
- **Eclampsia.** Dr. R.C. Brown, an obstetrical surgeon in England, linked intestinal toxemia with eclampsia.
- **Eye problems.** C.W. Hawley, M.D., treated many causes of eyestrain and disease with success by relieving intestinal toxemia.
- **Thyroid gland disease.** W.S. Revano, M.D., theoretically linked goiter to "a toxic process in the intestinal tract."

The science of soil organisms is exploding, and what we are learning is essential to good health. The ability of soil organisms to aid our quest for healing and maintaining good health is one of the most exciting breakthroughs in modern health.

The irony is that we are talking about soil organisms as old as the Earth. I would urge anyone with intractable autoimmune conditions, allergies, low energy, inability to gain weight, fibromyalgia, and chronic fatigue syndrome to take advantage of SBOs. Parents whose children have chronic middle ear infections would do well by their child to get him or her on SBOs. Regarding this, Dr. Brasco made these observations:

> The probiotic microorganisms found in soil-based organisms have been proven to be helpful for the enhancement of health and prolongation of life. Such proof has been shown ever since mankind inhabited the Earth. Primitive man absorbed the product's soil-based organisms from the environment in different ways; for instance, he buried meat and other food in the ground as a form of preservation. Such meat would combine with soil-based bacteria and be eaten to become a part of the human physiology, thus changing into what science now identifies as body-based organisms. Such friendly microorganisms, having established themselves in the human gut, create an environment for optimizing human nutrition.

> The microorganisms found in SBOs are unlike other probiotics or beneficial gut bacteria and can maintain intrepid health for modern men and women the way primitive man experienced it. Allow me to offer an illustrating case history. I had a patient named Marion Frome, an eighteen-year-old manicurist, consult with me for the treatment of Crohn's disease. She arrived after many forms of therapy had failed her. It was only after I prescribed the ingestion of soil-based organisms that her diarrhea came under control, abdominal cramping stopped, malabsorption corrected itself, and fistulae around the anus healed. She had an exceedingly positive response.

I'm a big believer in SBOs and have been now for many years.

Although they have been a part of the diet for centuries, product-specific studies of SBOs are fairly new. These studies have been accepted for publication in a special supplement of the peer-reviewed *Progress in Nutrition*.

The following are summaries of the studies from the journal in which three single-blind, placebo-controlled studies on soil organisms were conducted at the Dispensario Medico, Partido de la Revolucion Democratica, a medical dispensary in Irapuato, Mexico. The researchers wanted to find out whether SBOs could help people with high cholesterol and leukemia, as well as see if they made healthy test subjects feel more energetic and improved memory and concentration. Here are summaries of the results of the three studies:

High cholesterol:

Seventy patients with blood cholesterol counts higher than 300 milligrams per deciliter were given soil organisms or a placebo. Every subject given the soil organisms saw their total blood cholesterol count drop by 25 percent or more; the placebo subjects showed no change.

Energy levels, memory, and concentration:

Seventy patients with no known pathologies were given soil organisms or a placebo. Of the thirty-five subjects given soil organisms, thirty-three reported feeling more energetic. Vital hemoglobin (HGB) levels and red blood cell counts increased moderately in thirty-three subjects. In the placebo group, no subjects reported an increase in energy or vitality levels. Furthermore, in the placebo group, only two subjects out of thirty-three (two subjects dropped out of the study) saw their HGB levels increase. In only one subject did the red blood cell count increase. Conspicuous increases in memory and concentration were seen in twenty-eight out of thirty-five test patients, with only one patient improving in the placebo group.

Chronic lymphocytic leukemia stage II:

Thirty-five subjects with chronic lymphocytic leukemia were given soil organisms. The director of research reported that the soil organisms "attenuated the symptoms of approximately 80 percent of the treated patients." In 80 percent of subjects, white blood cell counts improved.

In a study conducted at Bio Inova Life Sciences Laboratories under the direction of Pierre Braquet, Ph.D., and Jean Michel Mencia-Juerta, Ph.D., researchers attempted to identify the antimicrobial properties of SBOs and found that the soil organisms were effective in inhibiting various pathogenic microorganisms, including *Pseudomonas aeruginosa*, a rare but life-threatening infectious agent.

Another study conducted at Bio Inova Life Sciences Laboratories evaluated the effectiveness of SBOs on the immune system. In this study, researchers looked at macrophage function and the production of cytokines such as interleukins and tumor necrosis factor. Macrophages are large white blood cells that also serve the immune system by killing foreign invaders. In the study, soil organisms were found to boost the immune system by enhancing macrophage function.

In another study at Bio Inova Life Sciences Laboratories, soil organisms were examined for inhibition of cancer cell lines. These were shown to inhibit the proliferation of cancer cell lines of the breast, liver, and lung.

In an open-label, 120-day clinical pilot study conducted at the Diabetes Resource Center by Dr. Ernesto Perez, M.D., researchers determined whether the soil organisms could help control blood sugar levels and decrease the risk of cardiovascular disease in people with type 2 diabetes.

Specifically, the researchers wanted to see if SBOs could aid in controlling blood sugar levels and lowering cholesterol and triglyceride levels. The study showed that using soil organisms and following the diet and lifestyle recommendations of the American Diabetes Association lowers blood glucose levels, lowers HbA1C (a long-term indicator of blood sugar control), lowers total cholesterol, and decreases triglycerides. Overall, the subjects using SBOs in the study lowered their risk of cardiovascular heart disease.

While the use of SBOs did result in improved blood sugar balance, the real standout results were in the reduction of high cholesterol and triglyceride levels. The most dramatic results occurred among a subgroup of patients having the highest cholesterol and triglyceride levels. Here are some of the study highlights:

- One woman patient with a starting total cholesterol count of 356 mg/dl experienced a 56 percent drop to 224 mg/dl, while her triglycerides went from 1106 mg/dl to 205 mg/dl, an 81 percent drop. Her coronary heart disease risk factors dropped 44 percent from 10.7 to 6.0.
- In another case, a female patient's total cholesterol went from 248 mg/dl to 181 mg/dl, a 27 percent drop, while her triglycerides went from 1,350 mg/dl to 167 mg/dl, an 88 percent drop. Her

coronary heart disease risk factor rating also dropped 53 percent from 9.5 to 4.5.

- A male with cholesterol levels of 313 mg/dl experienced a 30 percent decline to 219 mg/dl, while his triglyceride levels went from 436 mg/dl to 253 mg/dl for a 42 percent decline. His coronary heart disease risk factor rating went down 16 percent (from 9.7 to 8.1).

- Another male with a cholesterol level of 179 mg/dl experienced a 12 percent decline to 157 mg/dl and a 20 percent decline in triglycerides from 172 mg/dl to 138 mg/dl. His coronary heart disease risk factor rating declined 14 percent from 4.2 to 3.6.

- Another male had a cholesterol reading of 199 mg/dl, which declined 27 percent to 145 mg/dl, while his triglycerides went down 44 percent (from 217 mg/dl to 121 mg/dl). His coronary heart disease risk factor rating went down 23 percent from 5.3 to 4.1.

- Finally, a woman with cholesterol levels of 194 mg/dl experienced a 10 percent decline to 174 mg/dl and an 11 percent decline in triglycerides from 413 mg/dl to 369 mg/dl. Her coronary heart disease risk factor rating declined 14 percent from 5.1 to 4.4

In an open-label, 120-day clinical pilot study conducted by Paul A. Goldberg, M.PH, D.C., at the Goldberg Clinic in Marietta, Georgia, seventeen individuals suffering from complex digestive and immune system disorders were given SBOs for 120 days. The subjects' gastrointestinal and immune system disorders had been resistant to conventional and complimentary treatments. They also had a variety of chronic diseases that were unresponsive to medical intervention for a minimum of three years.

The subjects ranged in age from twenty to sixty-five. No dietary or lifestyle changes were made. Of the sixteen subjects, fifteen reported clinical improvements in their overall health. They had partial to full relief from troublesome bowel problems, decreases in asthmatic symptoms, increases in energy levels, improvements in skin conditions, improvement in chronic sinus infection, and general improvement in overall well-being. No subjects reported a worsening of their symptoms.

Eight of eight subjects with elevated yeast levels as verified by stool and/ or blood tests—in other words, 100 percent—had a significant reduction in candida yeast growth. Three subjects with asthma had a 50 percent or greater reduction in usage of inhalant medications and asthma symptoms.

Moreover, three subjects who suffered from long-term chronic constipation and had laxative dependency were able to move their bowels daily without the use of laxatives. Three subjects with chronic IBS showed between 25 and 100 percent improvement.

Four patients with chronic fatigue syndrome were completely free of symptoms by the end of the 120-day period. Before and after, blood tests and physical examinations showed that no subject experienced a worsening of conditions or exhibited any evidence of toxicity. Because this was not a placebo-controlled study, the results should be considered investigative and not scientific, but they deserve further research.

Now let's look at the results for some individual patients:

Subject 1: A fifty-three-year-old male with a twenty-seven-year medical history of progressive psoriatic arthritis and ulcerative colitis experienced symptomatic improvement during the first three weeks with improvements in bowel function and arthritic pains followed by an exacerbation with increases in joint inflammation and bloody diarrhea.

After consuming a regiment of SBOs, he reported that his bowel function improved 25 percent by the end of the study with occasional days of "near normal stools," which had not occurred for over five years. Improvements were also noted with less visible blood in his stool, better-formed stools, and reduced incidence of cramping. There was no improvement in overall stiffness/joint discomforts. His sedimentation rate fluctuated but, at the end of the study, remained close to what it had been at the start (55mm/hr). A follow-up of the stool microbiology showed a significant reduction in the stool yeast count.

Subject 2: A forty-two-year-old female radiologist with a five-year history of chronic fungal infection of the lungs also had significant (approximately 25 percent) loss of lung function. She had chronic chest pain upon breathing. Long-term use of an antifungal drug had not resolved the problem or allowed for any significant improvement. She also had chronic asthma and a significantly elevated serum yeast titer.

At completion of the study, the subject reported feeling significant improvement. Her asthma symptomatology had improved by 70 percent, as rated by subject. She reported greater ease in breathing, improved bowel function, and more energy. Yeast serum antibody testing performed on this subject at the completion of the study showed a marked drop in the titer from 900 to 438 U/ml. Therefore, it would appear that her infectious state had greatly improved, leading to improved lung function.

Subject 3: A thirty-six-year-old male with chronic psoriasis widespread over his scalp, elbows, face, torso, and legs improved with approximately 25 percent of the psoriatic lesions clearing and a lightening of the remaining affected areas.

Subject 4: A forty-six-year-old male with chronic IBS since childhood that interfered with social and work activities reported at end of the protocol a reduction in symptoms of cramping/diarrhea/irritable bowel of approximately 25 to 30 percent.

Subject 5: A thirty-five-year-old female with chronic constipation of seven years' duration and bowel movements that occurred once every three to four days reported in the third week of the protocol that her constipation had abated entirely with bowel movements occurring every one to two days. She reported an enhanced sense of well-being.

Subject 6: A forty-three-year-old female with chronic fatigue, constipation with laxative dependency, and depression reported significant improvement in energy levels, reduction of depression, and complete relief from chronic constipation of five years' duration with her laxative dependency ended. (Prior to protocol, this patient reported having a bowel movement once every three days. After the protocol, the patient reported a daily bowel movement without laxative usage.)

A ninety-day, seventy-patient, blind placebo-controlled clinical study, also published in *Progress in Nutrition*, evaluated the effectiveness of SBOs as a primary treatment for chronic digestive disorder and malabsorption syndrome. Thirty-one patients in the study group and fourteen patients in the placebo group completed the study. Some 52 percent of those taking SBOs achieved full remission of symptoms; 32 percent of the participants achieved greater than 60 percent; and the remaining 16 percent achieved a greater than 40 percent improvement of symptoms. No subjects had zero improvement or a worsening of symptoms.

According to the director of the study, SBOs qualify as an accomplished specific therapy with "significant efficacy" for treating chronic digestive disorders and malabsorption syndrome. "It is evident that the preparation triggers regulatory neuro-immune reactions, inducing healing processes of the herein indicated pathological conditions," the researchers noted.

In addition, a significant number of beneficial observations were made in the course of the study which, due to the fact that they were beyond the scope of the established protocol, regrettably could not be incorporated in the official reports published in *Progress in Nutrition*. Thus, these are presented here in an independent compilation:

- Fourteen patients (nine females, five males) reported remarkable increases in their energy levels beginning toward the end of the second month and continuing through the third month of treatment.
- Three female patients having suffered from chronic, recurrent migraine headaches reported total remission from their headaches by the end of the respective studies.
- Six patients (five females, one male), having suffered from varied grades of chronic skin rash, reported total remission of these symptoms.
- Six patients (four females, two males) reported significant vanishing of some of their facial wrinkles by the end of the study.

If my experiences can help one person, that's a blessing. Fortunately, as I've heard over the years from many people, they've been able to overcome their own health challenges with the help of SBOs, combined with adherence to the Maker's Diet. Hearing people tell me that makes what I went through worthwhile.

I must confess, however, that turning my health around, I had to face another major health challenge. This time it didn't involve me. Instead, my Grandmother Rose Menlowe, who was often my caretaker during my illness, was diagnosed with an aggressive cancer.

I'll tell you what happened next in my next chapter.

4

MANKIND'S MOST POWERFUL IMMUNE ENHANCER

The insurance industry is understandably dependent on statistics. Thus, both our average life span and the principal causes of premature death are continuously studied and monitored with the greatest care. Nonetheless, I have yet to meet the first statistician who can spell out the paramount cause of death among the human population, which is ignorance.

I'm not being cynical. There's some history here.

In the 19th century, the famed French scientist Louis Pasteur offered the world the wisdom that most diseases were caused by harmful microbes. In the wake of his discoveries nearly 150 years ago, research and development in conventional medicine has been and remains tightly focused on the theory that almost all pathology is brought on by germs, viruses, fungi, and macroscopic parasites. Thus, to fight diseases, the onslaught of such invading germs must to be terminated. In order to fight disease and cure the sick and ailing, pharmaceutical research has concentrated on developing potent medicines to destroy microorganisms.

While these compounds have succeeded in eliminating many forms of infections and saved untold millions of lives, there's a flip side to consider. What's being overlooked, in my opinion, is that many diseases are caused by a weak "terrain" inside the body that becomes a prime target for infectious microorganisms.

Even the great Pasteur himself echoed the same sentiment as a dying man. I've already mentioned the harm that indiscriminate antibiotic use poses to the gastrointestinal flora and populations of both beneficial and pathogenic bacterial species. Where I want to turn our attention to is how the misuse and overuse of antibiotics have contributed to antibiotic resistance, a circumstance that reduces or eliminates the effectiveness of antibiotics.

During my lifetime, we have witnessed the unequivocal repercussion and fiasco of antibiotics which, instead of delivering lasting solutions, have turned into a veritable menace. A consequence of the ever-more-potent antibiotics is that manifold strains of germs have mutated and acquired an iron-strong resistance to the medications developed against them.

Antimicrobial resistance has been recognized since the introduction of penicillin more than eighty years ago, when penicillin-resistant infections caused by *Staphylococcus aureus* rapidly appeared. Today, doctors and hospitals are facing unprecedented crises from the rapid emergence and dissemination of other microbes resistant to one or more antimicrobial agents.

Antibiotic resistance has become a major public health problem, with more than 2 million infections and 23,000 deaths annually caused by antibiotic-resistance organisms, according to a National Institutes of Health (NIH) report issued in 2016.

In testimony before the Senate Committee on Health, Education, Labor, and Pensions Subcommittee on Public Health and Safety, Anthony S. Fauci, M.D., director of the National Institute of Allergy and Infectious Diseases of the National Institutes of Health, presented his own disturbing views on the overuse of antibiotics:

> Many diseases are increasingly difficult to treat because of the emergence of drug-resistant organisms, including HIV and other viruses; bacteria such as *staphylococci, enterococci,* and *E. coli,* which cause serious infections in hospitalized patients; bacteria that cause respiratory diseases such as pneumonia and tuberculosis; food-borne pathogens such as salmonella and campylobacter; sexually transmitted organisms such as *Neisseria gonorrhoeae*; Candida and other fungi; and parasites such as *Plasmodium falciparum,* the cause of malaria. According to the Institute of Medicine (IOM),

the total cost of treating antimicrobial-resistant infections may be as high as $5 billion annually in the United States.

Consider the following facts:

- Strains of *S. aureus* resistant to methicillin and other antibiotics are endemic in hospitals.
- Infection with methicillin-resistant *S. aureus* strains may also be increasing in nonhospital settings. A limited number of drugs remain effective against these infections. *S. aureus* strains with reduced susceptibility to vancomycin have emerged in Japan and the United States. The emergence of completely vancomycin-resistant strains would present a serious problem for physicians and patients.
- Increasing reliance on vancomycin has led to the emergence of vancomycin-resistant enterococci, which are bacteria that infect wounds, the urinary tract, and other sites.
- *Streptococcus pneumoniae* causes thousands of cases of meningitis and pneumonia, and seven million cases of ear infection in the United States each year. Currently, about 30 percent of *S. pneumoniae* isolates are resistant to penicillin, the primary drug used to treat this infection. Many penicillin-resistant strains are also resistant to other antimicrobial drugs.
- In sexually transmitted disease clinics that monitor outbreaks of drug-resistant infections, doctors have found that more than 30 percent of gonorrhea isolates are resistant to penicillin or tetracycline, or both.
- An estimated 300 to 500 million people worldwide are infected with the parasites that cause malaria.
- Resistance to chloroquine, once widely used and highly effective for preventing and treating malaria, has emerged in most parts of the world. Resistance to other antimalaria drugs is widespread and growing.
- Strains of multidrug-resistant tuberculosis (MDR-TB) have emerged and pose a particular threat to

people infected with HIV. Drug-resistant strains are as contagious as those that are susceptible to drugs. MDR-TB is more difficult and vastly more expensive to treat, and patients may remain infectious longer due to inadequate treatment.

- Diarrheal diseases cause almost three million deaths a year—mostly in developing countries, where resistant strains of highly pathogenic bacteria such as *Shigella dysenteriae, Vibrio cholerae, Escherichia coli, Campylobacter,* and *Salmonella* are emerging. A potentially dangerous "superbug" known as *Salmonella typhimurium,* resistant to ampicillin, sulfa, streptomycin, tetracycline, and chloramphenicol, has caused illness in Europe, Canada, and the United States.

- Fungal pathogens account for a growing proportion of nosocomial (hospital) infections. Fungal diseases such as candidiasis and *Pneumocystis carinii* pneumonia are common among AIDS patients, and isolated outbreaks of other fungal diseases in people with normal immune systems have occurred recently in the United States. Scientists and clinicians are concerned that the increasing use of antifungal drugs will lead to drug-resistant fungi. In fact, recent studies have documented resistance of Candida species to fluconazole, a drug used widely to treat patients with systemic fungal diseases.

Consequently, many open-minded researchers are challenging the antibiotic theory of disease treatment and are seeking alternative solutions to the problems. Over time, two schools of therapeutic concepts have emerged. Traditional medicine and its proponents have completely accepted the notion that germs, viruses, and fungi bring on most diseases, and somehow these bacterial critters must be obliterated. They assert that this goal can best be achieved through the use of potent antibiotics and specific chemicals.

Needless to say, the pharmaceutical industry enthusiastically endorses this theory and supports all research leading to the development of such preparations. Considering that there are factually billions of different harmful microorganisms, an endless stream of medicines and drugs must be developed in order to fight all of them. This obviously generates many billions of dollars in profits, not only in manufacturing such products but also in research and development of the same.

I have a different view, however. I believe we need to go beyond this theory because of the problem of emerging antibiotic-resistant pathogens. We start by talking about a second school of thought that goes beyond the use of ever more toxic drugs to destroy microbes and the assumption that these are the sole cause of disease.

I begin by reminding you that our environment is literally teeming with billions of microorganisms, most of which are harmful. They thrive unchallenged in our air, water, and soil and even in our living tissues. Yet, thanks to the intricate and powerful design of our immune system, we are not only able to survive, but can actually thrive amidst such a continuous onslaught in spite of a global demographic explosion of our population. Why? It's because our proficient immune response keeps us alive.

The immune system operating in a healthy human body is perfectly capable of annihilating injurious microorganisms while leaving all benign and useful species undamaged. Thus, illness ensues when our immune system becomes defective and is unable to generate an appropriate immune response.

This also reveals why not everyone exposed to the assault of a given germ, virus, or fungus succumbs to its harmful effects. In other words, we must conclude that their vigilant immune systems are fully operational. Thus, the disciples of the second school of thought support the idea of continuously servicing and repairing the immune system by natural—that is, nontoxic—means, which enhance our body's inborn self-healing abilities.

It is quite obvious—to say the least—that the pharmaceutical industry does not encourage the spreading of such ideas because these generally must rely on the natural pharmacopoeia. Though likely to yield impressive health dividends, there is little profit to be generated by promoting a natural means of health maintenance and repair and in teaching healthy lifestyles. Getting down to basics, this probably explains, at least in part, why the pharmaceutical industry and the medical establishment frown on complementary and alternative therapeutic methods, often purporting that they involve quackery.

So with all these "miracle drugs" at our disposal, why is it that cancer—a disease characterized by the uncontrolled growth and spread of abnormal cells—ranks right up there with heart disease as the number-one killer of Americans under the age of eighty-five, which comprise 98.4 percent of the population? And why has this development occurred during the federal government's four-decade-old "War on Cancer," which has poured more than $50 billion into research, on top of the billions more that private industry has kicked in?

Despite the concerted scientific effort, about 1.7 million *new* cases of cancer were diagnosed in 2017, and approximately 600,000 died from the lethal disease. While one's eyes tend to glaze over from so many numbers, the stark reality is that half of all American men and one-third of American women will develop some type of cancer during their lifetimes.

The deadliest form of cancer is lung cancer, which kills around 160,000 Americans a year—more than breast cancer, colon cancer, and prostate cancer combined. Sixty percent of patients die within a year of diagnosis, and 87 percent of all lung cancer cases arise from those who stubbed their cigarette butts in ashtrays.

To be sure, cancer is a disease that preys on the old—about 77 percent of all cancers are diagnosed in people fifty-five years of age or older. Yet cancer's icy tentacles can attack at any age; leukemia, a type of blood cancer, is a known child killer, while breast cancer has buried too many mothers of young children. In addition, cancer is an equal-opportunity disease, striking Americans of all racial and ethnic groups, although the rate of cancer occurrence can vary from group to group.

Also troubling is that we are seeing increasing rates of cancer in children and for people living in highly urbanized and industrialized counties, especially for those living near and working in the vicinity of petrochemical, mining, smelting, and nuclear power plants.

What every medical school student learns is that cancer is a disease of the human cells caused by a breakdown in the immune system. The entire human body is comprised of cells, which, by definition, contain genetic material, or DNA, that tell the cell what to do. In a healthy body, cells divide at a controlled rate so as to grow and repair damaged tissues and replace dying cells. Any abnormal cells are quickly recognized by the body and removed before they can present harm.

Cells are constantly dividing and growing; these around-the-clock activities keep us in good health. When the body cannot check the growth of abnormal cells, however, these "bad" cells keep multiplying until a mass of tissue, called a growth or tumor, slowly emerges. Think of the entire process as something akin to stepping on an ant pile and watching an army of angry ants attack any skin in sight.

Tumors are either benign or malignant. While benign tumors are oftentimes no more than nuisances, it's the term *malignant* that strikes fear in our hearts because that means cancer has successfully invaded the body and taken a beachhead. Malignant tumors have the ability to metastasize (spread to other parts of the body), disrupt the normal function of the body, and assault other tissues.

This is how the *Encyclopedia of Nutritional Healing* describes what happens next:

> If a portion of a cell's DNA is damaged, the cell can become abnormal. When the abnormal cells divide, they form new cells that contain a photocopy of the damaged genetic material. This is an ongoing process occurring constantly within our bodies. Most of the time, our bodies have the ability to destroy these abnormal cells and maintaining a sort of cellular equilibrium. If a crucial portion of the DNA is destroyed, however, and the abnormal cells cannot be controlled any longer, cancer forms.
>
> All cancer cells have two things in common: they grow uncontrollably and they have the ability to metastasize. They can spread through the lymphatic system, the bloodstream, or avenues such as cerebrospinal fluid.

Different types of cancer behave differently in the body. Lung cancer and breast cancer, to name two of the most common, grow at different rates and respond to different treatments, which is why cancer treatments have become more specialized in the last twenty years. No matter what cancer is present in the body, however, you can be sure that cancer cells *will* travel to other parts of the body. Just remember that doctors always name the type of cancer from where it *began*, not where it has spread. For example, cancer that begins in the lungs before spreading to the liver will always be known as lung cancer.

Thus, the immune system plays a huge role in whether we develop cancer and live a healthy life—and whether we live or die. I truly believe that whichever pathology or disease we're facing—except for traumas or other conditions that can only be assisted by surgery—the only obvious and feasible solutions are those that endeavor the revival, modulation, and regulation of the immune and self-repair systems.

Until quite recently, the very idea to find substances capable of achieving such goals evoked a storm of indignant and scornful objections from the medical establishment. Times do change, however, and nowadays this very notion is at the forefront of the minds of both conventional and naturopathic practitioners. The development of a means for the enhancement of our immune responses has become a paramount priority. Whether embraced by the medical establishment or not, health-conscious consumers intuitively and intellectually grasp the importance of immune health.

⊙⊙

During the illness that nearly claimed my life more than twenty years ago, my maternal grandmother, Rose Menlowe, took care of me whenever my condition became too much for my parents and they needed relief. For instance, when I was hospitalized on two occasions, my grandmother slept in a chair next to the bed and was assuredly an angel who protected me and helped me to fight for my life.

So perhaps you can imagine how devastating the news was when just a few years after my own recovery, I learned my grandmother had cancer.

It all started in late spring 1999, when Grandma Rose was seventy-seven and began experiencing excruciating stomach pain. Then she started throwing up constantly. All of the laboratory tests kept coming back normal, however. My grandmother was still very sick, so my aunt and uncle asked her to come stay with them in Atlanta. But once in Georgia, she had to be carried out of bed and helped into the shower. She would need help in the middle of the night when she felt nauseous and had to throw up. When the stomach pain became unbearable, she asked my uncle (her son-in-law) to give her pills to end it all.

My uncle refused, of course. But grandma's condition worsened. Soon after, the pain became so wretched that the family rushed my grandmother to the emergency room in Atlanta, where she immediately was put under for major exploratory surgery. When she awoke, the doctor told her she had multiple malignancies including a goblet cell carcinoid in her appendix and stage IV ovarian cancer that had spread to her lymph nodes and portions of her small and large intestines.

Stage IV, by the way, is the most advanced stage of ovarian cancer. Growth of the cancer involves one or both ovaries and distant metastases (spread of the cancer to organs located outside of the peritoneal cavity) have occurred. Finding ovarian cancer cells in her pleural fluid (from the cavity surrounding the lungs) was also evidence of her stage IV disease.

The surgeon removed her ovaries, some of her lymph nodes, and portions of her small and large intestines, which were found to contain cancer. But the ovarian malignancy was extremely advanced, and we already had evidence that the cancer had spread to other sites. Though the larger tumors were removed, the chance of recurrence was high. Because of her age and weakened state, her surgeon suggested we regularly monitor her situation rather than going with follow-up chemotherapy and radiation.

I loved grandma, who was born in Poland in 1922 and lived on a farm in the country near Warsaw. As a child, her family consumed fruits and vegetables straight from the garden. The family had a mill where they pressed flaxseed and poppy seed into oil. "I used to eat lignan cakes as snacks with black sourdough bread," she recalled. "Oh, the bread was as hard as a rock but so delicious. You cannot find that kind of bread anymore. We used to break off pieces from the flax cakes and dip them in fresh oil right from the press."

By the time she was in her early teens, Europe was experiencing the devastating consequences of Nazism. "We were some of the last European Jews to arrive in America before the Holocaust," she explained. "I was twelve when we arrived—and, let me tell you, skinny, almost puny. In America, I fell in love with white bread and ate a lot of starchy things like cakes and doughnuts from the bakery."

Immediately after surgery, grandma became very depressed. She had the sense that she was going to die. She spoke of things in terms of having only limited time left.

Meanwhile, I was planning to be married in September 1999. Her surgery was in June, and all she hoped for was to live long enough to be at the wedding.

I wanted more than anything else for my Grandma Rose to not only be healthy enough to attend my wedding but also that she be healed of cancer and live many more fruitful years.

With that motivation, I began studying the body's immune system and natural methods of improving immune function, especially increasing the body's activity level of macrophages, natural killer cells, and cytokines (messenger chemicals). I decided that I had to somehow help strengthen grandma's immune response to suppress her cancer cells and promote healthy cells.

My grandmother needed her white blood cells and cytokines to be not only at optimal population levels but also highly activated. Sometimes—as researchers now know—our immune cells are numerous in number but have been rendered inactive or ineffectual by various chemicals that tumor cells secrete.

You see, a cancer cell wills itself to survive even if it causes the death of the host. To do so, the cancer cell produces a growth factor called transforming growth factor-beta (TGF-3). As immune cells come nearer to extinguish this invader, the TGF-3 causes the immune cells to become nonfunctional. TGF-3 inhibits proliferation of T cells, reduces the cancer cell–killing power of tumor necrosis factor, and inhibits the ability of macrophages, our immune system's first line of defense, to engage in phagocytosis. The body ends up thinking its forces are effectively attacking cancer cells, but they aren't any longer. In my grandmother's case, the key was to activate them by feeding the hungry cells of her immune system.

That research led me to studying chains of complex sugars known as polysaccharides or glyconutrients (nutrients from sugar) or, more specifically, polysaccharide peptides or glycoproteins (polysaccharides that are bound to proteins).

I learned that certain compounds, found in greatest abundance in edible fungi, enhance macrophage and natural killer cell production. This, in turn, enhances production of cytokines, which are immune cell secretions that facilitate cell-to-cell communications and fully optimize immune function. With glyconutrients, we might even be able to overcome some of the deceptive practices of TGF-3. Do not confuse these sugar-based compounds with commonly consumed sugars such as fructose or starches. I call these highly complex compounds the healing sugars.

I also learned that our primitive diet used to contain a lot of these compounds, but now due to our modern refined diets, our bodies are highly deficient in them. The richest source for these compounds is found in edible mushrooms, but, unfortunately, not the button mushrooms most of us buy at supermarkets.

Though our interest in edible fungi is limited in America, elsewhere in the world the healing powers of mushrooms have been known for more than 5,000 years. In the winter of 1991, hikers in the Italian Alps discovered the frozen remains of a man who had died some 5,300 years earlier. Apart from his knapsack and flint ax, the ancient man was carrying a string of dried mushrooms known as birch polypores (*Piptoporus betulinus*) and another as yet unidentified mushroom.

"The polypores can be used as tinder for starting fires and as medicine for treating wounds," wrote fungi expert Paul Stamets, author of *Growing Gourmet & Medicinal Mushrooms*. "Furthermore, a rich tea with immuno-enhancing properties can be prepared by boiling these mushrooms."

That mushrooms should possess significant healing powers is nothing new to Asian healing traditions. In the Orient, several types of mushrooms have been used for centuries to maintain health, preserve youth, and increase longevity. Although the healing aspects of mushrooms have been passed down through folklore, it has only been within our lifetimes that the scientific study of mushrooms and their healing properties has been initiated.

For instance, a medical article published in *Nutrition Reviews*, R. Chang of the Department of Medicine at Memorial Sloan-Kettering Cancer Center in New York City noted this:

Edible mushrooms…may have important salutary effects on health or even in treating disease. A mushroom characteristically contains many different bioactive compounds with diverse biological activity…In order of decreasing cultivated tonnage, *Lentinus* (shiitake), *Pleurotus* (oyster), *Auricularia* (mu-er), *Flammulina* (enokitake), *Tremella* (yin-er), *Hericium*, and *Grifola* (maitake) mushrooms have various degrees of immunomodulatory, lipid lowering, antitumor, and other beneficial or therapeutic health effects without any significant toxicity.

The complexity and variations in glyconutrients is truly mind-boggling. Each specific mushroom offers different combinations, involving far more complex and varied molecular structures than science has been able to identify or characterize. I also learned that various portions of the mushroom had different amounts of glyconutrients. For example, the mycelium of the mushroom, which is the seed of the mushroom, so to speak (not the fruiting body that we see above ground), is a particularly rich source of protein-bound polysaccharides (glycoproteins).

The way mushrooms are cultivated, and the way various grains and seeds are used, also influences mycelium glyconutrient content. Some mushrooms, like cordyceps found in the wild, actually use caterpillars as a growth medium. And, of course, we now know that organic production truly enhances potency of all foods, including mushrooms, while minimizing exposure to pesticides and heavy metals.

Not only was I fascinated by the burgeoning amount of research being conducted into glyconutrients, so were pharmaceutical scientists. Some of the most potent anticancer drugs being studied and tested these days are based on glyconutrients. These complex sugars are finding their way into other new applications such as wound and ulcer healing and cell transplantation (in diabetes). Another glyconutrient derivative is being heralded as a cure for influenza.

The commercial promise of glyconutrients eventually will lead to a new era of anti-inflammatory and anti-metastatic drugs. The future potential is enormous for the design of glyconutrient-based drugs.

No doubt, these drugs will be heralded as "new" breakthroughs. But are they really? After all, almost all synthetic drugs to be developed will be based on Nature's limitless molecular variations. I tapped into this mother lode when I began working with medicinal mushrooms. Certainly, the same glyconutrients on which the pharmaceutical drugs are being based are already making their presence felt in the world of natural health.

∞

I want to talk about something else I learned from my own illness. After studying and researching this issue, I realized people used to get much more reliable results from herbal medicines. Why? Because their digestive tracts, at one time, were far more able to utilize foods and herbs than today.

I'm afraid that most of us are walking around these days with digestive tracts that have been damaged to greater or lesser degrees from overuse of medications and poor dietary habits. Many herbs and other sources of natural healing agents, such as mushrooms, are fibrous and difficult for the body to break down. Some mushrooms contain as much as 60 percent fiber.

Grandma's diet had changed so much since moving from Poland forty years earlier that she needed a delivery system that would enable her to utilize the herbs I wanted her to start using.

I came up with a fermentation process that utilized more than fourteen species of SBOs and other lactic-acid–producing microorganisms and used it to predigest ten mushrooms, aloe vera, and cat's claw in a formula that would "unlock" the active ingredients.

This is important. There are records of traditional herbalism from the Orient and other cultures in the Far East dating back 1,500 years that talk about herbal remedies that were used to treat a variety of ailments. In the past, they provided very predictable, very effective, and very potent results. Yet today, we are not getting the same kind of healing response from these herbs.

The reason people today aren't being helped is not necessarily due to the lack of healing properties in the herbs themselves but is rather a direct result of an ultimate breakdown in the human digestive tract.

Said another way, the nutrients and phytochemicals contained in herbs are not being broken down and utilized properly by the body, primarily because people's guts have been destroyed from the overuse of prescription medications—antibiotics, corticosteroids, and other immune-suppressive drugs—as well as chlorinated and fluoridated water, ambient pollutants in our environment, and an overall poor diet coupled with a steady intake of junk foods.

I believe strongly that the application of a probiotic fermentation process is a fantastic way for the body to utilize all of the phytochemicals and phytonutrients available in these herbs, with very little stress on the digestive tract. This benefit is extremely important to those people undergoing chemotherapy and radiation, or those with the HIV virus or other immune disorders, who have very little digestive capability. This enzymatic "predigestion" process increases bioavailability and absorption of the medicinal compounds, which makes them "body-ready" for everyone, even those with compromised digestion.

In other words, the sickest persons, with the least ability to utilize fibrous herbs, receive a much greater boost from the probiotic fermentation process that the whole food concentrates and herbs undergo, making their healing constituents far more available to the sickened person's body. Especially relevant to what I wanted to accomplish with my grandmother was this discovery: Some mushrooms are comprised of more than 80 percent carbohydrates and thus lend themselves well to fermentation, which unlocks their healing powers and makes them available to be assimilated by the body.

This ancient method of bio-fermentation incorporates beneficial microorganisms (probiotics) and their enzymes into the foods to gently break them down into their most basic elements.

The probiotic fermentation process takes algae, seed, legumes, and grains and covers these natural foods with a mother culture for three to six weeks. (The typical fermentation process lasts one to four days.) The end result is a food that is nearly completely broken down and predigested with large amounts of probiotics, enzymes, B vitamins, and proteins.

Several novel phytochemicals that the body craves are also created, including the body's master antioxidant known as SOD, plus various immune-supportive beta-glucans and many other antioxidants—all created from the "alchemy" involved in fermentation.

Spirulina and grasses, which are part of this fermentation process, are a rich source of beta-carotene and chlorophyll. The body of a healthy person can convert beta-carotene into vitamin A or retinols, but unhealthy individuals cannot always make that conversion.

My grandmother began using a prototype medicinal mushroom and herbal formula that I developed immediately following her surgery. Not only did she gain weight and improve her energy level, but her physical appearance and general health improved to the point where she was the healthiest she felt in thirty years. Better yet, according to her latest CAT scan, she was cancer free—and she witnessed my marriage to Nicki with the biggest smile a grandmother can have.

On Labor Day 2001, at the Cancer Control Society's 26th annual convention in Universal City, California, grandma spoke before an audience of some 2,500 persons about her victorious battle with cancer. She described how the consumption of the medicinal mushroom and herbal formula that I formulated made all the difference in her fight against this deadly disease.

Grandma made an amazing recovery from a dire cancer prognosis, for which I was grateful. Her story didn't come as a surprise to Garry Gordon, M.D., D.O., M.D. (H.), who is called the "Father of Chelation Therapy" and is president of the Gordon Research Institute. His primary focus is researching natural products for every health problem, with particular emphasis on immune system support for heart disease and cancer.

"Let me tell you about my emerging views on cancer," he told me one time. "My main message is this: *Treat yourself for cancer before you get cancer*. In other words, we all have cancer at every moment in our lives. But why are we waiting for the expression of cancer before we do anything?"

For many cancer patients, the clinically visible signs of cancer are the result of processes that might well have begun years or decades earlier—processes that could have been stopped long before if the patient had only implemented a cancer treatment program before the cancer became clinically evident, Dr. Gordon said.

When Dr. Gordon speaks of treatment before the event, please understand he is not referring to chemotherapy, radiation, or surgery. Rather, he is referring to the use of botanical and nutritional supplements and other natural healing pathways long *before* the clinical signs of the disease emerge. This is when our natural pharmacy often works extremely well and gives us our best chance for delaying or completely eliminating expression of cancer in our lives.

"My program involves every aspect of your life—your diet, your exercise, your mind, your environment, and judicious use of nutritional supplements," Dr. Gordon said. "Now I know that it is difficult for everyone to take as many different nutritional supplements as is optimal, but I have been a practicing physician since 1958 and actively involved in the study of immune support and trace element research for nearly fifty years. I'm convinced that mushrooms such as cordyceps, ganoderma, coriolus, maitake, and shiitake have tremendous anticancer potential. These are routinely prescribed by doctors worldwide to complement cancer treatments," Dr. Gordon said.

Cordyceps sinensis (CS-4), he further explained, inhibits the production of DNA and RNA synthesis in cancer cells and has displayed antitumor activity on bladder, kidney, colon, and lung carcinoma as well as fibroblastoma cell lines. *Ganoderma lucidum* (reishi) inhibits leukemia cell lines. A mushroom known as *Trametes versicolor* is the source of the highly potent immune-enhancing extract PSK, an immuno-modulator used primarily in conjunction with chemotherapy, radiation, and surgical treatments for cancer.

Besides seeking out medicinal mushrooms, the use of cat's claw is also exceedingly important. But not just any cat's claw....

We start with a discussion of Peruvian traditional healing to learn why. According to the traditions of the Ashaninka Indians of the Cutivireni region of Peru, only high-ranking healer-priests are able to guide the harvest of the cat's claw herb. That is because, as Western scientists have learned, two distinct types of cat's claw grow in the wild, and they are almost impossible to differentiate. Though they could not characterize these differences with the use of modern analytical chemistry terms, the high priests of the Ashaninka tribe have been able to discern which plants contain the correct chemotype.

When the proper cat's claw is harvested and processed, it possesses an uncanny ability to know when to stimulate or "down-regulate" immune activity. That, in turn, plays a role in positive clinical results for persons with autoimmune conditions such as mixed connective tissue disease, rheumatoid arthritis, and allergies, where the immune system is overstimulated and attacking the host's own tissues.

In essence, this natural medicine is able to intuitively turn on or off the "switch" that caused either an under- or overactive immune state.

Finally, there is another little-known influence that mushrooms have on the human physiological process, and that's a tonifying effect. For example:

- Reishi (*Ganoderma lucidum*) alone has been shown to aid in blood sugar stabilization, normalization of blood pressure, and neuroprotection support.
- In Chinese medicine, cordyceps (*Cordyceps sinensis*) is utilized for circulatory, respiratory, immune, and sexual dysfunction, and other health problems. It is considered a tonic herb because of its ability to improve or normalize energy, stamina, appetite, endurance, and sleeping patterns.
- *Agaricus blazei's* glyconutrients (*polysaccharides*) activate interferon production to prevent viral infections.
- *Poria cocos* is used in Traditional Chinese Medicine with other herbs to promote blood flow and quell inflammation.
- Shiitake (*Lentinula edodes*) is the source of premiere anticancer agents used in Japanese medicine and is known for its cholesterol-normalizing benefits.

Summing up, your risk for cancer and your ability to recover are not etched in stone, as my Grandma Rose demonstrated. You should know that you can alter your cancer risk at any age, which is the positive and hopeful message I want to leave you with. Cancer is not something we are born with and predestined to be stricken. Prevention is possible.

If you are stricken with cancer, however, please know that there are options. We are fortunate to have powerful immune-boosting natural formulas in conjunction with modern cancer-fighting treatments available. I urge you to check them out.

5

ATTACKING THE SEVEN
CAUSES OF INFLAMMATION

*al-che-my: a power or process of transforming something common into
something special.*

—*Merriam-Webster's Collegiate Dictionary*

There is an alchemy that all of us seek in every aspect of life. Perhaps
it isn't the discovery of a universal cure for disease or the discovery
of a means of indefinitely prolonging life or transmutation of base metals
into gold, but if we accept a more modest definition of this wonderful
14th century term, I believe that the best herbalists and formulators today
seek to achieve a certain alchemy.

As for me and this idea of alchemy, I always try to study a problem
thoroughly and then go about solving it in a comprehensive fashion. That's
why I worked on a formulation to attack the major causes of inflammation.
My anti-inflammation formulation is a combination of chicken bone-broth
nutrients, collagen, and beneficial compounds blended with herbs, spices,
and enzymes. I'm happy with the results, and I know many people who feel
that they received relief from their issues with inflammation.

If you have been fortunate not to have inflammation, consider yourself blessed because it's a big deal. Most people think inflammation is
something that happens to your back after spending an entire Saturday

morning digging up weeds, but I'm talking about more than that. My focus is on inflammation that occurs internally as well.

Every day of your life, your body wards off gazillions of germs, which break down your immune system and make you more susceptible to health problems. Every day of your life (or so it seems), little "ow-ees" happen—a badly stubbed toe, mosquito bite, slight sunburn, pulled muscle, or nick while shaving your legs (for you gals) or your face and neck (for you guys). Whenever any of these scenarios happen, the body mounts an instantaneous defense, sending cells and natural chemicals to assault those nasty flu germs or repair the slight gash in your skin. Scientifically speaking, this response is known as *inflammation*.

When inflammation occurs, the liver produces a protein known as high-sensitivity C-reactive protein. This natural chemical is released into the bloodstream to help the body fight flu germs, for example, or repair itself after you pull a splinter out of your index finger.

"Inflammation has become one of the hottest areas of medical research," wrote Christine Gorman and Alice Park in *Time* magazine. "Hardly a week goes by without the publication of yet another study uncovering a new way that chronic inflammation does harm to the body. It destabilizes cholesterol deposits in the coronary arteries, leading to heart attacks...."

When I looked into producing an anti-inflammation formulation, I became aware that Stephen Rennard, M.D., chief of pulmonary medicine at the University of Nebraska Medical Center in Omaha, had conducted research on chicken soup—yes, good ol' chicken soup—acting as an anti-inflammatory because of the way the homemade soup apparently reduced the inflammation that occurs when coughs and congestion strike the respiratory tract.

I've become a big fan of chicken soup for the soul, as well as soup stocks made from meat, chicken, or fish. So I have a question: Is old-fashioned chicken soup or soup stocks missing from your diet? Do you consume chicken soup or soup stocks regularly? Perhaps you should. Wonderful health benefits are to be derived from our traditional recipes. There's a reason why Grandma Rose called chicken soup the "Jewish penicillin."

While chicken soup is often consumed in winter, few people go out of their way to slurp up soup stocks, however. This means you're missing out on the gelatinous substances like collagen found in soup stocks.

"A lamentable outcome of our modern meat processing techniques and our hurry-up throwaway lifestyle has been a decline in the use of meat, chicken and fish stocks," said Sally Fallon and Mary G. Enig, Ph.D., in their groundbreaking book, *Nourishing Traditions: The Cookbook that Challenges Politically Correct Nutrition and the Diet Dictocrats*. "In days gone by, when the butcher sold meat on the bone rather than as individual filets and whole chickens rather than boneless breasts, our thrifty ancestors made use of every part of the animal by preparing stock, broth, or bouillon from the bony portions." The authors added that stock "is also of great value because it supplies hydrophilic colloids to the diet. Raw food compounds are colloidal and tend to be hydrophilic, meaning that they attract liquids."

When cartilage deteriorates, you're left with bone against bone. But one of the beauties of traditional diets is that soup stocks made from whole chickens aid in rebuilding and maintaining cartilage by supplying high-quality gelatin and collagen, which are rich sources of glycosaminoglycans like chondroitin sulfate.

One thing collagen does is draw water to the joints, which, in turn, helps with cushioning. So, do eat chicken and beef stock.

I highly recommend the collagens in organic chicken and beef, which is why I traveled to France to source the collagen in my anti-inflammation support formulation. I wanted to work with farmers who don't farm chickens the way we typically do in America. The French farmers assured me that their chicken flocks received no antibiotics or mammalian remnants in their feed.

Whatever you eat or consume as a nutritional supplement, the integrity of the ingredients should be foremost in your mind.

⌬

One of the major causes of inflammation that gets overlooked is over-acidity in the body.

In fact, many experts consider over-acidity one of the major causes of inflammation, especially arthritic conditions. The body can only tolerate a small imbalance in blood pH, which is why alkalizing the body can be important for arthritis (especially gout) sufferers.

An interesting article in the *European Journal of Nutrition* stated that sodium chloride (NaCl) has been incorporated copiously into the contemporary diet, increasing the net systemic acid load imposed by the diet.

The researchers noted that their group "has shown that contemporary net acid-producing diets do indeed characteristically produce a low-grade systemic metabolic acidosis in otherwise healthy adult subjects, and that the degree of acidosis increases with age."

In a Russian-language medical journal, researchers studied changes in joint fluid acid–base balance in sixty-five rheumatoid arthritis patients. They found increasing acidity to be correlated with the severity of joint damage and inflammation. Russian researchers determined that whole body potassium is significantly lower in older arthritics and can sink to almost half of normal in some cases. This again tells us that the body is in an overly acidic state.

My anti-inflammation support formulation was designed to aid correction of acidosis and ameliorate those conditions. I would argue that any level of acidosis may be unacceptable, and indeed, that a low-grade metabolic alkalosis may be the optimal acid–base state for humans. For this reason, I made sure there were fermented alfalfa grass juices in my formula because they contain alkaline-forming minerals to help reduce acidity. A compound known as *Rhododendron caucasicum* helps to reduce acidic deposits, particularly in gout. Rhododendron is used as an effective treatment for gout throughout Russia.

If you suffer from chronic low-grade infections, then please know that the arthritis-infection connection is now well established. Infections are clearly associated with the body's inflammatory levels, which can be measured with a high-sensitivity C-reactive protein test. Many infections, however, do not manifest themselves as frank disease conditions such as the flu or common cold. They may simply cause minor symptoms like skin eruptions or fatigue or the more serious conditions such as arthritis and even heart disease.

In addition, compounds such as wild oregano concentrate and bayberry bark extract are premiere infection-fighting herbs that aid the body's health against pathogens.

Some people have an overactive immune system. I learned that a unique herb known as cat's claw has an almost intuitive ability to harmonize the body's immune system, quell an overactive immune response, and stimulate an underactive system. Many types of autoimmune arthritis or related inflammatory conditions (such as lupus) result from immune system dysfunction.

Are you taking arthritis drugs? So-called COX-2-inhibiting drugs designed to maintain the pain-reducing properties of traditional but stomach-harsh nonsteroidal anti-inflammatory drugs (NSAIDs) have proven to be problematic. Synthetic COX-2 inhibitors like Celebrex and Vioxx were found to come with their own side effects such as gastrointestinal distress and increased risk of heart attacks and strokes. Vioxx was taken off the market in 2004 and Celebrex had to add a warning label, so the former was dangerous and the latter is still problematic.

Natural COX-2 inhibitors, on the other hand, are safe. They also are effective. For instance, oregano contains rosmarinic acid, which has been reported in laboratory studies to have significant COX-2 inhibiting properties comparable to medical drugs such as ibuprofen, naproxen, and aspirin. Ginger and turmeric are also natural COX-2 inhibitors.

"In experimental studies, [ginger] has been shown to inhibit both the cyclooxygenase and lipoxygenase pathways and the production of prostaglandins, thromboxane, and leukotrienes, just as the NSAIDs do," wrote James B. LaValle, R.Ph., N.M.D., C.C.N, author of *The COX-2 Connection*. "Yet its clear advantage is that no significant side effects have been reported, unlike the NSAIDs, which can have quite serious side effects associated with their use."

Turmeric, closely related to ginger, is traditionally used to treat systemic inflammation. Researchers at New York Presbyterian Hospital and the Weill Medical College at Cornell University have shown that one of the major phytochemicals in turmeric has potent COX-2-inhibitory factors, as LaValle noted. Additional research at Vanderbilt University and the University of Leicester in England has further confirmed the powerful COX-2-inhibiting capabilities of this ancient herb.

Are you deficient in enzymes? Raw foods are an excellent source of enzymes and aid the body in maintaining the proper acid/alkaline balance, but most of us no longer consume adequate amounts of raw foods—vegetables, fruits, nuts, legumes, meats, and fish.

Of course, only the overly brave would consume raw meat due to the fear of bacterial contamination and mushy taste. (I've become a lover of raw fish in sushi, as have millions of Americans.) The downside of this precautionary approach to eating raw meats is that you can miss out on some of the most potent proteases.

Yet, enzymes can help to reduce circulating antibodies and have been shown to aid in all types of inflammatory processes. That's why I'm a big fan of inflammation-fighting enzymes, including proteases for protein digestion, lipase for fat digestion, amylase for carbohydrate digestion, and cellulase for the digestion of plant fiber.

Bromelain, an enzyme found in the stalk of pineapples, is effective in reducing inflammation in living tissue. On the other hand, papain, the enzyme found in unripe papaya, is useful to reduce sites of inflammation where dead or diseased tissue has been lodged.

If you're suffering from oxidative stress, then you'll be glad to know that the use of antioxidants will be recognized someday as one of the most significant contributions to modern health practices. While it's clear that you need basic vitamins and minerals as building blocks for structural support, antioxidants play an important role in fighting off the damaging effects of inflammation by quenching the devastating micro-cellular effects of free radicals that exert so much cumulative oxidative damage on joint tissues.

Another substance, *Rhododendron caucasicum,* is high in polyphenolic antioxidants that are similar to those found in green tea, grape seed, and pine bark extracts but is far more bioavailable. Turmeric and oregano are also powerful antioxidants that reduce oxidative stress.

Although we tend to think of inflammation almost solely in terms of arthritis, enhancing the body's healing response in cases of trauma and sports injuries, heart and circulatory disease, and virtually all other inflammatory conditions is something you want to strive for. Let me remind you that the consumption of anti-inflammation foods and herbs can do a body good.

By all means, I encourage you to take up the anti-inflammatory lifestyle.

6

YOU'RE NOT WHAT YOU EAT,
BUT WHAT YOU DIGEST

W e can't really talk about gastrointestinal health without discussing the digestion of our foods.

Digestion may be a most familiar household word. But what is far less commonly known is the complex and manifold process required to perform digestion in order to extract the necessary nutrients from our food. To understand these mechanisms and put their potentials in proper perspective, we first have to become familiar with a few basic principles.

What is digestion? Well, digestion entails the chemical breakdown of ingested food, programed and carried out with high precision. Digestion occurs without the need for central nervous system impulses. This, as mentioned, is the "law of the gut."

Thus, digestion is essentially a carefully executed decomposition process carried out by an independent ENS supported by an intricate array of interactive enzymes. The ingested food, however, yields only a small proportion of substances that the body is able to assimilate. The rest is eliminated as waste.

It's important to note that the body produces two fundamental kinds of waste—metabolic waste and digestive waste. Metabolic waste represents the cellular "household" waste and the breakdown of dead, discarded cells that are constantly being replaced in the body. Digestive waste comprises the breakdown of all matter that is not absorbed. It's interesting to note that less than 4 percent of our metabolic waste exits the body with our stool. About 96 percent is eliminated through the kidneys.

- Thus, to maintain its health and vitality, the human body requires a steady supply of many kinds of enzymes. Here again, before we continue, there are three basic tenets we'll have to become familiar with to understand why enzymes play a manifold role in our health.
- While there are thousands of different enzymes in Nature, they can be divided into two basic categories. The first is lytic enzymes, which exclusively break down substances for which they were specifically designed—such as the legions of proteolytic enzymes in charge of breaking down proteins.
- The other category consists of enzymes responsible for the manifold processes of synthesis in the body. In other words, these induce the building of molecules and, eventually, tissues such as the telomerases.
- The human body is able to produce most of the enzymes it needs, but not all of them. Certain enzymes such as cellulase, which is in charge of breaking down the fiber contained in plants, must be obtained from our food because the body has no mechanisms to produce them.

∞

According to a U.S. Surgeon General's report on nutrition and health, eight out of ten leading causes of death in the United States are diet related. Digestive problems comprise the number-one health problem in North America. Digestive complaints, including everything from hemorrhoids to colon cancer, result in more time lost at work, school, and play than any other health-related problem. What's even more disconcerting is that many of these digestive problems were rare or nonexistent less than a century ago.

How did this happen? Why now? Because, collectively speaking, we've dug ourselves a huge hole because of all the processed foods, fast-food stops, and junk food binges that are part and parcel of the way people eat today.

So how can we get back to the health of our ancestors? I believe part of the answer comes from consuming enzyme-rich foods and "live" enzyme supplements.

It's easy to understand that a stable supply of all enzymes is necessary for the human body and is of paramount importance. Alas, not only does our increasingly toxic eating habits deprive us of the enzymes we must import into our body, but our unhealthy lifestyles also deteriorate the organs in charge of producing the body's own enzymes. The progressive, overall depletion of enzymes leads to a situation in which we can neither digest the foods we eat nor can our bodies synthesize the materials required for cell repair and maintenance.

Therefore, not only general but also a partial, specific enzyme deficit is unquestionably responsible for many of the diseases that escalate in the wake of our relentlessly deteriorating lifestyle.

Summing up the situation, the result of our increasingly worsening enzyme deficiencies is a progressive failure to digest proteins, fats, sugars, starches, and other carbohydrates, which causes a great variety of diseases.

⚭

In the area of enzyme deficiency, I want to highlight the area of lymph gland blockage, a topic that should grab the attention of both health-conscious consumers and a wide range of health professionals.

Incompletely digested protein and/or carbohydrate molecules trigger a domino effect in which the fragmentary breakdown compounds produce a secondary carbohydrate known as polysaccharides. These then condense in the tissue fluids of the body and combine with excess proteins, forming a substance known as mucoproteins, which are aggregates of undigested proteins that form long chains of polypeptides. These adhere to unassimilated carbohydrates in a process called glycation.

Glycation then leads to overproduction of advanced glycation end products, which cause premature tissue aging. In a worst-case scenario, mucoproteins condense in blood plasma. The accumulation of such mucoproteins is the main cause of lymphatic congestion, which is the foremost trigger factor of a great variety of severe pathologies, blocking the lymphatic traffic in the interstitial tissues (i.e., the spaces between fine capillary vessels and cell structures).

This is important. And it's worth taking the time to explore the consequences of lymph gland blockage. The first thing you need to know is that the organs of the immune system, positioned throughout the body, are called lymphoid organs. The word *lymph* in Greek means a pure, clear stream—an appropriate description considering lymph's appearance and purpose.

The lymphatic system defends the body from foreign invasion by disease-causing agents such as viruses, bacteria, or fungi. The lymph system also contains a network of vessels that assists in circulating body fluids. Lymph bathes the tissues of the body, and the lymphatic vessels collect and move it eventually back into the blood circulation.

Lymph nodes dot the network of lymphatic vessels and provide meeting grounds for the immune system cells called upon to defend against invaders. The spleen, at the upper left of the abdomen, is also a staging ground and a place where immune system cells confront foreign microbes. Pockets of lymphoid tissue are in many other locations throughout the body, such as the bone marrow and thymus. Tonsils, adenoids, Peyer's patches, and the appendix are also lymphoid tissues.

Both immune cells and foreign molecules enter the lymph nodes via blood vessels or lymphatic vessels. All immune cells exit the lymphatic system and eventually return to the bloodstream. Once in the bloodstream, lymphocytes are transported to tissues throughout the body, where they act as sentries on the lookout for foreign antigens.

These vessels transport excess fluids away from interstitial spaces in body tissue and return these fluids to the bloodstream for eventual elimination. Lymphatic vessels also prevent the backflow of the lymph fluid. They have specialized bean-shaped organs called lymph nodes that filter out destroyed microorganisms. If your lymph system is malfunctioning, internal toxicity is quite likely.

This brings us to the next major problem resulting from enzyme deficiency—impaired immune function. This would be a good place for me to introduce an important acronym: GALT, which stands for gut-associated lymphoid tissue. It is the responsibility of the GALT to discriminate between nutritious components present in the transiting stool and possible antigens, in which case it would alert the immune system to stage an appropriate immune response. Without a properly functioning GALT, our immune health is compromised and toxins can escape from the colon into the bloodstream. The outcome of such conditions can generate manifold illnesses that may involve any organ and even the entire body.

It's important to keep digestive waste freely moving through the intestines. However, if the in-transit food is isolated from the GALT by layers of gluey and hardened food (as a result of enzyme deficiency), no discriminatory action will ensue and no immune responses will be alerted; consequently, large amounts of toxic substances will be absorbed by the body.

Certainly one of the keys to improving our health, especially unblocking the lymph system and maintaining healthy immune function in the gut, is to insure an optimal amount of enzyme activity in the body. Enzymes are catalysts in the body, and these protein-like substances help maintain the tissues, orchestrate the many functions of the body, and digest food.

But they are so much more, noted Dr. Edward Howell, a ground-breaking physician who devoted his life to the study of enzymes and one of the great enzyme scientists of the 20th century. Dr. Howell said to think of enzymes in this way—as the "labor force" that builds your body, just like construction workers are the labor force that builds your house, he says. "You may have all the necessary building materials and lumber, but to build a house you need workers, which represent the vital life element," Dr. Howell said. "Catalysts are only inert substances. They possess none of the life energy we find in enzymes. For instance, enzymes give off a kind of radiation when they work. This is not true of catalysts. In addition, although enzymes contain proteins—and some contain vitamins—the activity factor in enzymes has never been synthesized.

"Moreover, there is no combination of proteins or any combination of amino acids or any other substance which will give enzyme activity. There are proteins present in enzymes. However, they serve only as carriers of the enzyme activity factors. Therefore, we can say that enzymes consist of protein carriers charged with energy factors just as a battery consists of metallic plates charged with electrical energy."

Enzymes can be considered as important, if not more so, than perhaps any nutrient. This is because enzymes are responsible for nearly every facet of life and health. When we eat raw foods, we consume the enzymes in the foods. The foods are then digested easily by the body. When we eat cooked or processed foods, however, the body must provide the enzymes necessary to digest the cooked foods.

Unfortunately, food enzymes are destroyed at temperatures above 118 degrees Fahrenheit. Thus, all cooked and processed foods are devoid of food enzymes. This constant need for enzymes depletes our store of enzymes, strains the body, and causes the pancreas to enlarge.

We *need* enzymes in the worst way because without them, we're as good as dead. This is what Dr. Howell stated in his classic work, *Food Enzymes for Health and Longevity*: "After we have attained full mature growth, there is a slow and gradual decrease in the enzyme content of our bodies. When the enzyme content becomes so low that metabolism can't proceed at a proper level, death overtakes us."

Enzymes are not renewable resources. Once enzymes have completed their appointed task, they are destroyed. For life to continue, you must have a constant enzyme supply, and that requires continual replacement of enzymes. The best way to make sure your body receives the adequate number of enzymes every day is to consume a diet high in "live" raw and fermented foods and to consume a high-potency broad-spectrum digestive enzyme supplement.

Thus, supplementation with a powerful and comprehensive enzyme formula is an ideal solution to both prevent and treat such conditions as digestive-related lymph gland blockage and impaired digestive enzyme activity.

If you're at all skeptical about the effectiveness of these digestive enzymes, I challenge you to take an excellent plant-based digestive enzyme formula with each meal for about three to five days. Then stop taking this formula altogether for one to two days. You'll immediately notice the contrast as your body goes back to what you will now realize was your earlier sub-par state of poor digestion and low energy.

An excellent plant-based digestive enzyme has the power to break down the amount of food you are eating at the time. You need to take a nutritional supplement that contains a blend of proteolytic digestive enzymes, including peptidase, which aid in the digestion and utilization of dietary proteins.

In addition, the following digestive enzymes deliver specific nutrients necessary for muscle and tissue repair, as well as for vibrant immune system function:

- **Amylase** is digestive enzyme that digests starch and carbohydrates and acts in concert with proteases to stimulate immune system function. Amylase also acts in association with lipase to digest fragments of viruses and reduce inflammation and infections.
- **Lipase** is a digestive enzyme that digests fats, thereby aiding in weight control, maintaining and enhancing cardiovascular health, and helping support proper liver and gall bladder function.
- **Glucoamylase** breaks down carbohydrates, specifically poly-saccharides.
- **Malt diastase (maltase)** digests maltose, malt, and grain sugars and may help relieve environmental sensitivities and allergies.
- **Invertase (sucrase)** digests sugars and is beneficial in helping prevent gastrointestinal problems and discomfort.
- **Alpha-galactosidase** aids in the digestion of difficult-to-digest foods such as beans, legumes, and cruciferous vegetables such as cabbage, broccoli, and cauliflower.
- **Lactase** digests the milk sugar lactose and is extremely useful for individuals suffering from lactose intolerance. Lactase may be beneficial for those suffering from IBS and other digestive disorders in which a high percentage are adversely affected by dairy products.
- **Cellulase** digests fiber cellulose into smaller units, which include D-glucose. It helps remedy digestive problems such as malabsorption. Cellulase is an important enzyme because the human body cannot produce it on its own.
- **Xylanase** breaks down the sugar xylose.
- **Pectinase** breaks down carbohydrates such as pectin, which is found in many fruits.
- **Hemicellulase** breaks down carbohydrates called hemi-celluloses, which are found in plant foods.
- **Mannanase** digests the sugar known as mannose.
- **Phytase** breaks down carbohydrates, specifically phytates (phytic acid), present in many difficult-to-digest grains and beans. It is

especially useful for those suffering from serious bowel disorders that result in an inability to handle phytates from soy and gluten from wheat, oats, rye, and barley. Phytase may increase mineral absorption and the bioavailability of iron, zinc, calcium, and magnesium.

- **Beta-glucanase** breaks down polysaccharides and fibers known as beta-glucans.
- **Arabinosidase** digests the sugar arabinose.
- **Bromelain**, an enzyme from the stem of pineapples, breaks down protein and fights inflammation and reduces swelling. Bromelain may speed the recovery of injuries and swelling resulting from athletics, childbirth, and surgery.
- **Papain,** similar to the chymotrypsin, is a protein-digesting enzyme produced by the body that is used to treat chronic diarrhea and celiac disease as well as gastrointestinal discomfort due to intestinal parasites.

The following plants and spices have digestive benefits as well:

- **Barley grass** is one of Nature's richest sources of alkaline-forming minerals and antioxidant enzymes. Barley grass provides the mineral cofactors necessary to enhance the functions of the enzymes.
- **Ginger**, one of the most potent herbal digestive aids available, contains extremely potent protein-digesting enzymes. Ginger is frequently used to treat nausea and motion sickness.
- **Turmeric** is a popular Indian spice that is commonly used to improve digestion and reduce stomach discomfort.
- **Cat's claw**, once called the "opener of the way" by a physician who treated hundreds of people suffering from digestive problems, has been used for hundreds of years by native Peruvians as a treatment for digestive problems, UTI, and arthritis.

These enzymes and other whole foods not only effectively aid digestion in general, but also help to remove accumulated, sticky waste adhered to the lining of the intestines and colon—what some health experts term *mucoid plaque*—that originates a whole array of digestion-contingent diseases.

If you've been dealing with gastrointestinal distress, then look to digestive enzymes, essential prerequisites for great health.

7

CAPTURE THE POWER OF THE SUN

Completely regardless of how improbable it may seem, light definitely does exist within our cells. In fact, light may be the basis of cell-to-cell communication.

I thought of this when I was reading about the unending universal confusion among scientists regarding the exploration of the mechanisms that govern the immune response. The issue they were debating was this: How can so much information be processed so quickly throughout the body?

Biochemical reactions alone, the scientists believe, were too slow. Perhaps the answer was light, they hypothesized. Perhaps the body's communications themselves were carried out through biophotons at the speed of light.

In *The Whispering Pond: A Personal Guide to the Emerging Vision of Science*, author Ervin Laszlo gave a version of what turns out to be a fairly long-standing idea among scientists: Much of the physical world, and living Nature in particular, cannot be explained by current knowledge and that some form of unknown energy field is needed to explain it.

This concept dates back to the 1920s when the famous Russian professor of medicine and biophysicist Alexander Gurwitsch postulated that a system-wide force field, known as a morphogenetic field, generated various force fields of individual cells. Laszlo called this a fifth field, referring to the four accepted universal fields: the gravitational, the electromagnetic, the strong, and the weak nuclear fields.

This is deep stuff, and some wonder if morphogenetic fields might explain everything from the mysteries of the wave function in quantum mechanics to the remarkable synchronicity found in Nature or even psychic phenomena documented among people.

Gurwitsch was a pioneer of sorts, and back in the 1920s, he had already established beyond any reasonable doubt that living cells and tissues generate an extremely weak, yet biologically active, form of electromagnetic radiation in the ultraviolet range. The presence of this radiation is somehow intimately connected with the nature of living processes themselves. Basically, Gurwitsch was able to show evidence of a weak but permanent photon emission of a few counts (square centimeters squared) in the optical range from biological systems, pointing out that it stimulates cell divisions.

Gurwitsch was then led to his experimental demonstration of what he called "mitogenetic radiation" in a lawful and rigorous way, as a by-product of his attempts to hypothesize a universal biophysical principle which, among other things, would encompass the paradoxical but otherwise undeniable correlations between events of cell division (mitosis) and other events occurring in widely separated locations within a living organism.

After periods of neglect and even disregard, small groups in Russia, Australia, China, Italy, Japan, Germany, Poland, and the United States rediscovered ultra-weak light emissions from living tissues by use of modern photomultiplier techniques after World War II. The researchers likened these force fields to the power of ultraviolet light. Since then, numerous scientists in several parts of the world have unquestionably confirmed that in the core of living cells there is indeed perceptible light.

Eventually, after several decades of boisterous controversies, a team of German biophysicists irrefutably corroborated the postulate in 1975 under the direction of Professor Fritz-Albert Popp, conforming to the strictest requirements of the scientific method.

Popp, born in 1938 in Frankfurt, Germany, received a degree in experimental physics in 1966 at the University of Wurzburg (where Rontgen discovered X-rays) and received his Ph.D. in theoretical physics in 1969 at the University of Mainz. He has supervised approximately thirty diploma works and dissertations in physics, biology, and medicine and written approximately 150 publications on basic questions of theoretical physics, biology, complementary medicine, and biophotons.

In general terms, it is understood that the term *photon* refers to a "quantum of light." We know that a quantum constitutes the minutest and totally indivisible component of the universe. Popp, who placed the prefix bio- in front of photons, did so with the intention of suggesting that these may be emitted by living cells. Thus, he is the scientist who coined the expression *biophoton*.

Popp and coresearchers noted that while there is now agreement about the universality of this effect for all living systems, no agreement has been achieved in the area of interpretation. Meanwhile, a group of German physicists at the University Marburg hypothesized that biophoton emissions as a subject of quantum optics had to be assigned to a coherent photon field within the living system, responsible for intra- and intercellular communication and regulation of biological functions such as biochemical activities, cell growth, and differentiation.

In order to examine this hypothesis, consider that it has been shown that biophoton emission can be traced back to DNA as the most likely candidate for working as the main source, and that delayed luminescence (DL), which is the long-term afterglow of living systems after exposure to external light illumination, corresponds to excited states of the biophoton field.

In addition, all the correlations between biophoton emission and biological functions such as cell growth, cell differentiation, biological rhythms, and cancer development turned out to be consistent with the coherence hypothesis but could be only rather poorly explained in terms of free radical reactions.

Currently, there remain no doubts about the existence of such intracellular luminescence. (Not to be confused with the bioluminescence generated, for example, by glowworms.) Contemporary technology has developed powerful instruments capable of intensifying and measuring extremely minute light quantities, known as residual light, which prove unquestionably the existence of the biophotons.

It was also established that this biophysical force does not only pulsate in intensity but also in frequency. This explains quite satisfactorily the dynamics of its inherent mechanisms of interactions, which unfold among the different organs.

The question that remained to be answered was why do our cells emit light? Popp explained that "our organism must replace nearly ten million cells each minute."

That's a lot of cells.

It's becoming more and more obvious that the information required to achieve such a feat can only be processed at the speed of light. Apparently, such an overwhelming amount of signal traffic of data transference and processing within any living organism—be that human, animal, vegetal, or of insects—is achieved through biophotons with high precision. These minutest coherent rays of light are responsible for the maintenance and operation of the network of information linking all living cells in an organism, and they likewise allow the continuous, unobstructed, and intelligent updating of data.

So, how does all this scientific gobbledygook affect us? Strange as it may seem, every time we consume natural and fresh food, or their carefully preserved components, we also ingest light that—in one way or another—triggers certain activities in our system.

In other words, when we ingest fresh food, their individual components emit luminous signals that inescapably participate in the development and management of certain biochemical endogenous processes within the body. The greater the capacity of light storage in our nourishment, the more powerful will be their beneficial influence on our cells.

A German biochemist named Johanna Budwig was one of the first to postulate that we have lost touch with the powerful resonance whose source is linked to the photon-power of the sun. Back in the 1960s, she came out with a book called *Sonnenenergie und der Mensch ah Antenne* (*Solar Energy and Man as Antenna*). This seven-time Nobel Prize nominee also lectured widely.

Dr. Budwig first earned fame as a biochemist who developed key analytical techniques required for identifying types of fats. At one time, science was unable to identify key distinct fats in foods such as omega-3s (found in wild cold-water fish and flaxseed) from omega-6s (found in grains, certain seeds, and corn oil), and omega-9s (found in olive oil and avocadoes). Thus, the work of Dr. Budwig must be considered seminal in the advancement of nutritional science, particularly that of lipids.

However, Dr. Budwig's firmly grounded scientific work led her to hypothesize and later clinically validate much greater truths so profound that they bring together modern physics, biology, and even modern humanity's overall health.

"Sun rays reach the earth as an inexhaustible source of energy," she observed. "The sources of power in mineral oil, coal, green plant-foods, and fruits are based on the energy supplied by the sun's radiation."

Today, we know that the energy from the sun is in the form of photons, the fastest-moving, smallest units of elementary energy known. This concentration of the sun's energy is accomplished by ocean and land plants into the compounds that comprise their cells and tissues. The energy is then transferred into biophotons.

Our own health may be improved when we eat foods rich in electrons, which have themselves captured the power of the sun. A high amount of these electrons, which are on the wavelength of the sun's energy, are to be found in seed oils, observed Dr. Budwig.

"Scientifically," she explained, "the oils are even known as electron-rich essentially highly unsaturated fats."

The great leap Dr. Budwig made, however, was her insight that modern men and women lack the proper foods to adequately capture this elementary power of the sun for their vital health. It is intriguing that the most protective organ system in the human body, the central nervous system, requires the most unsaturated fatty acids, especially omega-3 fatty acids, for its cell membranes to function optimally. It is also interesting that Nature provides fatty acids in the *cis* form that bends fatty acids into the shape of a fish hook, rather than the *trans* form that would stretch the molecules into a more linear shape. The *cis* form intrinsically has more molecular electromagnetic tension than the *trans* form.

Could it be that the *cis* configuration is a way of storing within each molecule a special storage form of the sun's energy?

It has long been known that unless heroic preservation measures are taken, once seed grains are crushed they quickly turn rancid. Because of the high vulnerability of their electrons to oxidation, these precious oils, much like fruits or vegetables, are highly perishable.

The husks and germ of grains first began to be removed in the mid-1700s in Great Britain, extending shelf life but removing their vital contents, thereby precipitating overt B-vitamin deficiency diseases such as pellagra and beriberi. The vital powers of these photon-rich foods were lost.

Then, starting in the early 1900s, much of our wheat and other grain products were made into white flour by removing the bran and germ and along with them most of the nutrients.

Along came the corn oil craze in the 1950s. The producers of this commodity launched a massive public misinformation campaign, taking out full-page advertisements in the nation's medical journals. This campaign convinced medical doctors that corn oil, overloaded with omega-6 fatty acids, could prevent heart disease.

Another wrong turn occurred with the advent of hydrogenation, a process that turns vegetable oils into semisolid fats.

I believe that when one consumes certain foods rich in saturated fats such as meat and dairy products from animals that feed on greens and herbs, then we are getting a prepackaged rich source of these electrons. These fat-soluble activators, as they are often called, have been transformed by the animals' digestive tracts into highly usable health-promoting compounds.

Fats and oils treated to preserve them longer have their electronic structure changed—otherwise oxygen would try to grasp vulnerable electrons in the molecules. But this modified form is not the form useful to the body and may, in fact, be detrimental. The irony of modern society is that electron-rich foods, particularly the good fats such as those found in fish, grass-fed animal foods, and to some extent flaxseed, have become rare. No wonder we have much higher rates of heart disease, cancer, multiple sclerosis, and arthritis than primitive peoples!

When people began to process fats to make them keep longer on the supermarket shelves and when people began consuming refined polyunsaturated fats to such a great extent, no one stopped to consider the consequences to long-term health. What happened is that the vitally important electrons found in seed oils and healthy animal fats, with their continual movement and wonderful ability to capture the elementary power of the sun, were destroyed!

It's so much healthier to consume electron-rich foods, electron-rich seeds, healthy animal foods, herbs and spices, and vegetables and fruits that are rich in aroma and natural pigments from the color of the sunlight's photons. These all help the absorption, storage, and utilization of the sun's energy. The body's capacity to activate vital life functions is thus dramatically enhanced, resulting in extraordinary healing and rejuvenation.

It's important to note that these same principles begin to act—in fact, even more powerfully—when you consume food supplements that contain naturopathic factors that originate from biotechnological sources such as virgin plants, particularly seeds and sprouts, or even animal products and organs processed by special technical means that permit the preservation of their light-storing capacity and their ability to induce coherent biological light in their intracellular environments.

The physicist Popp declared this: "The human organism is not only a carnivorous, or vegetarian being, but also a consumer of light. In fact, it behaves like a luminivorous creature."

This is why I worked on a formulation rich in fermented grasses, herbs, sprouts, and seeds that were harvested at the point of optimal nutritional value. At the time, I did not understand all of the science behind what I was doing, but I wanted my formulation to be rich in seeds and chlorophyll-rich superfoods such as spirulina, chlorella, and dunaliella.

I also wanted young rye, wheat, barley, oat, and alfalfa grass as well as flax, sesame, sunflower, and pumpkin seeds. In my formulation, I knew that we needed a fermentation process to lock in the power of the phytonutrients. The fermentation process is an artisanal craft and not an industrial process. You have to remain steady at approximately 98.6 degrees and devote between three and six weeks to the process.

The fermentation process can be likened to the aging of a fine wine. Over the weeks of fermentation, wonderful flavors and aromas develop, not to mention the many health-enhancing compounds that the process generates. Once fermentation is finished, the material is dried at extremely low temperatures very quickly.

You see, the heat and solvents destroy the biophotonic energies of our foods and herbs. You don't want heat. You don't want irradiation, either, which is kind of like microwaving your ingredients.

Doing the fermentation process at low temperatures never exceeding 90 degrees Fahrenheit preserves their electron-rich nature.

And that's how you capture the power of the sun.

8

THE HEALING POWER
OF GREEN FOODS

I'm figuring by now that you expect the unexpected from me.

Well, here's another bit of advice that's outside the box: You should eat grass.

You'll be a lot healthier. And that's a promise.

Once, we recognized the value of grass, and I'm not talking about a backyard lawn or even "medical marijuana," which is now legal in a handful of states. I'm talking about wheat, rye, corn, rice, oats, barley, sorghum, millet, spelt, kamut, and even bamboo and sugarcane because, technically speaking, they are grasses.

Most of us today are either too busy or have no desire to contemplate the grass beneath our feet that softens the Earth and makes it so much more of a beautiful habitat. But grasses contain incredible and overlooked health benefits that enhance the value of consuming these type of "greens."

I like what popular writer Steve Meyerowitz has to say. He made this observation about grass:

> We step on it, sit on it, lay on it, jog on it, picnic on it, walk the dog on it, mow it, water it, in fact, we do most everything on it, for it, or with it except eat it! Wherever there is sun, water and earth, there is grass. From the outback Down Under to the one-inch thick Arctic tundra of Greenland…to the hundred-foot tall

tropical bamboo, grass is the most fundamental form of vegetation on the planet.

So yes, grass can be consumed. Let's explore why.

∞

In their ancient wisdom, our bodies crave grass. Though vitamin, mineral, and herbal supplements can be beneficial to our health, none match the nutritive value found in grasses. The reason grass is a superfood is because the powers of the sun that are trapped in its blades produce rich amounts of chlorophyll and other green photosynthetic pigments.

It is interesting to note that in 1936 cereal grass tablets were considered the first multi-nutrient in this country. Cereal grasses are the only foods in the vegetable kingdom that, even if consumed alone, enable animals to continually maintain weight, strength, and optimal health. Grasses are considered to be at or near the base of the terrestrial food chain.

So it really was in the 1930s when grass first got noticed by science and medicine for its stunning health benefits, by the American Medical Association. Then in 1939, the *Journal of the American Medical Association Council on Foods* announced that Cerophyl, a whole food concentrate made with young rapidly growing leaves of wheat, oats, and barley, would be "listed in the book of accepted foods."

The acceptance of grass was slowed during World War II, and then something else happened following the war when the concept of "better living through chemistry" took hold of the nation. Most of us forgot our ancient wisdom. Vitamins could be synthesized, and minerals could be isolated in the laboratory.

Yet, in spite of these wonderful technological advancements, the ancient wisdom of the grasses could not be duplicated within the test tube.

∞

Cereal grasses—known today as green superfoods—supply many nutritional factors that even today scientists cannot duplicate. Is it the chlorophyll—the trapped sunlight—that is the basis for life? Or is it the grass juice factor or enzymes in these plants that are thought to be found nowhere else? We can't deny this fact: Cereal grass is perhaps the most nutritious food on this green Earth.

Based on data from the U.S. Department of Agriculture Nutrient Data Laboratory, grasses are nutritionally rich in:

- calcium
- iron
- magnesium
- phosphorous
- potassium
- zinc
- copper
- manganese
- vitamin C
- thiamin
- riboflavin
- niacin
- vitamin B_6
- folate
- vitamin B_{12}
- carotenoids
- vitamin E

In the 1930s and 1940s, America's leading scientists, led by bio-chemist George Kohler, worked on grass research on the campus of the University of Wisconsin in Madison, Wisconsin. The Kohler team did remarkable work. They made the discovery of niacin (vitamin B_3), as well as the grass juice factor, a nutritive compound in grass that still can't be duplicated by vitamins or minerals.

In an experimental study, published in the *Journal of Nutrition*, Dr. Kohler and his team compared the growth of animals fed dried grass powder, lettuce, cabbage, or spinach. For eight weeks, young guinea pigs received only the combination of lettuce, cabbage, spinach, or dried grass powder.

The animals receiving the lettuce or cabbage lost weight. With spinach, the animals barely sustained their weight. But with cereal grass, the animals thrived and gained much weight. The researchers noted this: "The growth stimulating factor of grass was distinct from all the known vitamins." This study was confirmed in subsequent studies, published in the same journal or presented at the Cornell Nutrition Conference.

⌇

I believe you should eat fermented grass. Yes, I said fermented. The way fermentation works, it's a process in which a substance is broken down into a simpler substance. Microorganisms like yeast and bacteria often play a role in the fermentation process, creating beer, wine, bread, yogurt, and other foods. A similar fermentation process can be used with grass.

Most of us have never known the power of fermentation. We often think the superior way to consume veggies and fruit is raw. But this isn't always so. Sometimes proper food preparation methods release important compounds that would otherwise pass undigested and unused through our systems.

Fermentation is Nature's method of preparing foods for easy assimilation in the human body. But most of us don't even know that lactic acid fermentation is driven by beneficial microorganisms, producing enzymes that break down foods into usable compounds. Fanners—those who used to winnow grain in ancient times—knew this. So do cattle ranchers, who produce something called silage, which is fermented grass or hay, to feed to their cattle. This predigested grass allows the cows to get more nutrition from eating less grass. Farmers know that even cows with their multiple stomachs and strong digestive power can use a little help from our little probiotic friends.

Every long-lived culture in the world has consumed fermented foods with their meals. Some of the most common are fermented vegetables, dairy products, and meats. The Inuits (formerly known as the Eskimos) bury their walrus meat or fish in the ground and then pull these out later in the summer and consume this "rotten" meat to inoculate themselves against pathogenic organisms.

The aboriginal peoples of Australia bury sweet potatoes in the soil for months, remove them, and then eat sweet potatoes loaded with living microorganisms as a means of stimulating health. Even in this country our favorite condiments had their origins in lacto-fermented foods. Mayonnaise, mustard, ketchup, salsa, relish, guacamole, and jams all began as fermented foods replete with enzymes and living bacterial cultures that aid digestion and nutrient assimilation, as well as protecting people from pathogenic organisms.

Authors Sally Fallon and Mary Enig of *Nourishing Traditions* put it this way:

> It may seem strange to us that in earlier times people knew how to preserve vegetables for long periods without the use of refrigerators, freezers, or canning machines. This was done through the process of lacto-fermentation. Lactic acid is a natural preservative that inhibits putrefying bacteria. Starches and sugars in vegetables and fruits are converted into lactic acid by the many species of lactic-acid-producing bacteria. These lactobacilli are ubiquitous, present on the surface of all living things and especially numerous on leaves and roots of plants growing in or near the ground.
>
> The ancient Greeks understood that important chemical changes took place during this type of fermentation. Their name for this change was "alchemy"—like the fermentation of dairy products, preservation of vegetables and fruits by the process of lacto-fermentation has numerous advantages beyond those of simple preservation. The proliferation of lactobacilli in fermented vegetables enhances their digestibility and increases vitamin levels. These beneficial organisms produce numerous helpful enzymes as well as antibiotic and anti-carcinogenic substances. Their main byproduct, lactic acid, not only keeps vegetables and fruits in a state of perfect preservation but also promotes the growth of healthy flora throughout the intestine. Other alchemical by-products include hydrogen peroxide and small amounts of benzoic acid.
>
> A partial list of lacto-fermented vegetables from around the world is sufficient to prove the universality of this practice. In Europe, the principle lacto-fermented food is sauerkraut. Described in Roman texts, it was prized for both for its delicious taste as well as its medicinal properties. Cucumbers, beets, and turnips are

also traditional foods for lacto-fermentation. Less well known are ancient recipes for pickled herbs, sorrel leaves, and grape leaves.

In Russia and Poland, one finds pickled green tomatoes, peppers, and lettuces. Lacto-fermented foods form part of Asian cuisines as well. The peoples of Japan, China, and Korea make pickled preparations of cabbage, turnip, eggplant, cucumber, onion, squash, and carrot. Korean kimchi, for example, is a lacto-fermented condiment of cabbage with other vegetables and seasonings that is eaten on a daily basis, and no Japanese meal is complete without a portion of pickled vegetable.

American tradition includes many types of relishes—corn relish, cucumber relish, watermelon rind—all of which were no doubt originally lacto-fermented products. The pickling of fruit is less well known but, nevertheless, found in many traditional cultures. The Japanese prize pickled umeboshi plums, and the peoples of India traditionally fermented fruit with spices to make chutneys.

Lacto-fermentation, as I mentioned, is an artisanal craft that does not lend itself to industrialization. Results are not always predictable.

"For this reason," wrote Fallon and Enig, "when the pickling process became industrialized, many changes were made that rendered the final product more uniform and more saleable but not necessarily more nutritious. Chief among these was the use of vinegar for the brine, resulting in a product that is more acidic and not necessarily beneficial when eaten in large quantities; and of subjecting the final product to pasteurization, thereby effectively killing all the lactic-acid-producing bacteria and robbing consumers of their beneficial effect on the digestion."

After I overcame my health challenges, I worked on an organic super green formula that incorporated fermented grasses, beneficial microorganisms (probiotics), and their enzymes.

The end result was a food that was nearly completely broken down and predigested with large amounts of probiotics, enzymes, B vitamins, and proteins. My organic super green formula created several novel phytochemicals that the body craves, including the body's master antioxidant SOD, as well as various immune-supportive beta-glucans, and many other antioxidants—all created from the "alchemy" involved in the fermentation process I described earlier.

When looking for a super green formula to add to your smoothies, for instance, you want to find one with a blend of grasses, legumes, seeds, and key vegetables that provide a high concentration of nutrients like:

- chlorophyll, which aids in the elimination of harmful bacteria, promotes skin repair, transports oxygen, and deodorizes the intestinal tract
- polypeptide vegetable proteins, which enhance growth and immune function
- an abundance of bioavailable minerals and their cofactors gathered by the grasses' deep traveling roots
- unique enzymes for digestion and nutrient assimilation
- barley greens, which are anti-inflammatory and promote the growth of healthy tissue.

The vitamins and minerals in an organic super green formula may contain hundreds and possibly thousands of yet-to-be discovered nutrients.

A super green formula in powder form shaken with water or mixed into a smoothie is superb for optimal nutrition. In fact, if someone needs to be more economical, just one tablespoonful of a super green formula will often provide that person with the equivalent of five servings of vegetables and fruits. This type of excellent nourishment helps to repair the body by giving it whole food that's readily available for absorption.

Once you start having an organic super green food power drink in the morning, you won't be able to give up the habit.

PART II

THE MAKER'S DIET HEALING PROGRAM

9

RETURN TO THE MAKER'S DIET

Y ou would think if anyone would have developed excellent and lifelong healthy eating habits growing up, it would have been me. After all, my father was a trained naturopath. He was well versed in the hippocratic philosophy—*Let food be thy medicine.* He and Mom shopped for wholesome natural foods, and you couldn't find sugary cereals or store-bought cookies in our pantry. So naturally you would think my family's diet would have been great when I was a youngster.

We ate what we considered to be the healthiest foods. Although I slathered my bagels with cow's milk cream cheese, at least they were *whole-wheat* bagels. I ate turkey cold cuts instead of pork. And hold the sodium nitrite, please. I ate vegetables and whole grains instead of polished white rice or enriched flour. I had an apple, if not every day, every few days. We avoided the use of sugar and preservatives, and a special treat was a frozen yogurt at a nearby shop, covered with fresh berries. I thought my diet was pretty good.

Compared to most Americans' eating habits, mine were better than average—maybe way better than average. My diet wasn't what jaded nutritionists have coined as the SAD diet, referring to the acronym for the Standard American Diet. So even though I was eating a diet that made me nutritionally smarter than the average bear, that wasn't saying a whole lot. For most Americans, our diets are truly SAD.

I learned a lot about the importance of diet and what kinds of foods we should eat when I was sick, awake in bed and unable to do much of anything. During that lonely time, I read a lot of diet books, from *Dr. Atkins' New Diet Revolution* to *The Zone*. I also spoke to a lot of nutritional experts by phone or visited their clinics. One thing I learned from my struggle is that our dietary habits are the key to good health.

At the same time, though, I've also seen that so much of what we've learned about what constitutes a good diet is wrong—plain wrong—even from the so-called nutrition experts and from our highest-paid public health officials. During my lifetime, healthy eating has become politicized and commercialized—like pretty much anything during these hyper-partisan times. That said, our culture really has made far too many compromises that victimize our health.

It's a pity, too, that many of us suffer from eating sketchy foods. Our eating habits must change in many ways for us to reach the full potential of our health, which is why our eating habits are in desperate need of a complete overhaul. Most Americans simply do not eat the nutritious diets that our ancestors ate to remain healthy and live long, disease-free lives. That has to change.

What's happened is that we have strayed from the foods of our Creator, foods that at one time nourished the world's healthiest peoples. We have altered the Maker's intent and allowed food to become our idol, turning us into a fat, sick, and sedentary society.

I know that's a harsh assessment, but I also know it's true, and what all of us need today is a lot more truth and a lot less fluff. The kind of things that pass for food today—what we choose for table fare and snacking on—are absolutely pathetic!

Consider this: The common diseases of civilization—arthritis, cancer, diabetes, heart attack, high blood pressure, and strokes—are the top causes of death past the age of forty-five. These same diseases of civilization are becoming ever more widespread as civilization progressively becomes more industrialized. Certainly, our diets are a major factor in their spread. I say that with confidence because these were not common diseases—even among the oldest primitive persons—when we were maintaining a diet that was in keeping with the intent of our Creator.

First off, know this: I'm not about to tell you to toss off your clothes, put on a loin cloth, grab a long sharp stick, and spear some fish in the nearest body of water for lunch this afternoon—even if that is one of the ways our ancestors fed themselves back in the day. Just as the great 20th century novelist Thomas Wolfe once said, "You can never go back home again," so we can't go back to the old ways completely. But we can learn from the old ways and improve our modern lives. The old ways—by that I mean the primitive ways and heeding the word of our Maker—can help us to overcome modern diseases of civilization and provide the nourishment we need to make us strong and disease resistant.

Many cutting-edge researchers from major academic institutions as well as alternative medicine believe that a more primitive diet is superior in virtually all ways to the modern diet. But I want you to take a step further. I want you also to participate in the ultimate wisdom of the Maker's Diet.

Let me put it to you this way. Technology has advanced at far greater speed than our digestive tracts. We can process and preserve foods in ways that they will make them last for decades. It's all part of genetically modifying foods in the laboratory, which means taking genes from one organism and inserting them into another to make them grow higher, larger, denser, and more resistant to pests. What's been amazing to witness is how plants with genetically modified organisms (GMOs) have caught on since I became healthy more than twenty years ago. These days, GMO foods are everywhere, but that's not a good thing.

It's estimated that 60 to 70 percent of processed foods in grocery stores include at least one genetically engineered ingredient. Nearly 90 percent of soybeans and nearly two-thirds of the corn grown in this country come from crops that have been genetically engineered using the latest molecular biological techniques. Because many processed food products contain soybean or corn ingredients—and just think of all the juices and sodas sweetened with high fructose corn syrup—you can figure that genetically engineered foods have successfully penetrated the marketplace.

Too much technology is not advancing our health. For instance, we may be enjoying and using our amazing smartphones these days, but our bodies are still back in primitive times, six thousand years ago, meaning our bodies haven't changed. We will do better if we eat more like our primitive ancestors.

I also believe we should be eating foods as detailed in the Bible. I know this may sound outrageous to some readers, but whether you believe in the Bible or not, there is no denying that the Old Testament (or Tenakh, or Scriptures, as the Jews refer to it) describes the dietary habits of a group of people who were healthier than all of their neighbors.

This is why I'm confident in saying that there is wisdom in the Bible that goes far beyond the spiritual—especially when it comes to dietary considerations.

∞

Let's look a little more closely at an overview of the Maker's Diet with its religious underpinnings.

I begin in Genesis 1:29, where God tells us, "I give you every seed-bearing plant on the face of the whole earth and every tree that has fruit with seed in it. They will be yours for food."

Unlike our modern diet, the Maker's Diet provides a far greater amount of vitamins, minerals, protein, and healthy fats—as well as substances in plants that are neither vitamins nor minerals, known as phytochemicals—than other diet plans. The Maker is telling us that seed-bearing foods are healthy.

Fruits, vegetables, herbs, lentils, properly prepared whole grains are pretty much all good as long as we don't get fancy and impose too much modern technology on them. Rex Russell, M.D., the late author of *What the Bible Says about Healthy Living*, admonished readers with this bold statement: "Don't alter God's design."

On the same hand, the Maker's Diet contains no refined or processed carbohydrates and only a very small amount of healthy sweeteners. This is the opposite of our modern diet, which strays from God's design and delivers us all sorts of processed foods that are rich in calories, filled with refined carbohydrates, and devoid of adequate nutritional value. The

Maker's Diet fills us with foods from the Creator—unprocessed—replete with every healing miracle put on God's green Earth. On the flip side, the modern diet perverts the design of the Creator, strays from the wisdom of our ancestors, and overloads our bodies with adulterated fats and refined, simple sugars found in candy, baked goods, and certain grains.

Instead, our bodies will do better with the old school foods like:

- wild game instead of artificially fattened, estrogenized slabs of beef
- fermented raw dairy instead of antibiotic-rich, bovine growth hormone- and pesticide-contaminated pasteurized dairy
- wild fish with fins and scales instead of farm-raised antibiotic-laden fish
- nutritious fermented or sprouted whole-grain bread instead of Wonder white bread
- fermented relishes and condiments instead of sugary sauce substitutes

Lowering your risk for modern disease—arthritis, cancer, diabetes, heart attack, high blood pressure, and stroke—can be found in the simple truths of living healthfully and by following the Maker's Diet.

∞

It's hard to believe what I'm about to tell you, but it's largely true—our ancestors had some neat nutritional things going for them. So, let's drop the loutish, brutish, and savage stereotyping of our ancient predecessors here. There's a lot we can learn from them.

The biggest failing—if you can call it that—of our ancestors was simply that they did not have access to all of the technology that we have today. No neonatal units, no ICUs, and no antibiotics. As a result, many children died during infancy or quite young. In fact, infant mortality was 20 to 30 percent, which wasn't good and was ten to one hundred times greater than it is today. However, for those babies who survived the first two years of life, their likelihood of living past eighty in good health was many times greater than today.

Talk to anyone today, and the most common perception of our ancestors' more primitive lifestyle is that they were an undernourished group of filthy semi-human beings plagued by illness and their own stupidity. If that's what you think, think again. Our ancestors experienced robust health often until death. Our great, great-grandparents had no words for retirement or nursing homes. They lived a lifestyle and consumed a diet that was suited to their bodies and kept them strong and healthy well into the eighties and beyond.

We can learn more about the health of our ancestors by studying people who, even to this day, continue to consume a primitive diet and lead primitive lifestyles. We can also examine the records of anthropologists, explorers, and others who came into contact with primitive people during the 19th and 20th centuries.

While it is true that some primitive people did not live long enough to acquire cardiovascular diseases or cancer—the two leading causes of death in the United States and Europe today—we know that the ones who did live long acquired these diseases infrequently.

We know this, in part, because cardiovascular heart disease and cancer are relatively rare among those who eat a more primitive, ancestral diet today. Researchers made a survey of cardiovascular disease incidence and related risk factors among 2,300 subsistence horticulturists in the tropical island of Kitava, one of the Trobriand Islands belonging to Papua New Guinea. Their most important published findings were that sudden cardiac death, stroke, and exertion-related chest pain were nonexistent or extremely rare in the Kitavans. Infections, accidents, pregnancy complications, and senescence (deterioration with age) were the most common causes of death.

All the Kitavian adults had low diastolic blood pressure (all below 90 mm Hg) and were very lean. (Their weight decreased after age thirty, which is the opposite in today's culture.) Tubers, fruit, fish, and coconut were dietary staples in Kitava. The intake of Western food and alcohol was negligible. Salt intake was far lower, too. What was interesting to learn was that 80 percent of both sexes were daily smokers, which supports the concept that smoking alone is not sufficient to cause cardiovascular disease.

Michael Murray, N.D., a leading natural healing expert, has also written extensively about the absence of modern disease found in primitive cultures. He noted that among the aboriginal, primitive societies in

Australia, Africa, and South America that survived into the 20th century, the rates of cancer, rheumatoid arthritis, obesity, diabetes, osteoporosis, heart disease, and other conditions were remarkably low until they switched to modern diets.

Tragically, encroachment of modern civilization around the globe has led to the infiltration of once-isolated societies by modern culture. Today, few societies remain that have continued to consume the more primitive, simple diet of their ancestors. It seems that canned food, refined sugar, and white flour are consumed nearly everywhere on Earth—even in tiny isolated towns above the Arctic Circle in Alaska and Canada or remote stretches along the Amazon River. Almost every society has made the transition from the primitive diet to the modern diet.

But there is an historic record that tells us what we need to know about the virtues of the primitive diet. In 1913, Nobel Prize winner, medical doctor, and missionary Dr. Albert Schweitzer visited Gabon, Africa, and was astonished to encounter no cases of cancer among the natives two hundred miles from the coast. "I cannot, of course, say positively that there was no cancer at all, but, like other frontier doctors, I can only say that, if any cases existed they must have been quite rare. This absence of cancer seemed to be due to the difference in nutrition of the natives compared to the Europeans," wrote Dr. Schweitzer.

Explorer and anthropologist Vilhjalmur Stefansson kept meticulous diaries of his adventures in the Arctic. In *Cancer: Disease of Civilization,* Stefansson told readers that he searched in vain for cases of cancer among the Inuit peoples. (The Inuits were formerly known as the *Eskimos,* a derogatory term from the Cree language that means "he eats it raw.")

The Canadian explorer even cited the findings of a whaling ship doctor, George B. Leavitt, who found only a single cancer case in forty-nine years among the Inuit of Alaska and Canada. But by the 1970s, after the Inuit began consuming a modern diet of canned foods and provisions, breast cancer became a frequent form of malignancy. Today, we know that toxic chemicals from our modern foods and industries have contributed to this condition.

Down Under, once rare cases of diabetes among native Aborigines in Australia are now tenfold greater than among European arrivals, again due to dietary changes, noted Kerin O'Dea, a professor at Monash University in Melbourne, Australia. Interestingly, the Aborigines were once known for prodigious consumption of fermented sweet potatoes, a natural source of probiotics and soluble fiber that fed the good bacteria of the gastrointestinal tract and thought to markedly reduce risk of blood sugar imbalances.

∞

Dr. Weston A. Price, a Harvard-trained dentist, has been called the "Isaac Newton of Nutrition" because of his groundbreaking research showing how the modern Western diet caused nutritional deficiencies that in turn caused dental issues and health problems.

It all started in the 1910s and 1920s when Dr. Price was practicing dentistry in the Cleveland area and was alarmed by the number of cavities, crooked teeth, and deformed dental arches he saw in his young patients. Even though we're talking about a time that was a hundred years ago, people were eating a lot of sugary foodstuffs as well as enjoying newfangled "soft drinks" and "sodas" that didn't do their teeth any favors. Hence, all the cavities needed filling.

Dr. Price wondered if these abnormalities were caused by nutritional deficiencies. The Cleveland dentist believed, and rightfully so, that dental health was a good indicator of physical health. He rightfully understood that deformed dental arches, crooked teeth, and cavities were signs of physical degeneration and a vulnerability to diseases such as heart attacks and cancer, which has been confirmed by science in the last century.

In his search for the causes of dental decay and the physical degeneration he observed in his dental practice, the inquisitive Dr. Price turned from test tubes and microscopes to researching evidence among human beings.

With his wife, Florence, he left his Ohio home in the early 1930s and embarked on a six-year journey that took him to primitive societies on five continents. Wherever Dr. Price went, he photographed and studied the inhabitants' teeth. He made detailed notes about diet of these primitive peoples, the state of their health, and their way of life.

Dr. Price chose an opportune time to undertake his study. In the 1930s, the last remaining societies in the world where people ate a primitive diet were making the transformation to the modern diet. Dr. Price had a chance to compare people, sometimes in the same family or household, who had grown up with the primitive *and* the modern diet.

Dr. Price traveled the world over to study isolated human groups, including sequestered villages high up in the Swiss Alps, Gaelic communities in the Outer Hebrides, Eskimos and Indians (as they were known back then) of North America, Melanesian and Polynesian South Sea Islanders, African tribes, Australian Aborigines, New Zealand Maori, and the Indians of South America. Wherever he went, Dr. Price found that beautiful straight teeth, freedom from decay, stalwart bodies, resistance to disease, and integrity of character were typical of primitives subsisting on their traditional diets, rich in essential food factors.

Dr. Price sought the factors responsible for fine teeth among the people who had them—the isolated "primitives." The world became his laboratory. As he traveled, his findings led him to this conclusion: that dental caries and deformed dental arches resulting in crowded, crooked teeth and unattractive appearance were a strong sign of physical degeneration, resulting from what he had suspected—nutritional deficiencies.

Dr. Price reported his findings in an extraordinary book titled *Nutritional and Physical Degeneration.* He posited that primitive people who were cut off from the modern diet had very little tooth decay and perfectly formed teeth and jaws.

They say that a picture is worth a thousand words, and in his book, the photographs he took were astonishing. The narrow faces, misshapen jaws, and crooked teeth of primitive people who ate the modern diet were shown in stark contrast to the wide faces, perfect teeth, and perfectly formed dental arches of their fathers, mothers, sisters, and brothers who ate a primitive diet.

What accounted for primitive people's good physical health? It could only be their diet, Dr. Price concluded. Wherever the American dentist went, he noticed that people who ate the modern diet suffered from physical degeneration. Moreover, Dr. Price suggested that dietary deficiencies may cause poor brain development and lead to social disorders such as juvenile delinquency and high crime rates.

At a time when primitive people were disparaged and sneered at, Dr. Price made the startling suggestion that modern humans could learn something from primitive people. He advocated returning to the primitive diet that had made our ancestors so healthy and said we could learn much from some of their practices as well, especially those pertaining to child rearing and child development. Dr. Price wrote this:

> No era in the long journey of mankind reveals in the skeletal remains such a terrible degeneration of teeth and bones as this brief modern period records. Must Nature reject our vaunted culture and call back the more obedient primitives?

Next, Dr. Price analyzed the foods used by isolated primitive peoples and found that they provided at least four times the water-soluble vitamins, calcium, and other minerals, and at least ten times the fat-soluble vitamins found in animal foods such as butter, fatty fish, wild game, and organ meats.

The importance of good nutrition for mothers during pregnancy has long been recognized, but Dr. Price's investigation showed that in primitive cultures they understood and practiced preconception nutritional programs for both parents. Many tribes required a period of premarital nutrition because pregnancies often happened quickly once they were together, and children were spaced to permit the mother to maintain her full health and strength, thus assuring subsequent offspring of physical excellence. Special foods were often given to pregnant and lactating women, as well as to maturing boys and girls preparing for future parenthood. Dr. Price found these foods to be very rich in fat-soluble vitamins A and D, nutrients found only in animal fats.

These primitives with their fine bodies, homogeneous reproduction, emotional stability, and freedom from degenerative ills stand forth in sharp contrast to those subsisting on the impoverished foods of civilization—sugar, white flour, pasteurized milk, and convenience foods filled with shelf-life extenders and additives.

Dr. Price performed a nutritional intake comparison between those primitive groups that demonstrated resistance to dental caries and freedom from degenerative processes with the diets of modernized groups who had forsaken their native diets for the foods of commerce, consisting largely of white flour products, sugar, polished rice, jams, canned goods, and vegetable oils.

Here are some observations from his book *Nutrition and Physical Degeneration*, which was published on the eve of World War II in 1939:

- On Switzerland: "The isolated groups dependent on locally produced natural foods have nearly complete natural immunity to dental caries, and the substitution of modern dietaries for these primitive natural foods destroyed this immunity…."

- On the Outer Hebrides Islands: "I was advised that in the last fifty years the average height of Scotch men in some parts decreased four inches, and that this had been coincident with the general change from high immunity to dental caries to a loss of immunity in a great part of this general district. A study of the market places revealed that a large part of the nutrition was shipped into the district in the form of refined flours and canned goods and sugar."

- On Alaska: "We neither saw nor heard of a case [of arthritis] in the isolated groups. However, at the point of contact with the foods of modern civilization, many cases were found, including ten bed-ridden cripples in a series of about twenty Indian homes. Some other afflictions made their appearance there, particularly tuberculosis, which was taking a very severe toll on the children who had been born at the center."

- On the Tongan Islands: "Following the war [World War I], the price of copra [aged dried coconut meat] went from $40 per ton to $400, which brought trading ships with white flour and sugar to exchange for the copra. The effect of this is shown clearly in the teeth. The incidence of dental caries among the isolated groups living on native foods was 0.6 percent, while for those around the port living in part on trade foods was 33.4 percent. Now the trader ships no longer call, and this forced isolation is very clearly a blessing in disguise. Dental caries have largely ceased to be active since imported foods became scarce after the price of copra fell back to $4 a ton again."

- On Ethiopia: "In one of the most efficiently organized mission schools that we found in Africa, the principal asked me to help them solve a serious problem. He said there was no single question asked them so often by the native boys in their school as why it is that those families that have grown up in the mission or government schools were physically not so strong as those families who had never been in contact with the mission or government schools."

- On New Zealand: "Whereas the original primitive Maori had reportedly the finest teeth in the world, the whites now in New Zealand are claimed to have the poorest teeth in the world."
- On Australia: "The rapid degeneration of the Australian Aborigines after the adoption of the government's modern foods provides a demonstration that should be infinitely more convincing than animal experimentation. It should be a matter not only of concern but deep alarm that human beings can degenerate physically so rapidly by the use of a certain type of nutrition, particularly the dietary products used so generally by modern civilization."

At times, Dr. Price writes rhapsodically about primitive people—their endurance, their stamina, their physical strength, and their natural beauty. For sure, they did not suffer from obesity, heart disease, digestive problems, or cancer at the rates we do. Thanks in large part to their diet, they enjoyed a vibrant health that has been lost to modern civilization.

But some folks have called Dr. Price's work biased, as if he cherry-picked the peoples he wanted to study. So let's go to the anthropologists and archaeologists to see what we can glean from their scientific work. I think you will find their body of evidence entirely supports the work of the late great Dr. Price.

When we study the skeletons and teeth of primitive people for evidence of vitamin and mineral deficiencies, here's what we learn: The evidence suggests that humans before the advent of modern agriculture were stronger, bigger, and healthier. Generally speaking, whenever our primitive ancestors took to agriculture as their primary food supply, their health declined.

The Illinois Valley is one of the few sites in the United States containing an intact mortuary record dating back to when Native Americans first populated the area. In addition to skeletal remains, a large amount of archaeological dietary evidence has also been recovered. This enables us to draw conclusions on health and disease as it relates to subsistence during the various cultural components.

One site, the Dickson Mounds in Illinois, provides ample data to show a correlation between increasing primary food production and overall health level. The three components represented by sufficient data are the Late Woodland period (AD 950–1100), the Mississippian Acculturated/Late Woodland period (AD 1100–1200), and the Middle Mississippian period (AD 1200–1300).

The Late Woodland component is associated with a generalized hunting-and-gathering economy. From the appearance of the first people at the Dickson Mounds, there is a general increase in the reliance on maize as the primary food crop. The number of skeletons with nonspecific skeletal infections greatly increases as the maize dependence increases. By the Middle Mississippian period, the infection rate more than doubled. Decreased host immunity resulting from severe iron-deficiency anemia due to the maize-based mono-diet probably is responsible for the great increase in infection rates. Iron-deficiency anemia greatly inhibits the ability of the body's immune system to stave off infection because iron plays a key role in the function of the immune system.

Similar findings have been reported from ancient cultures elsewhere in the Americas. In East Georgia, maize cultivation occurs only after AD 1150. After this time, there is a progressive increase in habitation site density and distribution. There is an increase in overall bone infections for the agricultural-based people. The decrease in bone size, robusticity, and stature for the agriculturists is also evident. The fact that people became smaller can be attributed to the change in subsistence practices. When people became sedentary, it greatly decreased their physical stress. As a result, their size and stature decreased.

Another equal factor in this reduced size is nutritional- and disease-related stress. Before the advent of widespread modern agriculture, the human diet consisted mostly of fruits, vegetables, wild grain and seeds, fish, and meat from wild animals. No matter how far we have progressed socially and technologically, our bodies crave the foods of our ancestors.

Our genetic constitutions and nutritional requirements were established during our past. Those people were optimally adapted to the types of foods that they could gather, and there's no evidence to suggest that modern humans are any different. We are literally designed to eat the same foods in the same proportions as those who lived thousands of years ago.

Our physiology and biochemistry cry out for a primitive diet with its plentiful amounts of healthy meat, fish, fruit, vegetables, and nuts. We have departed so far from the wisdom of our forefathers that most of the American diet is "new food" not eaten by our ancestors.

∽

So how do you do it? How do you move from the modern diet to the Maker's Diet? Let's look in detail at some of the components of the Maker's Diet.

Fruits and Vegetables

Primitive humans ate three times more of a wide variety of fruits and vegetables than we do. Fruits and vegetables (along with legumes and nuts) provided a startling 50 to 65 percent of daily calories and up to 100 grams of fiber a day—five times today's level. Vitamins, minerals, and antioxidants were supplied in amounts people now get only through supplements. Modern research clearly shows that heavy consumers of fruits and vegetables have less cancer, heart disease, diabetes, high blood pressure, and other chronic ills.

Grass-Fed Meat

Our not-so-distant ancestors consumed 35 percent of their calories in protein. The difference, though, is this: their protein came from pasture-fed animals, wild game, and fish, which also supplied highly beneficial omega-3 fatty acids that protect against modern diseases like cancer, diabetes, and heart problems.

On the other hand, our ancestors ate less of the following:

Grains, Cereals, Pasta, and Bread

The overconsumption of grain products is a huge problem in our world today. Grains contain nutrient inhibitors that prevent us from utilizing many minerals. Grains also contain disaccharides or sugars, which are difficult to digest and can lead to the growth of undesirable microorganisms in the gut. The overconsumption of carbohydrate foods, particularly grains, can lead to the overproduction of insulin, which may be a major cause of many metabolic disorders and other illnesses.

Most grains today are improperly prepared or refined and no longer supply important vitamins, minerals, and phytochemicals. Some research has linked grains, notably wheat, to arthritis, gastrointestinal problems, headaches, and depression, perhaps indicating subtle allergic food reactions.

Refined Sugar

Rather than honey and fruit, today's main sweets come from the 120 pounds of refined sugar the average person consumes in a year. Evidence shows sugar drives up blood levels of insulin, glucose, and triglycerides, which are known factors in diabetes and heart disease.

Processed Oils

Modern processing techniques have led to a dramatic change in the types and kinds of oils we now consume. Today, we consume highly refined, nutrient-poor vegetable oils and shortening, which cause our bodies to become overloaded with polyunsaturated fats and artificially created hydrogenated and trans fats that promote cancer, inflammation, abnormal types of cholesterol, and heart disease.

Watch Out for Refined Carbohydrates

The simple, refined carbohydrates we commonly call sugar are the primary modern fuel for the body. Anyone who has gone through a bout of sugar cravings in the middle of the afternoon and found himself munching on a candy bar knows how intimately sugar governs alertness, mood, and all of our mental powers.

Listen, every cell of your body needs sugar. Your need for sugar is instinctual and genetic. After all, in primitive times our bodies knew that when we tasted something sweet it was coming from a ripened fruit or vegetable, replete with all of its nutritional bounty.

But today modern food processors have learned how to trick our brains and exploit these ancient instincts. Hence, the lure of the candy bar or an after-dinner bowl of ice cream when we are feeling lethargic or desiring to top off a meal is irresistible. But we are being nutritionally deceived. Instead of receiving the nutritional bounty of God's fruits and sweeteners, our body is simply receiving the empty calories of a Snickers bar.

Refined carbohydrates like those found in candy, baked goods, and other processed foods are preferred by the pathogenic bacteria in our gastro-intestinal tract. Eating too much of them can cause imbalances in the ratio of pathogenic-to-friendly microorganisms. They can also cause abnormal fermentation, which interferes with digestion. In addition, refined foods are almost identical to table sugar. They cause blood sugar levels to spike and then go down rapidly, exacerbating diabetic and prediabetic conditions. Foods rich in refined carbohydrates are also nutritionally depleted and are substituted in our diet instead of more nutritious wholesome fare.

In addition, refined carbohydrates lead to hormonal imbalances. As most of us know, hormones are messenger proteins that regulate bodily functions ranging from sexual maturation to tissue growth and sleep patterns. When you eat large amounts of carbohydrates, your body produces too much insulin. Not all of us with glucose/insulin problems suffer from overt diabetes. Most of us with such imbalances would not even be considered diabetic.

According to the experts, however, a lot more people are on the borderline of blood sugar disorders than are typically clinically diagnosed. Many such persons suffer from Syndrome X and have relatively serious blood sugar problems—though not diabetes. Fortunately, blood sugar imbalances can be positively influenced by the Maker's Diet.

Pure, organic fruits, vegetables, and a small amount of soaked, fermented, or sprouted whole grains, nuts, and seeds—grown and processed minimally as our Maker intended—should be our source of carbohydrates, not candies, bread, pasta, baked goods, and table sugar.

As in the Bible, our primitive ancestors did not eat sugar, either. Their source of sugary sweetness was the rare find of raw wild honey, but even honey, notes the Bible, should be consumed as a treat and not a staple. This is nothing to take away from honey which, when unheated, raw, and unprocessed, is a wonderful source of trace minerals, vitamins, and many other nutrients—especially amylases, which are enzymes that aid in the digestion of carbohydrates. Nevertheless, we are told in Proverbs 25:27, "It is not good to eat too much honey."

Another insidious form of refined carbohydrates comes from the way we process grains. I know what I'm telling you is probably difficult for some to digest (no pun intended). After all, the cultivation of grain is one of the hallmarks of the agrarian society, which archaeologists say represents the dawn of modern civilization. Indeed, the tillage of grains—especially wheat and corn—is at the heart of almost every civilization's agricultural practices. The invention of the millstone—consisting of two circular stones used for grinding grain—is heralded as one of the great agricultural advancements of early humans.

Many anthropologists believe that our ancestors first stockpiled grains as a storable food source. Interestingly when their grains got wet, they sprouted. People found that if the sprouted grain was planted, then it yielded yet more seeds.

Perhaps our primitive ancestors realized intuitively that when they sprouted, germinated, or fermented grains, their phytonutrients became far more bioavailable. We now know sprouting grains and seeds unlocks their vitamin content, especially the B vitamins, and increases enzyme activity by eightfold.

Another advantage of sprouting and fermenting is that phytic acid and other enzyme inhibitors in grains are neutralized. Phytic acid, known as a great nutritional robber, is found in the bran of all grains. If ingested in high amounts, phytic acid can rob the body of important minerals such as iron, calcium, and magnesium and prevent their absorption. Soaking and fermenting grains also limits enzyme inhibitors that interfere with the body's digestive enzymes, as well as breaking down the difficult-to-digest disaccharides found in the starch of the grain.

Once again, the Bible provides us with the wisdom our bodies require for the proper assimilation of grains. Take for example the word *pulse*. In Daniel 1:12, in the King James Version, Daniel told Ashpenaz, the head of King Nebuchadnezzar's court in Babylon, "Prove thy servants, I beseech thee, ten days; and let them give us pulse to eat, and water to drink."

So what happened? In Daniel 1:15 (KJV), we are told, "And at the end of ten days their countenances appeared fairer and fatter in flesh than all the children which did eat the portion of the king's meat."

There are generally two definitions of pulse. In the first, we think that pulse is a sprout. In the second, we believe that pulse refers to rye grain. Perhaps in biblical use of the word *pulse*, we have sprouted rye. This makes sense.

Through much of history, a person's social station could be discerned by the color of bread they consumed—the darker the bread, the lower the social station. This was because whiter flours were more expensive to produce and harder for millers to adulterate with other products. Because of their relatively high cost, these whiter flours were most coveted by the wealthy members of ancient society, but as I like to quip, "The whiter the bread, the sooner you're dead."

Today, we have seen a reversal of this trend when darker breads are more expensive and highly prized for their taste as well as their nutritional value. My advice is to go easy on or, better yet, eliminate pastas and regular breads. I know they seem like they are pretty innocuous foods, but they aren't. Most are highly refined grains and not keeping with the primitive diet nor the Maker's wisdom.

If you're a bread eater, I truly believe your health will improve tremendously if you switch to sprouted or properly prepared sourdough bread made from whole organic grains. In health food stores and natural grocers, a typical healthful bread contains organic sprouted wheat, sprouted barley, sprouted millet, sprouted lentils, sprouted soybeans, sprouted spelt. You'll also find several sprouted breads baked by following the recipe found in Ezekiel 4:9, which goes like this in Scripture: "Take thou also unto thee wheat, and barley, and beans, and lentiles, and millet, and fitches, and put them in one vessel, and make thee bread thereof" (KJV).

Researchers estimate that 20 to 40 percent of our ancestors' diet was made up of protein-rich food, whereas today the percentage of our diet made up of protein is generally around 15 percent. That's quite a difference, and

I think that's why, in some respects, our nation's people are getting so fat. We eat way too many carbohydrates and not enough protein.

Consider that protein along with fat is an essential macronutrient. Believe it or not, the body can live without carbohydrates. If no carbohydrates are consumed, the body will covert proteins and fats into carbohydrates. Proteins are actually made up of long strings of amino acids. We ingest proteins from plant and animal foods and the enzymes in our digestive tract split these into smaller molecules, such as peptides and individual amino acids.

These are then used or combined by other enzymes to form important messenger substances in the body—such as hormones, growth factors, cytokines, and antibodies—that play key roles in muscle building and tissue repair, as well as immune function. You can see that protein is essential to life.

The body can produce certain amino acids. But others—the essential amino acids—must be obtained exclusively from our diet. Although vegetables and fruits provide proteins, they are incomplete sources of proteins because they lack one or more of the essential amino acids. Beef, chicken, fish, eggs, and dairy are complete protein sources, providing all essential amino acids.

Unfortunately, most of what passes for meat today is pathetic. Farm animals are often raised inhumanely in crowded conditions, fattened on growth stimulants, given subtherapeutic levels of antibiotics, and even fed remnants of other warm-blooded creatures.

In these stifling, politically correct times, I have a different take on protein than a lot of other people. Although I am a complete believer in the humane treatment of all God's creatures, I don't ascribe to a vegetarian diet. I know PETA (People for the Ethical Treatment of Animals) and other vegetarian groups oppose consumption of animal foods. Some groups even claim that a true biblical diet shouldn't contain any animal products. But two entire chapters in the Bible, Leviticus 11 and Deuteronomy 14, are devoted solely to the consumption of animal foods—which to eat and which to avoid.

We know that Jesus consumed and provided flesh foods with His disciples. In Matthew 15:36, we learn, "Then he took the seven loaves and the fish, and when he had given thanks, he broke them and gave them to his disciples, and they in turn to the people." And in Luke 24:42, upon Jesus' resurrection, we are told that His disciples, "gave Him a piece of a broiled fish and some honeycomb" (NKJV).

As for the supposed dangers of consuming animal foods, our primitive ancestors received most of their protein from meat, fish, eggs, and cultured dairy products but rarely experienced heart disease. I know this may be confusing to some readers because we have all been taught that meat—especially beef—is the cause of many major illnesses, including colon cancer and heart disease. We have even been told that the saturated fat in meat causes clogged arteries and is implicated in heart attacks and stroke.

This couldn't be further from the truth. In fact, the preferred fuel source for the heart *is* saturated fatty acids. In primitive times, meats were an important source of heart-protective omega-3 fatty acids and even conjugated linoleic acid. They provided the kinds of fats that kept blood flowing smoothly, fought the ravages of cancer, and aided metabolism so that folks didn't get rolls of abdominal fat.

This was possible because in the old days, animals grazed on grasses and bio-accumulated these important fatty acids. Today, however, animals are kept in pens or otherwise confined and fed foods that are deficient in omega-3 fatty acids and abundant in omega-6 fatty acids (more on that later).

As for dairy, the milk came from cows, goats, or sheep that were strictly free-range and grass-fed, although it must be said that goats eat leaves, herbs, and bark as well. Raw, cultured, and rich in beneficial bacteria, enzymes, and other important substances, these milks did a body good.

When it came to fish, they came from the ocean or freshwater streams and lakes. The fish were unpolluted, not factory farmed or contaminated with mercury.

Wild meats eaten by our ancestors also contained healthier fats than modern farmed cattle, explained Loren Cordain, author of *The Paleo Diet* and a tenured professor at Colorado State University. He and his colleagues have shown that meat from buffalo, wild elk, deer, and antelope contain more beneficial types of fat than meat from today's grain-fed cattle.

Cordain and his team at Colorado State compared the muscle, brain, bone marrow, and fat of wild animals with those of domestic cattle. A wild steak has 2 percent total fat as opposed to the 10 to 15 percent in commercially available lean beef. Wild meat also contains more omega-3 fatty acids, which are present in oily fish and have been linked to a reduced risk of heart disease and cancer. Meat from pasture-grazed cattle resembles wild meat more closely than meat from cows fed corn and sorghum. "We should try and raise our meat so it emulates wild meat," Cordain said.

Try to purchase only grass-fed beef, buffalo, lamb, and venison and free-range or pastured chicken and poultry. Free-range chickens have a natural diet of grass, seeds, and insects. The meat from these chickens as well as their eggs are far richer sources of all-important omega-3 fatty acids including docosahexaenoic acid (DHA), an omega-3 fatty acid critical to brain development.

Also, be sure to avoid toxic meat sources. In Leviticus 11:3, God says, "You may eat any animal that has a divided hoof and that chews the cud." In 11:9, we are told, "Of all the creatures living in the water of the seas and the streams you may eat any that have fins and scales." And in verse 47, we learn, "You must distinguish between the unclean and the clean, between living creatures that may be eaten and those that may not be eaten."

Scientists have confirmed the wisdom of distinguishing between the clean and unclean flesh foods. Dr. David Macht of Johns Hopkins University conducted a study in which he took all of the clean and unclean foods recommended in the Maker's Diet and compared them for toxicity. He did so by taking a growth culture and adding the flesh to it. If the flesh substance reduced the culture's growth rate below 75 percent, it was considered to be toxic. Above 75 percent was considered nontoxic.

In all cases, the flesh of the biblically clean animals tested nontoxic and the flesh of the unclean animals was toxic. The blood of all animals was more toxic than the flesh. We find similar results with clean fowl such as goose, chicken, coot, duck, pigeon, quail, swan, and turkey when compared to the unclean fowl, including cormorant, crow, eagle, falcon, hawk, heron, ibis, and raven.

The findings are pretty remarkable. Clean animals such as calf, deer, goat, ox, buffalo, and lamb were all rated 82 percent or higher. Unclean animals such as swine (pork), bear, camel, cat, guinea pig, dog, fox, groundhog, hamster, horse, opossum, rabbit, rat, rhinoceros, and squirrel rated from 39 to 62 percent. So remember, the next time you are tempted to have a rhinoceros burger with cheese, I suggest you pass.

In Leviticus 11:4-8 (NKJV), we are told by our Maker:

> Nevertheless these you shall not eat among those that chew the cud or those that have cloven hooves: the camel, because it chews the cud but does not have cloven hooves, is unclean to you; the rock hyrax, because it chews the cud but does not have cloven hooves, is unclean to you; the hare, because it chews the cud but does not have cloven hooves, is unclean to you; and the swine, though it divides the hoof, having cloven hooves, yet does not chew the cud, is unclean to you. Their flesh you shall not eat, and their carcasses you shall not touch. They are unclean to you.

Perhaps no dietary commandment is as widely flaunted as that which cautions against consumption of pork. But, again, even in these modern times, there is good reason to heed our Maker's wisdom. Researchers from the Department of Animal Hygiene and Prophylaxis at the Agricultural University of Szczecin in Poland, noted that, "Pork and its products are still the main cause of human trichinellosis in Poland."

Sadly, many cases of trichinellosis remain undetected. The rate of *Trichinella spiralis* infection in swine throughout Bolivia is considered to be very high. Although few cases of trichinellosis are reported among swine or humans, a high percentage of people have tested positive for exposure to this parasite. Many people also report various symptoms of trichinellosis, such as headaches, fever, and swelling in the extremities. Clearly, many people are made ill from this parasite, though it remains underdiagnosed.

The Maker warned against consumption of creatures of the sea without fins or scales. Why are we warned against shellfish consumption? Again, these foods are likely to carry dangerous pathogens. A friend of mine who served on the seafood safety committee of the National Academy of Sciences told me that committee members considered the odds to be about one in 300 that anyone eating raw or cooked shellfish in America today will become seriously ill with infectious disease. That's actually a very high rate of potential for serious illness.

Shellfish are a source of cholera as well as diseases involving paralysis. The reason why the flesh of shellfish is tainted is because they are bottom feeders who "filter" water by consuming the collective wastes they swim in. While they help to purify their environment, shellfish accumulate pathogens and other contaminants.

Many caretakers of ponds and other bodies of water know the best way to purify a freshwater pond or lake is to throw loads of scallops—another bottom feeder—into the murky water and wait a few days. The lake will be purified, and the scallops will float to the top. The same can be said of other scavengers such as oysters, clams, shrimp, and lobsters.

The scavengers that the Maker warned us against play a critical role in our environment. But, remember, our Maker told us to eat only certain flesh foods—animals with cloven hooves and that chew the cud and certain fowl. As for the rest, this question is posed in Job 14:4: "Who can bring a clean thing out of an unclean? No one!"

$$\infty$$

There is no question of the importance of protein in our diet. But when I began my search for the ultimate protein with which to supplement our diet, the task was more difficult than I first thought. Nearly every producer of protein powder on store shelves makes the product from nonorganic, highly processed cow's milk or soy milk. Due to the fact that I consider both sources inadequate at best, I began to search for alternatives. Then it happened, and I found what I consider to be the world's finest protein powder ever offered—one suited for infants, the elderly, and even professional athletes. I'm talking about a protein powder made from goat's milk.

Goat's milk is the most widely consumed dairy beverage in the world. Fully 65 percent of the world's population drinks goat's milk. Goat's milk has been a staple in much of the world since biblical times.

For people with intestinal disorders, goat's milk and goat's milk products have the potential to heal. Whereas cow's milk requires up to three hours to be absorbed, goat's milk requires only twenty minutes. This is because the protein molecules in goat's milk are half the size of those in cow's milk and have thinner, more fragile membranes. For that reason, they are easier to absorb through the wall of the small intestine.

Here are some of the other advantages of drinking goat's milk:

- Goat's milk is less allergic than cow's milk because it doesn't contain the protein complexes in cow's milk that stimulate allergic reactions. Children who have allergic reactions to cow's milk have seen their allergies improve after switching to goat's milk.
- Goat's milk doesn't produce gas or bloating as readily. Because goat's milk is digested quickly, it doesn't remain in the small intestine and ferment. It contains 7 percent less lactose than cow's milk.
- Goat's milk is high in the medium-chain fatty acids that inhibit candida.
- Goat's milk is not mucus forming.
- Goat's milk is a rich source of selenium. This mineral is believed to be an immuno-regulator. It quickens a sluggish immune system but quiets an overactive one. In this way, selenium keeps the immune system in tune and well balanced.
- Goat's milk doesn't contain the *Mycobacterium avium* subspecies *paratuberculosis* (MAP) microorganism.

The clinical nutritionist and chiropractic physician Bernard Jensen, Ph.D., D.C., stated this in the *Journal of the American Medical Association* (JAMA) under the heading of Dietetics and Hygiene:

The goat is the healthiest domestic animal known. Goat's milk is superior in every way to cow's milk. Goat's milk is the ideal food for babies, convalescents, and invalids, especially those with weakened digestive powers. Goat's milk is the purest, most healthful, and most complete food known.

A goat's milk protein powder is a highly concentrated source of amino acids in both their peptide and free forms. Among the components in goat's protein powder are the biologically active amino acids cystine, glycine, and glutamic acid. These three are precursors to glutathione formation by the body. As is generally known, glutathione functions as a principal antioxidant, scavenging free radicals and environmental toxins such as lipid peroxides that often damage and destroy healthy cells. Anyone suffering from oxidative stress, with its resultant nervous system, immune system, and endocrine system dysfunctions accompanied by fatigue, undergoes marked loss of physiological glutathione.

Goat's milk protein powder also provides immunoproteins such as albumin, lactalbumin, and lactoferin, which have been proven to stimulate immune response. Additionally, it's a balanced combination of whey protein and milk proteins that offers a favorable ratio of amino acids.

Goat's milk furnishes the growth materials each person requires for tissue repair, energy, the production of hormones, enzymes, antibodies, cellular components, amino acids, immunoglobulins, and every other part of the human physiology. As an animal source, it contains complete protein unlike any vegetable protein such as soy, and goat's milk is much less allergenic than cow's milk.

"The fat particles in goat's cream are five times smaller than those in cow's milk and much less hard on the liver," Dr. Jensen said, adding, "Goat's milk is sometimes superior to mother's milk because goat's milk contains food elements that mother's milk does not contain."

Gloria Gilbere, N.D. and author of *I Was Poisoned by My Body*, knows about the nutritional superiority of goat's milk. "Goat protein powder has been special in my practice because almost exclusively I put my attention on chemically induced immune disorders and leaky gut syndrome. Most of the patients who consult me for treatment are so chemically sensitive that most of the time they're unable to assimilate any kind of food except perhaps vegetable juices and wild rice. This same circumstance happened to me too from my being affected by multiple chemical sensitivity.

"That's why I moved to an out-of-the-way but pristine environment, Bonners Ferry, Idaho, located ninety miles south of the Canadian border, sandwiched between Montana and Washington State. Along with avoiding chemicals of all types, eating a purely natural and nontoxic diet, and taking various nutritional supplements containing no binders, my personal treatment involves drinking copious quantities of goat's milk in the form of a powder that I can add to smoothies, shakes, cooked oatmeal, muffins, and other delicious foods."

As the medical director of the Naturopathic Health and Research Center in Bonners Ferry, Dr. Gloria Gilbere administers to patients who come see her in person or consult with her via Skype. She described her inspiring tale of immunological restoration from multiple chemical sensitivities in this way:

> People who are nutritionally deprived or those who suffer from livers overburdened with immune system breakdown due to their excessive use of prescription drugs, street drugs, overindulgence of alcohol, environmental toxins, eating overly processed diets, or just engaging in bad lifestyle choices, do reach a point where protein can't be handled any more.
>
> By ingesting goat's milk protein powder the way I do in a smoothie, shake, or in cooked but cooled cereal, the concentrated protein becomes available so that their bodies can use all of it. That way they avoid anaphylactic shock and still receive excellent nourishment.
>
> Since this goat's milk protein is bioavailable, it's easy on the digestive system and brings on absolutely no disturbance to serious gastrointestinal disorders such as Crohn's disease, IBS, leaky gut, and other conditions that lock people into acute states of chemical sensitivity.
>
> Remember, in my practice I deal strictly with people who are highly sensitive to almost anything. Items such as nightshade foods, soy, cow's milk, wheat, and gluten set them off. They are predisposed to respond adversely with serious symptoms such as skin rashes, gastrointestinal refluxes, anaphylaxis or some other negative reactions. When I recommend that they use goat's milk protein powder and they do, I never need to worry about negative reactions to their bodies.
>
> One time I treated a surgical nurse, age fifty-four, who had moved into a recently constructed hospital facility and became chemically sensitive almost overnight from the new building materials. The overriding symptom was her inability to eat anything—no appetite at all. Within a couple of months, her body weight dropped by

over 35 percent to just ninety-two pounds. She became a shadow of her former self. Her weakness prevented the performance of any meaningful activity, and she certainly could not work in surgical nursing or do her housekeeping chores.

Immediately I began my patient on a detoxification program because she failed to eliminate her body wastes. She was experiencing just one bowel movement per week, and that was accomplished only with much concentration. She would spend large amounts of time in the bathroom trying to eliminate and often without result. But the goat's milk protein powder along with other components of my program changed all that.

After finding that the nurse could not tolerate even the blandest vegetable juices, I introduced her to a goat's milk protein powder combined with rice milk as a smoothie drink. She took to this protein drink well and relied on it as almost the only thing ingested. She put on twelve pounds in five weeks without any gastrointestinal cramping. Her bowels became more normal with a movement occurring every second day. It's now a year later, and my patient experiences two bowel movements daily.

She currently supplements any form of protein she ingests with goat's milk protein powder because even today, this surgical nurse is unable to eat any other animal-derived products—no yogurt, cow's milk, eggs, fish, shellfish, meat, or poultry. Moreover, the patient is highly lactose-intolerant, but she finds goat's milk protein powder to be quite digestible as the mainstay of her diet.

Here's something else about goat's milk: nanny goats produce milk that almost duplicates human breast milk. I find it interesting that the nanny's natural function is to feed her kid (a baby goat) weighing between seven and nine pounds, which is the size of a human baby.

In contrast, the cow's newborn calf weighs as much as 90 pounds so that bovine milk's chemicals, including its fat and protein, are tailored to fit the needs of a baby animal quite different in size from a newborn human. Molecules of the cow's milk protein are overly large for digestion and absorption by human infants, and for this reason, among others, cow's milk frequently incites allergic responses in children.

When injected with bovine growth hormone (bGH) or bovine somatotropin (bST), a dairy cow can produce 12 gallons of milk daily as opposed to the goat, which can produce only up to 2 gallons a day. The bGH stimulates a cow's mammary glands to secrete excessively, but the hormone is absorbed in the animal's dairy product. There is risk associated with endocrine imbalance caused by cow's milk. In contrast, goats graze on pasture and are fed chemical-free feed, meaning their milk is free of hormones, antibiotics, and pesticides.

Here are some thoughts to ponder: The English word *protein* comes from the Latin *proteus*, which means of primary importance. The vast number of amino acids found in goat's milk protein are essential for normal growth and give rise to all connective tissues, enzymes, hormones, antibodies, muscles, skin, bones, hair, nails, heart, teeth, blood, brain, biochemical activities, and the entire nervous system. Protein deficiency is responsible for the lowering of immune function and for much of the immune system suppression diseases that the medical community is currently confronting.

Goat's milk protein powder is ideal for those who prefer not to eat meat because of its hormonal content. Athletes who must maintain an anabolic state (the building of tissue) certainly wish to avoid residues of hormones in meat. But most cattle are fed or injected with female hormones for purposes of producing greater amounts of meat.

Leigh Erin Connealy, M.D., who founded the Center for New Medicine in Irvine, California, where she serves as the medical director, said, "Most patients who consult me show signs that they are not getting an adequate amount of protein in their diets. I understand there is controversy as to what should be the main source of protein—meat, fish, cow's milk, eggs, soy, whey, etc. Because there is so much genetically altered protein, which often contains too many additives, that I decided to solve the controversy for myself. After conducting my own research, my recommendation is that a person's main protein source should be goat's milk from organically raised goats. I am definitely not an exponent of soy because of its carcinogenic aspects for the breast—and because it usually tastes bad. If people must eat soy, they should take it from an organic source. But my rule is to generally avoid soy and other types of designer proteins.

"As the mother of three children, it was my standard practice to feed them liquid goat's milk or use goat milk's protein powder, which is an excellent protein supplement," said Dr. Connealy. "I advise my patients to make a shake with the powder and add fruit, nuts, seeds, and other foods, especially peaches, berries, and so forth that they wish to include. Such combinations are highly nutritious and taste wonderful."

America has feared fat for a long time.

Sure, we know that the wrong fats will cause you to gain weight, clog your arteries, and promote cancer. But too little fat is also a killer, and people don't know that.

Most people have it all wrong when it comes to fat, and that comes from studies done in the 1950s that concluded all fats to be bad—saturated, monounsaturated, or polyunsaturated—and all the fat we were consuming was turning unsuspecting folks into heart attack risks. The trouble is that the original researchers failed to distinguish between different kinds of fat.

When it comes to cardiovascular health, I believe the real culprits in heart disease are obscenely elevated intakes of human-made trans-fatty acids, polyunsaturated fats high in omega-6 fatty acids, and the overconsumption of carbohydrates.

Let's go to Greece for a moment and get a clearer picture of this good fat versus bad fat concept. In Greece, the typical diet consists of 40 percent fat, which happens to be the same percentage as in the United States, but Greek men and women have significantly lower rates of heart disease, prostate, and breast cancer.

That's why I say that fat per se is not the enemy—but the type of fat. You see, the Greek diet is loaded with omega-3 and monounsaturated (omega-9) fatty acids, conjugated linoleic acid (CLA), as well as healthy saturated fats. These are the *good fats* that come from salmon, walnuts, purslane, olives, lamb, and goat meat; goats' and sheep's milk and cheese; and other properly prepared dairy products. These are fats that we don't get enough of from our American diet anymore. The trouble is that most people have decreased their consumption of natural, unadulterated essential fatty acids and drastically increased their consumption of refined and adulterated fats and oils.

Our ingestion of omega-6 fatty acids has skyrocketed with the advent of seed extraction technology during the Industrial Revolution. Oils such as sunflower, safflower, peanut, and corn oil are dominant in omega-6 fatty acids, while being virtually void of beneficial omega-3 fatty acids.

Saturated fats are solid at room temperature. They are stable and do not go rancid even when they are heated, which makes them ideal for cooking even at high temperatures. Saturated fats are found mostly in animal and dairy products, as well as tropical oils such as coconut, palm, and palm kernel oils. These saturated fats also contain healing short-chain and medium-chain fatty acids that are very important to our health.

Traditional foods contain appreciable amounts of other beneficial fats, including CLA, caprylic acid, lauric acid, butyric acid, and omega-3 fatty acids. These fatty acids are extremely beneficial to the health of the immune system and digestive tract. They can supply a significant portion of our energy requirements. But today, our cloven-hoofed friends are fed terrible diets, rarely graze on grass, and, as a result, no longer contain appreciable amounts of beneficial omega-3 fatty acids or other healthy fats.

Dramatic scientific research shows that excess amounts of trans-fatty acids (which are human-made molecules created from hydrogenating vegetable oils) are killers, increasing risk for heart disease, cancer, diabetes, and other age-related maladies. You'll find these bad fats in margarines, many baked goods, and other processed foods.

Until World War II, much of the added fat or oil in the diet, other than the animal, poultry, and dairy fats, came either from small presses such as those used for flaxseed oil in Eastern Europe or larger presses used for olive oil. But following World War II, the food industry capitalized on its ability to turn liquid oils, which were plentiful but not sufficiently marketable, into solid fats for the budding fast-food industry and for the expanding baking and snack food industries.

It was the beginning of a nutritional disaster. Profits made in the ensuing years came at the expense of public health. Scientists' main concern about their health effects arose because of the structural similarity of these isomers to saturated fatty acids. Today, researchers consider trans-fatty acids to be a major cause of heart disease. Trans-fatty acids also increase circulating levels of lipoprotein(a), a non-dietary-related risk of atherogenesis.

If the ingredients list on a food includes partially hydrogenated vegetable oil, then the food contains trans fats. Trans fats are found only in foods that have been altered, and they conform neither to the primitive diet nor the intent of our Maker.

On the other hand, accumulating evidence from molecular and cellular biology experiments, experimental studies, and human clinical trials suggests omega-3 fatty acids, as well as short- and medium-chain fatty acids, may potentially confer important health benefits related to cardiovascular disease, cancer prevention, and reducing inflammation.

These potential health benefits are consistent with epidemiological evidence that rates of heart disease, various cancers, bone fractures in people with osteoporosis, and menopausal symptoms are much less prevalent among populations that consume diets rich in omega-3, short- and medium-chain fatty acids.

Omega-3 fatty acids fight heart disease by lowering dangerous LDL cholesterol and triglycerides, as well as decreasing the viscosity of thick blood. They also reduce the buildup of atherosclerotic plaque on artery walls.

"Population studies demonstrate that people who consume a diet rich in omega-3 oils from either fish or vegetable sources have a significantly reduced risk of developing heart disease," said Dr. Michael Murray, one of the world's leading authorities on natural medicine. "Over sixty double-blind studies show that either fish oil supplements or flaxseed oil [both rich in omega-3 fatty acids] are very effective in lowering blood pressure."

Unfortunately, modern processing has eliminated the good fats from our diet. Lalitha Davis, author of *10 Essential Foods*, said, "Most researchers describe a healthy balance of omega-6 to omega-3 oils as anywhere from 1:1 to 3:1 or 4:1. You probably won't be surprised to learn that the actual balance of these two essential fatty acids in the body of the average American is about 20:1! This basic nutrient imbalance of much more omega-6s than omega-3s is caused by a diet high in processed and refined foods, grains, and grocery store vegetable oils that are highly refined with toxic chemicals, and domestic animal meats fed mostly grain."

I want to go beyond simply telling you about omega-3 fatty acids because, truthfully, many other fats are also important to your health and many people know next to nothing about them.

As I mentioned, modern health experts tell us to avoid fat and especially saturated fat. Modern health experts tell us fat consumption is responsible for heart disease, obesity, and cancer. They have been especially harsh on the use of tropical oils such as coconut, palm, and palm kernel oil.

"While this claim has been widely disproved in many scientific studies and journals, unfortunately this perception is still around," noted Dr. Enig, the coauthor of *Nourishing Traditions* and a researcher known for her unconventional positions on the role saturated fats play in our health.

"The tropical oils were very popular in the [United States] food industry prior to World War II. With the war and the shortages of imported tropical oils, an effort was made to promote local oils like soybean and corn oil. The [United States] is the largest exporter of soybeans. Studies were done to show that coconut oil, and all saturated fats, were bad for one's health because they raised serum cholesterol levels. However, these studies were done on hydrogenated coconut oil, and all hydrogenated oils produce higher serum cholesterol levels, whether they are saturated or not. Recent research shows that it is the presence of *trans fatty acids* that causes health problems, as they are fatty acid chains that have been altered from their original form in nature by the oil refining process."

Among saturated fats that have taken the worst beating is butter, although the pendulum is swinging in the other direction in recent years. Now it's coconut oil that's on the hot seat. A report from the American Heart Association released in 2017 advised against its use, saying that coconut oil increases LDL cholesterol, a cause of cardiovascular disease.

These are the same folks who've told us that soy, corn, canola, safflower, sunflower, and cottonseed oils are just fine, and these are the oils that major food companies use in zillions of products today.

This is why margarine is king in this country. Since the 1950s we've been told that margarine is healthier. Once again, our so-called nutritional and health experts have steered us upon a bitter course. Even though butter, coconut oil, and animal fats have nourished human beings for thousands of years, these healthy foods have been relegated and replaced by concoctions of questionable nutritional value.

Saturated animal fat is and should be an essential and vital part of many diets. The Maasai, and related tribes in East Africa, consume a diet almost completely composed of beef, milk, and blood (which neither the Bible nor I recommend). At some parts of the year, a typical Maasai warrior will consume up to 10 quarts of whole, raw cow's milk a day. The Maasai are noted for their tall stature and great endurance. Heart disease, obesity, diabetes, osteoporosis, and cancer are unknown to the Maasai. The Maasai are also the most feared warriors, as they are healthier than virtually any of their surrounding neighbors who eat a much more vegetarian diet.

The Inuits are another good example of a people who have historically thrived with a diet comprised largely of animal products, including huge amounts of blubber (fat) from various marine animals. Given the harsh, icy climate they live in, the Inuits are not frequent consumers of grains, fruits, or vegetables. Inuits who have not abandoned their native diet have virtually no incidence of heart disease, cancer, arteriosclerosis, osteoporosis, or diabetes. Some studies have appeared in recent years attempting to show that Inuits suffer from bone loss due to their high protein diets, but such studies have been discredited when researchers note that only those Inuits who abandoned their native diet for "civilized" food—and alcohol—suffered from calcium loss.

More examples could be provided to prove that saturated fat consumption, even when very high, is not implicated in heart disease or cancer. Despite this, the prevailing dietary opinion is that saturated fat is bad and should be avoided.

I strongly disagree. Let's take a closer look at sources of some of the healthy saturated fats.

Butter

As an excellent source of fat-soluble vitamins, butter is rich in lecithin (needed for fat metabolism), trace minerals (particularly selenium), arachidonic acid (needed for prostaglandin production), and short- and medium-chain fatty acids that the body uses for energy. Two of these fatty acids, butyric and lauric acids, have antitumor, antifungal, and antimicrobial properties.

Studies have shown that vitamins and minerals from vegetables are better absorbed when eaten with butter. Butter also provides the intestines with the fatty material needed to convert carotenes from plants into vitamin A. It's best to choose butter that is from goat's or sheep's milk or from cow's milk from grass-fed animals and free of growth hormones.

Lamb and Beef

Mostly found in lamb and beef tallow, stearic acid is the preferred fuel source for the heart. Despite current dietary wisdom telling us that saturated fat is bad for the heart, the heart excels at converting fatty acids into energy for itself. Lamb tallow is also rich in oleic acid, another beneficial fat for the cardiovascular system. Palm oil and olive oil are also rich in oleic acid.

Extra Virgin Coconut Oil

Extra virgin coconut oil is perhaps the most-avoided miracle food, which is a shame. Coconut oil has been used as cooking oil for thousands of years. Popular cookbooks advertised it at the end of the 19th century. Then came the campaign against saturated fats and in favor of vegetable-sourced polyunsaturated fats such as canola, soybean, safflower, corn, and other seed and nut oils, plus their partially hydrogenated counterparts such as margarine.

Although saturated fats have never been linked to heart disease in well-designed, honest epidemiological studies, nearly all commercial foods today avoid saturated fats, instead relying on polyunsaturated or partially hydrogenated vegetable fats. These may be "all vegetarian" or "no-cholesterol" foods, but they're not necessarily better for your health. Indeed, for the last five or six decades, Americans have *increased* their consumption of unsaturated fats and partially hydrogenated fats and *decreased* their consumption of saturated fatty acids and butter. At the same time, the rate of deaths caused by heart disease has increased, as has obesity and many immune system disorders.

Here's why I recommend coconut oil:

- Foods cooked in coconut oil taste better and taste better longer. If left at room temperature unsaturated oils turn rancid fairly quickly, but even after one year at room temperature, coconut oil shows no evidence of rancidity. Coconut oil is packed with antioxidants, and it also reduces the body's need for vitamin E.

- Coconut oil stimulates thyroid function which, in turn, stimulates conversion of production of low-density lipoprotein cholesterol into the antiaging prohormones and hormones pregnenolone, progesterone, and dehydroepiandrosterone (DHEA). These valuable agents support the fight against heart disease, senility, obesity, cancer and other diseases associated with premature aging, as well as chronic, degenerative diseases.

- Another benefit from coconut oil's unique ability to support thyroid function is weight loss. In the 1940s, farmers tried coconut oil to fatten their animals but discovered that it made them lean and active and increased their appetite. Whoops! Then they tried an antithyroid drug, which made the livestock fat with less food but was found to be a carcinogen (cancer-causing drug). Whoops! Farmers then discovered that they could fatten their herds by simply feeding their animals soybeans and corn, which is why we are where we are today.

- Coconut oil protects against cancer. Generally speaking, animals fed unsaturated oils develop more tumors.

- Coconut oil has tremendous antiviral properties. Coconut oil contains medium-chain fatty acids such as lauric, caprylic, and capric acids. Of these three, coconut oil contains 40 to 55 percent lauric acid, which has the greatest antiviral activity of these three fatty acids. Lauric acid is so adept at fighting viral pathogens; it is present in large quantities in breast milk. The body converts lauric acid to a fatty acid derivative (monolaurin), which is the substance that protects infants and adults alike from viral, bacterial, or protozoal infections.

It's important to prefer extra virgin coconut oil using fresh coconut meat and not add chemicals or use a high heating process when refining coconut oil.

The method used in the Philippines to produce extra virgin coconut oil from coconut milk is fermentation. The coconut milk expressed from the freshly harvested coconuts is fermented for twenty-four to thirty-six hours. During this time, the water separates from the oil. The oil is then slightly heated for a short time to remove moisture and become filtered. The result is a clear coconut oil that retains the distinct scent and taste of coconuts.

This is a traditional method of coconut oil extraction that has been used in the Philippines for hundreds of years. Laboratory tests show that this is a high-quality coconut oil with the lauric acid content being 50 to 53 percent. This oil is not mass produced but is made by hand just as it has been done for hundreds of years. Because the producers of the coconut oil live in the community where the coconuts grow, they are assured of using the best organic coconuts available in producing their extra virgin coconut oil, being careful that no chemicals whatsoever are used in the growing or processing of the coconuts.

Most commercial grade coconut oils are made from copra, which is the dried kernel (meat) of the coconut. Copra is made by smoke drying, sun drying, kiln drying, or a combination of these methods. If standard copra is used as a starting material, the unrefined coconut oil extracted from copra is not suitable for consumption and must be further refined. This is because the way most copra is dried is very unsanitary.

Most of the copra is dried under the sun in the open air, where it is exposed to insects and molds. The standard end product made from copra is RBD coconut oil—RBD standing for refined, bleached, and deodorized. Both high heat and chemical solvents are used in this method. The RBD oil is also often hydrogenated or partially hydrogenated, which means it's not a good product.

Another difference between extra virgin coconut oil and refined coconut oils is the scent and taste. Extra virgin retains the fresh scent and taste of coconuts, whereas the copra-based refined coconut oils have no taste at all due to the refining process.

Promising studies have been done on patients suffering from immune deficiency diseases and their use of coconut oil, which is why I'm a big fan of the healing properties of coconut oil. As you will read in the protocol section, I recommend virtually everyone consume coconut oil on a daily basis. I truly believe that coconut oil is the best widely available oil to use for cooking and baking and is even great when used externally to promote smooth and supple skin. It's also great for hair. If your hair is dry or longer, like past your shoulders, work a little dab of coconut oil through the bottom half of it when wet, after washing, for softer, healthier hair.

Dairy Products

Another important source of fats in the diet is dairy. Although not all peoples of the world have consumed dairy products in abundance in the past, primitive nomads drank the milk of their cattle, goats, and sheep. Primitive people also fermented milk products as a means of preserving them. Archaeologists have found Sumerian tablets dating to six thousand years ago that explain how to ferment milk to prepare cheese.

Yogurt has been a food staple of the Middle East and Caucasian Mountains for many thousands of years. The godly men of the Bible were shepherds and herdsmen. Abel, Job, Abraham, Isaac, Jacob, Jacob's twelve sons, David, and many others all had very large numbers of livestock. In fact, in biblical times the amount of wealth and stature one had was measured in the number of livestock kept. Jacob's entire household was in the profession of animal husbandry. That is why they settled in Goshen for the Egyptians did not like being keepers of animals. No doubt, the chosen people of God ate and enjoyed dairy products, as well as meat.

The biggest difference between our milk and the milk that primitive people drank can be seen in the destructive processes of pasteurization, homogenization, and the removal of fat or the skimming process. Today, the nonorganic milk that most people drink comes from cows that have been fed hormones and antibiotics.

A century ago, a Holstein, a popular breed of dairy cow, produced 400 to 500 pounds of milk annually. Today, the average Holstein produces 20,000 to 30,000 pounds in a year! This high milk production is due in part to use of bovine growth hormone and other factory farm methods. Such hormone-treated cows produce milk that is high in a protein called insulin-like growth factor-1 (IGF-1). This protein stimulates cell growth and has been associated with certain kinds of cancer, especially prostate cancer. Cows are often raised in close quarters and are therefore subject to infectious diseases. Due to excessive milking, their udders are usually excoriated and infected. For these reasons, cows are fed antibiotics.

Because of the way milk is commercially sold these days, most people cannot conceive of drinking milk or taking any milk product unless it has been pasteurized. Pasteurization is named for Louis Pasteur, the French scientist who invented the process. In pasteurization, milk is heat treated to destroy disease-causing bacteria. Some have argued that stainless steel tanks and other sanitizing innovations in the milk production industry have made pasteurization unnecessary. Nonetheless, there are some drawbacks to consuming pasteurized milk:

- Like antibiotics, pasteurization kills good as well as harmful bacteria. Raw milk contains lactic acid-producing bacteria. Lactic acid can kill certain pathogens and thereby prevent disease.
- Pasteurization kills the enzymes in milk. The lack of these enzymes makes milk harder to digest.
- Pasteurization lowers the potency of some vitamins in milk, chiefly vitamin C and B_{12}. The process also makes calcium, magnesium, phosphorus, and sulfur less bioavailable.
- The U.S. government reports that 30 percent of commercial milk samples contain measurable levels of contaminants such as pesticides and antibiotic residues. Pasteurization does not rid milk of these contaminants from industrial milk production.

Only California and twelve other states currently permit raw, unpasteurized milk to be sold commercially, but even in those states finding raw milk is difficult. In many areas of this country, however, one can find people raising goats and selling fresh, raw goat's milk. Raw milk is delicious and has a consistency closer to cream than milk. Mixed with fruit, it makes a delicious dessert. For reasons explained throughout this book, I am a huge advocate of consuming goat's milk instead of cow's milk.

Raw milk, by the way, is fresh milk. The pasteurized milk in grocery stores is probably three to four weeks old because the milk has to go from the dairy to a processor to a wholesaler and then to the retail grocery store, where it is sold.

On the bright side, you can find some cheeses, especially imported ones, made with raw milk. Look for "raw milk" on the label.

The best dairy products are the lacto-fermented kind—yogurt, kefir, hard cheeses, cultured cream cheese, cottage cheese, and cultured cream. People who normally can't consume dairy products because they are lactose-intolerant can oftentimes tolerate fermented dairy products because the enzyme lactase is produced by the lactic acid bacteria found in those products. This enzyme can break down and digest lactose, the milk sugar found in dairy products. What's more, properly prepared cultured dairy products should contain little or no residual lactose because the bacteria feeds on this sugar during the fermentation process. In its wake, the bacteria leave galactose, an easy-to-digest monosaccharide-type sugar.

Fermentation increases vitamin B and C content of milk. Most importantly, fermentation is good for intestinal health because of the way it supplies beneficial bacteria to the intestinal tract and produces lactic acid, a substance that aids the absorption of calcium, copper, iron, magnesium, and manganese.

By acidifying the gut and making it easier for proteins to be absorbed in the small intestine, the *Lactobacillus* bacteria in fermented dairy products make minerals more bioavailable. Some *Lactobacillus* strains in fermented dairy products produce natural antibiotics that are useful against infections.

The best dairy source of all is goat's milk.

Fiber

Also known as roughage, fiber is the indigestible remnants of plant cells in food. Fiber is made chiefly of plant cellulose, but these substances are also fibers: hemicellulose, pectin, lignans, gums, and mucilages.

Sources of fiber include vegetables, fruits, whole grains, and beans. Fiber is necessary for regular bowel movements and prevents constipation. Fiber increases the elimination of waste matter in the large intestine and pressures the rectum muscles to loosen and expel waste.

There are two kinds of fiber—insoluble fiber cannot be broken down at all, whereas soluble fiber dissolves in water. Most fibrous foods contain both types of fiber. Insoluble fiber is believed to reduce the risk of colon cancer. Weight-loss programs recommend fiber because it gives people the feeling that they are filled up without contributing more calories to their diet.

Primitive people ate far more fiber than we do. Although Americans are constantly being reminded to eat more fiber, the average American eats approximately eight grams per day. In 1850, the average American ate 20 to 30 grams daily, which happens to be what the National Cancer Institute recommends eating.

In pioneering studies made in the 1970s, a British missionary surgeon named Dr. Denis Burkitt observed that rural Africans who ate high-fiber diets had far less colon cancer than people in the West. The native people had almost no diabetes, constipation, or IBS as well. Dr. Burkitt observed that Africans who ate a Western diet suffered from these diseases, concluding that the Africans' high-fiber intake accounted for their good intestinal health.

Dr. Burkitt's studies marked the beginning of "the fiber hypothesis," the idea that eating large amounts of fiber and decreasing fat intake can prevent colon cancer as well as diverticulosis, hemorrhoids, and colonic polyps. For thirty years, the fiber hypothesis was considered the gospel truth, but the hypothesis has been refined in recent years.

First of all, fiber is a carbohydrate. Many people, eager to improve their health by eating more fiber, eat high-fiber, high-carbohydrate foods such as bran, fibrous breakfast cereals, whole-wheat bread, brown rice, and potatoes. As I've pointed out time and time again, however, the over-consumption of these carbohydrates is a primary cause of intestinal and other diseases.

The kind of fiber that promotes colon health is found as low-carbohydrate, high-fiber foods such as broccoli, cauliflower, celery, lettuce, soaked or sprouted seeds and nuts, berries, and other small fruits. Fruits and vegetables with edible skins are especially high in fiber. Besides providing fiber, these foods are rich in vitamins, minerals, and antioxidants.

Meanwhile, mucilaginous fiber decreases transit time—the amount of time that food spends in the colon before it is expelled. Lowered transit times mean that food has less time to ferment or putrefy in the colon. Toxins are quickly flushed out. Mucilaginous fiber, which soothes inflamed tissue in the lining of the gut, can be found in psyllium seeds, marshmallow root, slippery elm, chia seeds, and flaxseed.

Unfortunately, many people with gut disorders have a hard time with fiber, particularly insoluble fiber. Usually cooking, juicing, pureeing, or fermenting vegetables and fruits is necessary before they can be eaten. I recommend going to the extra trouble to prepare vegetables in one of these ways because they are a healthy source of fiber.

Condiments and Salt

Go into most restaurants and you will see a selection of condiments on the table—salt, pepper, ketchup, mustard, and maybe Sriracha sauce. Most people keep a small supply of these condiments in their pantry or refrigerator.

Condiments have been a part of the human diet for many centuries, but their purpose has been lost in modern times. Originally, condiments were digestive aids and meant to be taken in small amounts with a meal to encourage proper digestion. Unlike the condiments of today, almost all the original condiments were fermented.

The next time you are dressing up your hamburger at the neighbor's barbeque, consider the pedigree of ketchup. From the Chinese *ke-tsiap*, ketchup started out as a fermented fish-brine sauce. Sailors brought it from China to England, where the locals added pickled cucumbers, kidney beans, and oysters to the mix. New Englanders made tomatoes the chief feature of ketchup in the late 1700s. Sadly, our modern commercialized ketchup is no longer fermented. Today's ketchup, however, is loaded with sugar and corn syrup. That's why it's captured the American palate.

Lacto-fermentation is difficult to achieve on an industrial scale. For that reason, the makers of modern condiments use vinegar in the brine, but this makes condiments more acidic. Worse, many condiments are pasteurized, which kills the beneficial lactic acid bacteria that naturally occur in properly prepared condiments.

These days, condiments have ceased to be aids to digestion and are used to dress up prepared food and give it a little more tang. Ironically, dietitians recommend cutting back on condiments, the foods that people ate originally to promote good health.

It's possible to make your own lacto-fermented condiments, so be sure to read *Nourishing Traditions* by Sally Fallon with Mary Enig, which shares fantastic recipes.

More so than any other condiment, most people reach for the shaker and sprinkle lots of salt on their food. Salt is one of the oldest food additives. Even people who lived far from the ocean obtained salt by burning sodium-rich grasses and mixing the ash into their food. Some have argued that salt raises blood pressure, but this contention is still open to debate.

These good things can be said about salt:

- Salt provides chloride for the manufacturing of hydrochloric acid, the stomach acid that breaks down food.
- Salt stimulates salivation.
- Salt is an enzyme activator.
- Salt is required for proper functioning of the adrenal gland.
- And, of course, salt makes food taste better.

The downside to conventional table salt, like the kind you buy in most stores, is that it's processed. Aluminum compounds are added to keep the salt dry. The trace minerals and iodine salts that occur naturally in sea salt are removed during processing. To make the salt a pristine white, it is exposed to bleaching agents.

That's why I recommend a natural, unrefined salt called Celtic sea salt. This light-gray salt comes from the Brittany region in northwest France, where it is gathered in clay-lined ponds as part of a 2,000-year-old tradition. Celtic sea salt is high in organic iodine from plants and the tiny skeletons of ancient marine life and includes many trace minerals, including sodium chloride and magnesium salts.

Herbamare, a combination of sea salt, spices, herbs, and vegetables all steeped together for over a year, is a favorite seasoning of mine. I've consumed Herbamare for years and never tire of it.

Regarding other fermented foods, the Austrians and Germans have sauerkraut. The Japanese have pickled ginger. There is kefir and a porridge called podji. In the United States, our best-known fermented foods are catsup, mayonnaise, and sourdough bread.

In one sense, for all its benefits (and there are plenty) for fermented foods, we can also say the miracle of refrigeration has ruined the health of modern men and women. Refrigeration, at least in modern societies, has replaced our need for fermented foods, and so have modern processing methods that no longer allow for the fermentation of foods. In spite of technological advancements, our bodies still cry out for such healthy foods as well as the enzymes they contain.

Enzymes are proteins that act as catalysts for chemical reactions in the body. They are the labor force of the body. They speed up the rate of chemical reactions. They initiate chemical reactions but are not themselves changed by those reactions. Enzymes take the foods we eat and turn them into chemical structures that are able to pass through the cell membranes of the small intestine and into the bloodstream. Enzymes are found in all living organisms.

Raw food contains enzymes that assist with digestion. As soon as you put raw food in your mouth, the enzymes begin digesting it, and they continue to do so in the cardia (upper) portion of the stomach after the food is swallowed. These digestive enzymes—*proteases* to digest protein, *amylases* to digest carbohydrates, and *lipases* to digest fat—break down food so it can be absorbed in the small intestine.

Our primitive ancestors knew the value of raw food to digestion. Not only did primitive people eat raw fruits and vegetables, they ate raw meat. The Inuits, for example, ate raw fat from seals, whale blubber, and raw fish. These foods contain an abundance of the enzyme lipase. Some Pygmies devouring the decomposing carcass of a dead elephant in equatorial Africa, when asked how they tolerated such unsavory food, replied that they were eating the meat of the elephant, not its odor.

Does eating raw meat seem repulsive to you? In genteel Victorian London, physicians prescribed sandwiches made from raw thyroid glands to aging patients to help rejuvenate them.

The fact of the matter is that prolonged heat over 118 degrees Fahrenheit kills all enzymes. Therefore, cooking destroys the digestive enzymes in raw food. So does food processing methods and pasteurization. Seeing as most people eat cooked food, processed food, or pasteurized food, the modern diet is empty of vital enzymes. Raw food, however, is alive. Unless you make a point of eating more raw food, you lose the benefits of live food and its digestive enzymes.

In his classic book, *Enzyme Nutrition,* Dr. Edward Howell proposed the idea that everyone is born with a finite store of enzymes. Enzymes, he noted, fall into three classes:

- metabolic enzymes that direct body functions
- digestive enzymes secreted by the pancreas for digesting food
- enzymes found in raw foods that assist with digestion

Dr. Howell believed that eating too much cooked food depleted the body's store of finite enzymes. To digest cooked food, the body must draw upon its own enzymes, which leaves fewer enzymes for other functions, like operating the brain, muscles, organs, and tissues. Dr. Howell believed in eating more raw food in order to keep the body's store of enzymes from being depleted. Consider what he wrote here:

> A certain amount of raw, uncooked food in the diet is indispensable to the highest degree of health. Assuming that the proteins, fats, carbohydrates, minerals, and vitamins are equally available for nutrition in raw and cooked food, any demonstrable nutritional superiority of raw food must then be ascribed to the "live" quality of raw food, and when this live quality is subjected to analysis, it is shown to consist of...no other property than that possessed by enzymes.

The enzymes in fruits and vegetables fully develop when the fruits and vegetables are ripe. A ripe banana, for example, has far more digestive enzymes than a green banana. For this reason, you should try to eat naturally ripened fruits and vegetables that have not been truck- or gas-ripened. What's more, some seeds and nuts contain enzyme inhibitors. These substances prevent seeds and nuts from sprouting until they are nestled deeply enough in the soil. Enzyme inhibitors serve an important role in Nature, but they also make the enzymes in fruits and nuts unavailable. You can, however, free the enzymes in seeds and nuts by soaking them before eating.

Besides eating raw food, consider taking digestive enzyme supplements. In my experience, digestive enzyme supplements help people with gastrointestinal disorders immensely because of the way they aid digestion and reduce inflammation in the colon.

Stocks, Broths, and Gelatin

Unfortunately for our health, stocks, bone soups, and broths, which require several hours of careful simmering, are no longer an important part of the modern diet. People believe they are too busy to make these foods, but that sort of thinking is shortsighted because stocks and bone broth are some of the most nutritious foods you can eat. "Good broth resurrects the dead," according to a South American proverb. Stocks, broths, and non-pork gelatins are a folk remedy for colds and the flu in almost every culture. There's a reason for this.

Stocks and broths are especially beneficial to people who have intestinal diseases because they are high in nutrients the gastrointestinal tract can absorb without having to do a lot of work. Gelatin, the odorless, tasteless substance extracted by boiling bones, animal tissues, and hooves, is especially easy to digest. Broth from meat and animal bones is an excellent source of many important minerals, including iodine, chloride, sodium, magnesium, and potassium. Iodine is especially plentiful in stock made from fish bones and heads.

Dr. Francis Pottenger, a physician who intentionally applied the principles of Dr. Weston A. Price in his treatment of respiratory disease such as tuberculosis, asthma, and allergies, believed that stocks, broths, and gelatin were easy to digest because they contain hydrophilic colloids. Colloids are large molecules. Hydrophilic means "water-loving." Normally, the colloids in cooked food are the opposite of hydrophilic—they are hydrophobic, meaning they don't attract liquids. But stocks, broths, and gelatins, although they have been cooked, attract digestive liquids. This explains why they are easier to digest than other cooked food.

Beverages

The modern diet is insufficient in water, and the beverages that are in the diet are often more harmful than healthy. In most cases, our primitive ancestors were able to obtain drinking water straight from the source—from a river, creek, or spring. Natural water is extremely healthy. This water is mineral-rich and "structured." That is, the water has a strong electrical charge and low surface tension.

Naturally structured water isn't as dense as conventional tap water. No one knows precisely why people in some cultures live, on average, longer than others, but many attribute longevity to drinking copious amounts of healthy water.

Whenever possible, it is important to consume such structured waters. Structured water facilitates the activity of enzymes and has a high solubility for the body's minerals and vitamins. Structured water tends to go from the digestive tract and bloodstream into the tissues much more efficiently.

What about other beverages? Soda pop is marketed aggressively to the young and rightfully called a "sweet poison." Girls in their early teens who drink soda pop often have an increased risk of getting fractures and osteoporosis. The culprit is probably the phosphoric acid in soda pop, which impedes the absorption of magnesium and calcium. Soda pop represents yet another inroad made by sugar into the American diet.

Soft drinks are often blamed for the increase in obesity among children, which has been steadily rising since I became very sick.

One of the common ingredients in carbonated drinks—a preservative known as sodium benzoate—has the ability to switch off vital parts of DNA, which could lead to diseases like cirrhosis of the liver and Parkinson's disease. Professor Peter Piper, a professor of molecular biology at Sheffield University in Great Britain, tested the impact of sodium benzoate on living yeast cells in his laboratory, and what he found alarmed him. The benzoate had the ability to "cause severe damage to DNA," he said.

In order to avoid the calories imparted by sugar, many soda drinkers are turning to sugar-free beverages. Aspartame, the artificial sweetener found in most sugar-free soda pop brands, may be worse than sugar, however. Aspartame has been implicated in seizures, depression, and neurological disorders such as dizziness and muscle aches. In an American Cancer Society study of 78,000 women, those who consumed artificially sweetened foods gained more weight over a one-year period than those who consumed sugar-sweetened products. The researchers speculated that the sugar substitutes may have stimulated the women's appetites.

The other beverage that has gained in popularity in recent years is coffee, thanks to coffee shops like Starbucks and Peet's on every street corner. Drinking coffee not only does a number on the stomach and esophagus, but it also relaxes the sphincter muscle that controls the passage of food from the esophagus to the stomach and may permit hydrochloric acid from the stomach to splash into the esophagus and cause heartburn.

On account of its caffeine content, coffee can tax the adrenal glands, which can lead to adrenal gland exhaustion, a condition in which the adrenal glands fail to release adrenaline. Some believe that adrenal gland exhaustion weakens the immune system and makes the body more susceptible to disease and infection. Coffee also raises blood pressure and impairs one's ability to cope with stress (probably via its effects on the adrenal glands).

Concentrated fruit juices and sports drinks are better avoided as well because they contain copious amounts of sugar. These drinks present all the problems that a diet high in sugar presents, causing a sudden surge of blood sugar that disrupts hormonal functions that can contribute to diabetes and other health problems.

By the way, almost as important as what to drink is *when* to drink. I think you should avoid drinking liquids with meals because the fluid may dilute digestive enzymes. Drink between meals instead. Avoid ice-cold beverages as well. Traditional societies simply did not drink ice-cold beverages. You don't want to drink cold beverages because the body must use enzymes to raise the temperature of ice-cold beverages before it can absorb them. Ice-cold drinks may shock the system and temporarily shut down digestion. In Asian cultures, cold drinks are almost never consumed.

Instead, think teas and vegetables juices. Teas such as maitake, ginseng, green tea, and teas made from other herbs have a wonderful tonifying and relaxing effect on the body and are much healthier than coffee, soda pop, or even fruit juices. Vegetable juices made from low-sugar vegetables such as greens, celery, or spinach mixed with super green foods such as chlorella, spirulina, and wheat grass are also good choices.

10

THE MAKER'S DIET IN YOUR DAILY LIFE

Although some people feel that we live to eat, I believe we eat to live. Believe me, when you follow the Maker's Diet, you will eat to live *and* eat well. To get us going in the right direction, you'll see that I've ranked foods Extraordinary, Average, or Trouble in descending order based on their health-giving qualities.

Obviously, listing every type of food is impossible, but you can follow this rule of thumb to determine which category a food belongs in: If foods are overly processed, nonorganic, or altered in any major way from the way they were created, you can be pretty sure that they belong in the "Average" or "Trouble" category.

The best foods to serve and eat are what I call "Extraordinary," which God created for us to eat and will give you the best chance to live a long and happy life. Foods that fall in the "Extraordinary" category are highly nutritious and life giving and have kept people healthy and disease free for thousands of years. They supply the body with the building blocks it needs to heal itself and maintain vibrant health.

In their organic form, "Extraordinary" foods contain little or no residues from pesticides, herbicides, hormones, or antibiotics. The utmost care is taken in their growth in accordance with self-sustaining agricultural practices.

I selected each food on the "Extraordinary" list according to its level of vitamins, minerals, healthy fats, enzymes, and probiotics. These foods truly exemplify the principles of the Maker's Diet. Generally speaking, the foods in this top category are well tolerated even by people with gastrointestinal diseases, food allergies, and food sensitivities and have a moderate amount of calories per serving.

That said, I believe it's best to consume foods from the "Extraordinary" category more than 75 percent of the time.

The next list comprises foods that I call "Average," which should make up no more than 25 percent of your daily diet. Many foods in the "Average" category should be avoided altogether or consumed in strict moderation while following the Maker's Diet.

The final list are foods I've relegated to the "Trouble" category, which should be consumed with extreme caution. You would be wise to avoid these foods completely.

Eating any of the "Trouble" foods will significantly increase your risk of illness or, if you've been ill, a relapse. If you do consume these foods, it is prudent to consume extra digestive enzymes and increase your consumption of probiotics for three days after the food is eaten. That's why I recommend carrying digestive enzyme supplements with you at all times. This way, when you eat at someone else's house or in a restaurant that offers only "Average" or "Trouble" foods, you can take the enzymes and hope to digest the food properly.

Eating sketchy foods is a reminder that our bodies were not designed to operate at optimum levels after consuming junk food, fast food, prepackaged food, or any of the genetically modified, antibiotic-laden, and growth hormone-laden meals that most Americans eat today.

You're going to be far better off shopping for organic foods, which give you a higher percentage of nutrients and a lower amount of residual pesticides, no antibiotics, no growth hormones, no GMOs, and an opportunity to live a much healthier life.

Disclaimers Regarding Raw Dairy, Raw Eggs, Raw Fish, and Raw Juice

The following are government-issued warnings for the consumption of raw or undercooked foods and beverages.

- Raw milk products may contain disease-causing microorganisms. Persons at highest risk for disease from these organisms include newborns and infants, the elderly, pregnant women, those taking corticosteroids, antibiotics and antacids, and those having chronic illnesses and other conditions that weaken their immunity.

- Consuming raw or undercooked eggs may increase your risk of food-borne illness.

- Consuming raw or undercooked seafood may increase your risk of food-borne illness.

- Juice that has not been pasteurized may contain bacteria that can increase the risk of food-borne illness. People most at risk are children, the elderly, and persons with a weakened immune system.

Extraordinary Foods

Meat (grass-fed organic is best)

- meat bone soup or stock
- liver and heart (must be organic)
- lamb
- buffalo
- elk
- venison
- beef
- goat
- veal
- jerky (with no chemicals, nitrates, or nitrites)
- beef or buffalo sausage (with no pork casing)
- beef or buffalo hot dogs (with no pork casing)

Fish (wild- or ocean-caught is best, and the fish must have fins and scales)

- fish soup or stock
- salmon
- halibut
- tuna
- cod
- scrod
- grouper
- haddock
- mahi-mahi
- pompano
- wahoo
- trout
- tilapia
- orange roughy
- sea bass
- snapper

- sardines (canned in water or olive oil only)
- herring
- sole
- whitefish

Poultry (pastured and organic is best)

- poultry bone soup or stock
- chicken
- Cornish game hen
- guinea fowl
- turkey
- duck
- chicken or turkey bacon (with no pork casing)
- chicken or turkey sausage (with no pork casing)
- chicken or turkey hot dogs (with no pork casing)

Lunch Meat (organic, free range, and hormone free is best)

- turkey
- chicken
- roast beef

Eggs (high omega-3/DHA or organic is best)

- chicken eggs (whole with yolk)
- duck eggs (whole with yolk)
- fish roe or caviar (must be fresh, not preserved)

Dairy (organic is best)

- homemade kefir made from raw goat's milk
- homemade kefir made from raw cow's milk
- raw goat's milk hard cheeses
- raw cow's milk hard cheeses
- goat's milk plain whole yogurt
- organic cow's milk yogurt or kefir
- raw cream

Fats and Oils (organic is best)

- oil, coconut, extra virgin (best for cooking)
- oil, olive, extra virgin (not for cooking)
- oil, butter (ghee)
- butter, goat's milk, raw (not for cooking)
- butter, goat's milk
- butter, cow's milk, raw, grass fed (not for cooking)
- butter, cow's milk
- avocado
- coconut milk/cream (canned)
- oil, unrefined flaxseed (not for cooking)
- oil, unrefined hemp seed (not for cooking)
- oil, expeller-pressed sesame
- oil, expeller-pressed peanut

Vegetables (organic fresh or frozen is best)

- raw fermented veggies (no vinegar)
- squash (winter or summer)
- broccoli
- artichokes (French, not Jerusalem)
- asparagus
- beets
- cauliflower
- Brussels sprouts
- cabbage
- carrots
- celery
- cucumbers
- eggplant
- pumpkins
- garlic
- onions
- leafy greens (kale, collard, broccoli rabe, mustard greens)
- salad greens (radicchio, escarole, endive)
- okra

- lettuce (leaves of all kinds)
- spinach
- mushrooms
- peas
- peppers
- string beans
- tomatoes
- sprouts (broccoli, sunflower, pea shoots, radish, etc.)
- sweet potatoes
- sea vegetables (kelp, dulse, nori, kombu, and hijiki)
- white potatoes
- corn

Fruits (organic fresh or frozen is best)

- blueberries
- strawberries
- blackberries
- raspberries
- lemons
- limes
- apples
- apricots
- grapes
- melons
- peaches
- oranges
- grapefruit
- pears
- plums
- kiwis
- pineapples
- bananas
- mangos
- papayas
- dried fruits (no sugar or sulfites)

- raisins
- figs
- dates
- prunes

Grains and Starchy Carbohydrates (organic is best, and whole grains and flours are best if soaked for six to twelve hours before cooking)

- sprouted Ezekiel-type bread
- sprouted Essene bread
- fermented whole grain sourdough bread
- sprouted whole grain cereal
- quinoa
- amaranth
- buckwheat
- millet

Sweeteners

- unheated raw honey
- date sugar

Beans and Legumes (best if soaked for twelve hours)

- miso
- lentils
- tempeh
- natto
- black beans
- kidney beans
- navy beans
- white beans
- pinto beans
- red beans
- split peas
- garbanzo beans
- lima beans

- broad beans
- black-eyed peas
- soybeans (edamame)

Nuts and Seeds (organic, raw, and/or soaked is best)

- almonds (raw or dry roasted)
- pumpkin seeds (raw or dry roasted)
- hemp seeds (raw)
- flaxseeds (raw and ground)
- sunflower seeds (raw or dry roasted)
- almond butter (raw or roasted)
- tahini (raw or roasted)
- pumpkin seed butter (raw or roasted)
- hemp seed butter (raw)
- sunflower butter (raw or roasted)
- walnuts (raw or dry roasted)
- macadamia nuts (raw or dry roasted)
- pecans (raw or dry roasted)
- hazelnuts (raw)
- Brazil nuts (raw)

Condiments, Spices, and Seasonings (organic is best)

- salsa (fresh or canned)
- tomato sauce (no added sugar)
- guacamole (fresh)
- soy sauce (wheat free, tamari)
- apple cider vinegar
- raw salad dressings and marinades
- herbs and spices (no added stabilizers)
- Herbamare seasoning
- Celtic Sea Salt
- Real Salt
- sea salt
- mustard
- ketchup (no sugar)

- salad dressings (no canola oil)
- marinades (no canola oil)
- omega-3 mayonnaise
- umeboshi paste
- flavoring extracts such as vanilla or almond (alcohol based, no sugar)

Snacks

- healthy food bars
- goat's milk protein powder
- flaxseed crackers
- raw food snacks
- healthy macaroons
- healthy trail mix
- organic cocoa powder
- organic chocolate spreads
- carob powder

Beverages

- purified, nonchlorinated water
- natural sparkling water, no carbonation added (i.e., Perrier)
- unsweetened or honey-sweetened herbal teas
- raw vegetable or fruit juices
- lacto-fermented beverages
- coconut water

Average Foods

Foods in the Average category are just that—average. Again, foods from this list should make up less than 25 percent of your daily diet.

Dairy (organic is best)

- goat's milk
- cheese (cow, goat, or sheep)
- cow's milk cottage cheese
- cow's milk

- plain sour cream
- cream cheese
- heavy cream
- cultured whole soy yogurt
- Amazake
- low-fat yogurt
- fat-free yogurt
- almond milk
- oat milk
- rice milk
- soy milk

Fats and Oils

- sunflower oil
- soy oil
- safflower oil

Vegetables (organic is best)

- canned vegetables

Nuts, Seeds, Beans, and Legumes (organic is best)

- tofu
- peanuts (dry roasted)
- peanut butter (roasted)
- cashews (raw or dry roasted)
- cashew butter (raw or roasted, in small quantities)
- soynut butter (in small quantities)

Condiments, Spices, and Seasonings (organic chemical and preservative free is best)

- ketchup
- mayonnaise
- salad dressing
- marinade
- pickled ginger
- wasabi

Fruits

- canned fruit in its own juices

Grains and Starchy Carbohydrates (whole grains and whole-grain flours are healthiest if soaked for twelve hours before consuming)

- brown rice
- oats
- kamut
- spelt
- barley
- corn
- white potatoes
- whole grain pasta (wheat, kamut, or spelt)
- wheat
- rye
- whole-grain dried cereal

Sweeteners

- honey
- Stevia
- organic dehydrated cane juice
- maple syrup
- agave nectar
- xylitol
- barley malt
- brown rice syrup

Beverages (organic is best)

- pasteurized vegetable juices
- pasteurized fruit juices (not from concentrate)
- fresh ground coffee (limit to one cup per day)

Snacks

- healthy popcorn
- baked corn or rice chips
- milk or whey protein powder from cow's milk
- rice protein
- soy protein (non-genetically modified)

Trouble Foods

Foods in the Trouble category should be consumed with extreme caution and should be completely avoided, if possible.

Meat

- pork
- ham
- bacon
- sausage (pork)
- rabbit
- ostrich
- emu
- imitation meat products (soy)
- veggie burgers

Fish and Seafood

- fried or breaded fish
- all shellfish, including
  - crabs
  - oysters
  - clams
  - mussels
  - lobsters
  - shrimp
  - scallops
  - catfish
  - eel
  - squid (calamari)
  - shark

Poultry

- fried or breaded chicken

Lunch Meat

- ham
- corned beef
- soy lunch meat

Eggs

- imitation eggs (i.e., Egg Beaters)

Dairy

- soy cheese
- rice cheese
- homogenized milk
- low-fat or skim milk
- commercial ice cream with sugar
- processed cheese food
- American cheese (singles)
- yogurt with sugar or artificial sweeteners
- any dairy product with added stabilizers, preservatives, sugars, or artificial sweeteners

Fats and Oils

- lard
- margarine
- shortening
- canola oil
- corn oil
- cottonseed oil
- any partially hydrogenated oil

Nuts and Seeds

- nuts roasted in oil
- honey-roasted nuts

Condiments, Spices, and Seasonings

- all spices that contain added sugar or preservatives

Fruits

- canned fruits in syrup

Beverages

- commercial beer and wine
- sodas

- chlorinated tap water
- fruit juices or drinks with artificial flavors
- fruit juices or drinks made from concentrate

Grains and Starchy Carbohydrates

- bread or crackers made with white or unbleached flour
- pastas made with white or unbleached flour
- white or unbleached flour
- dried cereal with sugar
- white rice
- instant oatmeal
- pastries
- baked goods

Sweeteners

- sugar
- corn syrup
- high-fructose corn syrup
- all artificial sweeteners, including
  - aspartame
  - sucralose
  - acesulfame K
  - sorbitol
  - maltitol

Miscellaneous

- snack foods with sugar, partially hydrogenated oils, artificial sweeteners, or unbleached flour.

A Sample Eating Plan

Many people are wondering what they should eat during the day. To give you an idea, I've prepared a three-day sample eating plan for the Maker's Diet.

Of course, please feel free to substitute foods from the Extraordinary category as you see fit.

Day 1

7 a.m.: cleansing beverage (spring water, herbal infusion, or cultured whey) or a green juice or fruit smoothie

9:30 a.m.: cleansing beverage (spring water, herbal infusion, cultured whey, or green juice)

12 p.m.: green salad with mixed greens, tomatoes, avocado, carrots, cucumbers, celery, red cabbage, red peppers, and red onions topped with three ounces of canned high omega-3 tuna, two ounces of raw cheese, and one ounce of sprouted sunflower seeds.

For the salad dressing, mix extra virgin olive oil, apple cider vinegar, and high-mineral sea salt, herbs, and spices, or you may mix one tablespoon of extra virgin olive oil with 1 tablespoon of organic store-bought dressing.

3 p.m.: cleansing beverage (spring water, herbal infusion, cultured whey, or green juice)

3:30 p.m.: organic protein bar

6 p.m.: a dinner consisting of organic meatloaf, quinoa, green beans

Dessert: fresh fruit with a cleansing beverage (spring water, herbal infusion, cultured whey, or green juice)

Day 2

7 a.m.: cleansing beverage (spring water, herbal infusion, or cultured whey) or a green juice or fruit smoothie

9:30 a.m.: cleansing beverage (spring water, herbal infusion, cultured whey, or green juice)

12 p.m.: salad with organic chicken or beef with avocado and carrot sticks

3 p.m.: cleansing beverage (spring water, herbal infusion, cultured whey, or green juice) and organic almonds, cashews, or your favorite nuts

6 p.m.: lemon garlic chicken, baked sweet potato, sautéed veggies, and green salad with mixed greens, tomatoes, avocado, carrots, cucumbers, celery, red cabbage, red peppers, red onions, and one ounce of sprouted pumpkin seeds.

For the salad dressing, mix extra virgin olive oil, apple cider vinegar, and high-mineral sea salt, herbs, and spices, or you may mix one tablespoon of extra virgin olive oil with one tablespoon of organic store-bought dressing.

Dessert: goat's milk yogurt or kefir with sprouted cereal

Day 3

7 a.m.: cleansing beverage (spring water, herbal infusion, or cultured whey) or a green juice or fruit smoothie

9:30 a.m.: cleansing beverage (spring water, herbal infusion, cultured whey, or green juice)

12 p.m.: green salad with mixed greens, tomatoes, avocado, carrots, cucumbers, celery, red cabbage, red peppers, and red onions topped with three ounces of organic steak, raw jack cheese, and one ounce of sprouted sunflower seeds.

For the salad dressing, mix extra virgin olive oil, apple cider vinegar, and high-mineral sea salt, herbs, and spices, or you may mix one tablespoon of extra virgin olive oil with one tablespoon of organic store-bought dressing.

3 p.m.: cleansing beverage (spring water, herbal infusion, cultured whey, or green juice) and organic protein bar

6 p.m.: blackened sea bass, purple potatoes browned in coconut oil, and fresh veggies

Dessert: fruit smoothie. Mix the following in a high-speed blender:

- one cup goat's milk yogurt or kefir
- one tablespoon organic raw honey
- two organic pasture-raised eggs (see disclaimer)
- one cup fresh or frozen fruit

Shopping Tips

When it comes to following the Maker's Diet, you'll want to do the bulk of your grocery shopping at natural food markets like Whole Foods, Sprouts, Wild Oats, Lazy Acres, and Trader Joe's. If you can get into the habit of shopping at local farmers' markets or, even better, local farms, then you'll really be shopping from "farm to fork."

If you've never shopped in a natural grocer or a health food store before, I wouldn't blame you if you felt totally confused upon walking in the first time. You may have no idea where to begin, or you may not know how to read the food labels. You may not even be sure that everything in the store is truly healthy for you—and you'd be right about that. Don't worry. I have some advice for you.

First, I highly suggest you ask the "associates," "team members," or "crew" for advice and assistance. They are almost always informed, friendly, and eager to help. Second, your guiding principle is to shop for fresh organic fruits, vegetables, beans, and legumes, as well as wild-caught fish, pastured poultry, and eggs.

I understand that organically raised meat and fish and organic fruit and vegetables are expensive. Do your best to stay within your budget and look for weekly specials. You'll be surprised that there are some deals out there. If you have to make compromises, I would reluctantly recommend compromising on organic fruits and vegetables before grass-fed meat and free-range poultry. In other words, it is better to spend the money on high-quality meat than on organic fruit and vegetables.

If you simply can't afford organic produce, the next best thing to organic is to apply a vegetable wash to your conventionally grown vegetables and fruits. Keep in mind that it's much better to consume conventionally grown fruits and vegetables than not to eat them, even if they are not organic. That said, many traditional grocery stores now carry certified organic produce and sometimes there are good sales, so be on the lookout.

Consuming Healthy Fruits and Vegetables

Certified organic fruits and vegetables have an incredible amount of nutrients—vitamins, minerals, live enzymes, antioxidants, and many other beneficial compounds. Depending on what season it is, there are different fruits and vegetables available, but every fruit and vegetable has something unique to offer. Let's take a closer look at some of the healthiest foods on the planet:

Berries such as strawberries, blueberries, blackberries, and raspberries are all high in antioxidants and some of the most important fruits you can consume. Antioxidants are beneficial compounds found naturally in the body and in plants such as fruits and vegetables—especially berries. Of course, buying your berries fresh is best, but frozen berries are a great source of antioxidants year-round.

Check out these amazing berry benefits:

Blueberries are prized as a high source of antioxidants with great overall health benefits.

Cranberries, usually consumed seasonally, are another great source of antioxidants. They are excellent for urinary tract health and come to a harvest peak in November—thus their association with Thanksgiving.

Raspberries contain ellagic acid, which is an antioxidant with immune-boosting properties and excellent benefits for female health. They are also high in pectin, which makes them an excellent thickener in homemade jellies and jams.

Pineapple contains bromelain, an enzyme that aids digestion of protein. Eat pineapple fresh or frozen, not canned.

If you eat dried fruits, avoid the kind with sulfite preservatives. Sulfites, or sulfur-based preservatives, are added to hundreds of foods to stop spoilage, but these can be toxic to the human body. Some studies have shown that sulfur additives may contribute to digestive upset. So choose your pineapple and all other dried fruits sulfite and preservative free.

Avocado, a much-maligned food, is a fruit, not a vegetable. Avocados contain high-quality fats as well as vitamin E and are a great source of fiber and potassium. Avocados contain monounsaturated fats, similar to those found in olive oil.

Lettuce comes in several varieties and is high in fiber. The more colorful varieties are great sources of antioxidants. Americans are used to consuming iceberg lettuce, but today there are many great mixed green blends. These mixed green blends contain organic baby lettuces, including green oak leaf, organic baby spinach, red and green chard, and arugula. They're prewashed, and they're easy for people who don't have a lot of time on their hands. These greens contain virtually every mineral and trace element and large amounts of beta-carotene, which fits into the nutritional category of carotenoids, a class of very important antioxidants that give fruit and vegetables their bright colors.

Cabbage is excellent for the digestive tract, particularly when fermented or juiced. It contains something called vitamin U, which is known as the antiulcer vitamin. Cabbage is also extremely effective as sauerkraut, making it very bioavailable.

Mushrooms are high in nutrients, particularly the mineral selenium, which works with vitamin E as an antioxidant and binds with toxins in the body, rendering them harmless. Mushrooms have over 90 percent water and are high in biotin, one of the B-complex type vitamins.

Mushrooms are one of those foods that should be eaten organically because of where they are grown. Mushrooms pick up many nutrients from the soil and the trees they grow on. If they are grown in a nonorganic environment, however, they are often high in heavy metals, so you need to be careful about eating nonorganic mushrooms. Despite what you hear, eating mushrooms does not contribute to yeast overgrowth in the body. Some people who are yeast sensitive, however, have cross-sensitivities to mushrooms and should proceed with caution.

Peppers are rich in antioxidants, which prevent oxidative damage to the body. Green peppers may be more difficult to digest than other colored peppers, so if you have complicated digestive problems, you should eat yellow, orange, or red peppers. The different colors are rich in different nutrients as well. Red peppers are substantially higher in vitamins C and A than green peppers.

Sweet potatoes are one of the highest sources of beta-carotene. Sweet potatoes also contain vitamin C, calcium, potassium, carbohydrates, and fiber.

Eggs contain all the known nutrients except for vitamin C. They are good sources of the fat-soluble vitamins A and D as well as certain carotenoids that guard against free-radical damage to the body. They also contain lutein, which has been shown to support ocular health. But please note that when it comes to healthy kinds of eggs, not just any old egg will do.

What kind of eggs should you look for in your health food store? Organic pasture-raised, high omega-3 eggs. They are nature's perfect food. When possible, try to buy eggs from farms where the chickens are allowed to roam free and eat their natural diet. Eggs produced from chickens in their natural environment contain a healthy balance of omega-3 fatty acids to omega-6 fatty acids and docosahexaenoic acid (DHA), which is good for the brain and eyes. High omega-3/DHA or organic eggs have six times the vitamin E and nine times the omega-3 fatty acids as regular store-purchased eggs.

You may have heard that you should watch how many eggs you eat because they are high in cholesterol. The myths about cholesterol are completely unfounded. Eggs are a healthy addition to anyone's diet.

Consuming Healthy Poultry and Fish

I recommend **organic, pasture-raised chicken, turkey, and duck**. When purchasing poultry, look for chicken and turkey that has been raised on a soy-free diet. Poultry is healthiest when consumed in a soup or stock. Dark meat has more nutrients than the white meat.

For seafood, eat only fish with fins and scales caught in the ocean or freshwater lakes and streams, not farm-raised fish. **Salmon, halibut, tuna, cod, sea bass, and sardines** are highly recommended, but don't eat shellfish and crustaceans because they contain abundant toxins from their water-bound scavenging habits. In fact, scientists gauge the contaminant levels of our oceans, bays, and rivers by measuring the biological toxin levels in the flesh of crabs, oysters, clams, and lobsters.

Wild salmon, with sockeye being one of the best varieties, is loaded with healthy protein, omega-3 fatty acids, vitamin D, and the antioxidant astaxanthin, which has been extensively studied and shown to benefit the entire body with its powerful antioxidant effects. Fish is also rich in vitamins A and D and provides zinc and iodine, two minerals that are found in abundance in the ocean but have been depleted from the soil.

Attention, though: Mercury is an issue in the case of deep-water fish. Wild Pacific salmon, red snapper, cod, and halibut, however, are four types of fish known to be relatively low in mercury.

Believe it or not, you can find very healthy seafood in a can. The big key is whether the can is marked "wild caught" rather than "farm raised." You want to choose the former. The good news is that when you are looking for salmon, sardines, and even herring, canned is almost always going to be wild.

High-quality sardines are one of the world's greatest foods, although many people hold their nose just thinking about them. Whole, canned sardines are an extremely rich source of omega-3 fats and contain as much calcium as a glass of milk. Make sure to obtain sardines that contain edible soft bones and organs of the fish, which make it a total package.

I also recommend wild-caught canned tuna, but it would be wise to restrict canned tuna to one or two cans a week based upon their possible contamination with heavy metals and PCBs. Research shows chunk light tuna contains less mercury than other types because the natural oils contained in fish are detoxifiers of heavy metals.

So, when consuming tuna, try to eat chunk light. You can also look for high omega-3 tuna, which is a more premium product coming from younger, fattier fish. Look for tuna canned in spring water with a high amount of fat (6 to 8 grams) per serving. Tuna higher in fats are usually lower in toxins such as heavy metals. The advantage of buying tuna in a health food store is that the product doesn't contain additives or preservatives. The fewer ingredients, the better.

Omega-3 fatty acids—the fats we lack the most in our diet—are critical in negating the effects of the overabundance of omega-6 acids and hydrogenated fats found in the standard American diet. The ratio of omega-3 fatty acids to omega-6 fatty acids can be balanced by consuming more omega-3 foods such as ocean-caught fish with fins and scales (salmon, tuna, and sardines) and eggs high in omega-3 fats.

Consuming Healthy Grains

When on the Maker's Diet eating plan, you can include grains such as **amaranth, millet, quinoa, buckwheat, and brown rice**, as well as cereal and breads made with sprouted grains. Feel free to enjoy whole organic grain products in your diet as long as they have been properly prepared through soaking, sprouting, or fermenting.

When choosing bread, look for the term *sprouted* on the label. Varieties such as Ezekiel and Essene-style breads are extremely high in fiber and can be very nutritious. You can tell a good whole-grain sourdough bread when the label lists a handful of ingredients such as whole-grain spelt, water, and sea salt and has the designation as a "whole-grain yeast-free bread." When you buy bread made from sprouted organic grains or whole-grain sourdough bread, you can be assured that you're getting the highest quality products.

White bread is totally devoid of any nutritional properties and should never be eaten—never. In fact, a diet high in white bread, white rice, and white potatoes puts women at much higher risk of pancreatic cancer, especially if they are overweight and don't get adequate exercise, according to the National Cancer Institute.

Whole-grain sourdough and sprouted breads and cereals are healthy grain foods for most people, unless you have a known intolerance to gluten. Before the advent of modern food processing technology, it was common for our ancient ancestors to soak their grains overnight and then allow them to dry in the open air until they sprouted. Many times they allowed their grains to go through an ancient leavening process that resulted in whole-grain sourdough bread.

Be aware that white rice is just like white bread, meaning that it is a high-glycemic carbohydrate that is absorbed quickly into the bloodstream and can raise insulin levels rapidly. As a result, white rice causes a spike of blood sugar and a surge of insulin. Instead, try whole-grain brown or wild rice, amaranth, millet, quinoa, buckwheat, or oats soaked overnight. Instant oatmeal is processed and refined and is much less healthy than slowly cooked whole oats. Puffed or flaked wheat, oats, and rice have been processed by high heat and pressure. They also shoot your insulin levels way up.

Some of the largest sources of mineral-depleting nutrients are contained in the sugary breakfast cereals lining the shelves of America's grocery stores. Studies show these cereals can have even more detrimental effects on blood sugar than refined sugar and white flour.

As a healthier alternative, I recommend hot cereals made from soaked or sprouted whole grains. They are not processed and do not have preservatives, artificial flavors, added colors, added synthetic vitamins, hidden sugars, or artificial sweeteners.

Consuming Healthy Oils, Spices, Condiments, and Salt

When it comes to oils, I suggest cooking and baking with saturated fats, which are stable, healthy fats. The two best fats to cook with are **extra virgin coconut oil** and **organic red palm oil**. These fats can withstand high heat without oxidizing.

Coconut oil promotes a healthy microbial balance and supports healthy digestion and immune system function. High-quality extra virgin coconut oil produced through natural fermentation should have the aroma of a fresh coconut.

Margarine is a human-made fat produced by using bleaching agents, deodorization, and high heat, destroying nearly all of its nutrients. Margarine contains harmful hydrogenated oils. These hydrogenated oils contain trans-fatty acids and are the real culprits behind many of our nation's health problems.

Olive oil is extremely healthy, but olive oil should be used only on food and never heated. Look for certified organic extra virgin olive oil in a dark bottle because light coming into clear bottles can decrease some of the important health properties of the oil as well as its freshness. Extra virgin olive oil is produced from the first cold pressing of the olives, and that's where you'll get the most antioxidants and other nutrients. Choose a colorful oil with a rich aroma. Stay away from the hydrogenated vegetable oils and polyunsaturated oils, especially when cooked, as well as soy, sunflower, canola, or safflower oils.

When choosing cooking oil, your first choice should be **extra virgin coconut oil** that's been certified organic and chemical free. Extra virgin coconut oil is a great choice for frying just about anything—from meat to veggies to leftovers.

What about extra virgin olive oil? Well, it's not as stable under heat as coconut oil, so it's best used in salad dressings. Processed oils like corn oil, canola oil, soybean oil, safflower oil, and cottonseed oil contains unstable fats that should not be used when cooking. Here's another thing about processed oils: They are subject to rancidity. Most include deodorizing chemicals that disguise their rancidity. When you heat processed oil as you fry food, you release chemicals into the air—unhealthy chemicals.

Read the labels of the food you buy because fats and oils are frequently key ingredients in packaged foods. Many contain artificially processed fats and oils that are hydrogenated and partially hydrogenated oils that contain trans-fatty acids. The processing they undergo makes them more stable, enabling them to sit on a shelf for years at a time, but this process can damage our bodies.

The best spices are organic because they don't contain caking agents and other preservatives that you may find in nonorganic spices. Flavored blends are combination seasonings with a variety of organic herbs and spices. Some other favorite seasonings include unrefined sea salt seasonings. You can use them in cooking and add them to your favorite foods.

Cultured veggies and **spicy kimchi** are condiments par excellence. Be brave and give them a try. This would also be a good time to clear your refrigerator and pantry of any commercial ketchup, mustard, mayonnaise, pickled relish, or other common condiments. Organic versions of these popular condiments are readily available these days, even in supermarkets. They come without refined sugar and unhealthy preservatives.

Regular table salt is highly refined with chemicals and high temperature processes. These processes remove many of the valuable minerals, use harmful and potentially toxic additives, and employ bleaching agents to make the salt pristine white. **Unrefined sea salt**, however, has many important minerals, and can be slightly gray or pink in color. Celtic Sea Salt and Real Salt are recommended brands.

Consuming Healthy Sweeteners

We've all seen the pink, blue, and yellow packets on restaurant tables. Stay away from those artificial sweeteners! Though the FDA has approved the use of artificial sweeteners like aspartame, saccharin, and sucralose in drinks and food, these chemical additives may prove to be detrimental to your health in the long term.

The best sweetener to use is **raw, unheated honey**, which is a rich storehouse of naturally occurring enzymes. My second favorite sweetener is evaporated coconut nectar, also known as coconut sugar. Some other acceptable sweeteners are **organic cane sugar** and **organic maple syrup**.

Consuming Healthy Nuts and Seeds

When blood sugar levels fall, many reach for a candy bar or soda for a quick "pick me up." These commercially produced snack foods are loaded with sugar, preservatives, and artificial ingredients that can rob you of your good health.

Some of the most convenient and healthiest snacks are **nuts and seeds**, which are great sources of fiber, healthy fats, and nutrients. If properly prepared, they are extremely nutritious. "Properly prepared" means raw, soaked, or sprouted. Make sure they are organic. Try **almonds, walnuts, pecans, pumpkin seeds**, and **sunflower seeds**. The most nutritious seeds are **flaxseeds** and **chia and hemp seeds**, all loaded with omega-3 fatty acids and fiber.

Raw nut butters, made from almonds, cashews, and sunflower seeds, are something worth checking out. They're better, in my opinion, because when they're raw—not roasted or heated—they're easy to digest and still have their vitamins, minerals, and enzymes. Nut butters can be used as a veggie dip or spread onto sprouted bread or fresh fruit.

It is worth noting that the phytates found on the covering of grains and seeds "grab" minerals in the intestinal tract and block their absorption. The sprouting process effectively removes these phytates from the outer covering of the natural grain. Germination initiates a chemical transformation in the seed grains that neutralizes the phytates, causing them to come alive, making all of the nutrition within the seed available for digestion.

Dining Out Tips

Eating healthy and following the Maker's Diet isn't easy when you're home, but traveling out of town will present you with a new set of difficulties. If you're shopping for food, I recommend using Google Maps and looking for natural grocers like Whole Foods and Trader Joe's, where you are more likely to find "Extraordinary" foods to purchase and eat. Finding a decent restaurant will be more problematic, however. Sure, a Google search or Yelp reviews can help, and there are restaurant chains like Native Café that serve delicious vegan food and mock-meat dishes.

But oftentimes, especially for business people on the road, they are invited to meet their clients at restaurants where "Average" and "Trouble" foods are on the menu. If you find yourself in that situation, stick with the proteins—fish, chicken, and beef. Wild-caught fish—and it should say so on the menu—is usually the best chance to get protein from the "Extraordinary" category. Be sure to ask the waiter if your entrée is cooked in butter or margarine and always ask for butter and order vegetables instead of potatoes.

If you're the one choosing the restaurant, and your budget allows for it, opt for a higher-end restaurant because it is more likely to offer healthy entrées, such as wild-caught salmon or grass-fed burgers, than a fast-food restaurant. And keep this thought in mind: The simpler the meal, the better it usually is for your health.

Here are some meal suggestions for tourists and business travelers:

Breakfast: Eggs, fruit, and lean meats such as breakfast steak are the best choices. Ask the waiter if the eggs are prepared in margarine or shortening, and if they are, avoid them. Skip the traditional toast and hash browns that are served in many roadside diners.

Lunch: Salads, lean meats, fish, and fresh fruit are available on most luncheon menus. Stay with olive oil–based dressings. That means no ranch or thousand island or similar sweet-tasting dressings. These dressings usually contain added sugar, or worse.

Dinner: Ask for seafood or a lean organically raised meat as the main course, and remember to keep it simple. Avoid rich sauces. As a side dish, get the steamed vegetables or have a salad.

Be sure to pack digestive enzyme supplements when you are on the road. No matter where your travels take you and what food you eat, digestive enzymes can help you digest the food. They make it less likely that you will suffer heartburn, diarrhea, or worse.

Here are some other tips when you eat out:

1. Opt for water as your beverage of choice, preferably spring or filtered (not chlorinated). Avoid alcohol, juice, and soda and consume only organic tea or herbal infusions.

2. Don't reach for the bread or chips at the table. This includes dinner rolls, bread sticks, sliced bread, muffins, and tortilla chips.

3. Avoid appetizers as much as possible. Eat your salad before eating your entrée.

4. When ordering soup, make sure no sugar is added. Avoid the use of toppings such as crackers, croutons, bacon, cream cheese, or cheese.

5. Choose the house salad over the Caesar salad or other salads with numerous ingredients and toppings. The plainer the salad, the better.

6. Make sure the salad dressing is really simple: balsamic vinegar and extra virgin olive oil. Other dressings are full of hydrogenated oils and sugars. It is safer to just order the balsamic vinaigrette as the waiter may not know exactly what is in the other dressings. Also, avoid the croutons.

7. Ask your server how the food is prepared. To avoid some hidden traps in your meal, inquire about the butter, margarine, cream, or oil that may be used in preparing that item. Have your meal cooked in olive oil or butter. Look for the words *grilled, poached, baked, roasted,* or *broiled* on the menu.

8. Request that your food be prepared without monosodium glutamate (MSG) or sugar.

9. Avoid entrées with a lot of ingredients. Avoid foods that have the following descriptions: fried, buttery, creamy, rich, au gratin, scalloped, béarnaise, Newburg, BBQ, sweet and sour, teriyaki, or breaded.

10. For your main entrée, use the following pecking order when choosing a protein:
    - wild fish
    - wild game (venison or bison)

- lamb (most lamb is raised well in Australia or New Zealand and fairly well in the States)
- beef (best if organic or pasture raised)
- farm-raised fish (not the healthiest food by any stretch, but still an okay option for dining out)
- chicken (by far the worst of the biblically clean, conventionally raised animals due to the way factory-farmed poultry is treated and processed)

11. Don't be afraid to make special requests. Most restaurants are willing to accommodate your dietary needs when possible. Order steamed vegetables instead of mashed potatoes, French fries, or coleslaw.

12. There is no need to dress your food up with salt. Most foods already have salt added to them while being cooked.

13. If you order eggs as your main dish, mix it up by requesting diced tomatoes, peppers, and onions—but no ham, please.

14. If you are eating a light dinner, try a salad with grilled wild fish, topped with olive oil and balsamic vinegar for the dressing.

Foods Essential for Healing

The last part of this chapter concerns foods that are essential to healing and good health. You are encouraged to fall in love with these foods. They can be your best friends. These foods are nutritious and soothing to the gastrointestinal tract which, after all, is the center of your health universe. They have been eaten since primitive times for their nutritional qualities, not to mention their good flavor.

Cultured Goat's Milk Products

Goat's milk yogurt that has been fermented for thirty hours is a rich source of probiotics, enzymes, and short-chain fatty acids. This type of yogurt is virtually free of lactose, which means that people who are lactose-intolerant can consume it. It is a rich source of selenium. It does not contain *Streptococcus thermophilus*, the bacterial strain that has been known to exacerbate certain autoimmune disorders, or MAP, the microorganism that some believe may be involved in the development of Crohn's disease.

Not only does goat's milk yogurt have no negative effects, but it's beneficial for a healthy immune system. Everybody who can obtain this excellent healing food should take full advantage of it. I have consumed cultured goat's milk products for more than twenty years, and I believe it was one of the secrets that helped me overcome my own illness.

High Omega-3 Eggs

Eggs from chickens, turkeys, and ducks who are truly free to roam and eat a diet high in insects and worms, as well as eggs from chickens fed certain strains of algae, contain large amounts of important omega-3 fatty acids.

Eggs from these birds usually contain a ratio of omega-3 to omega-6 fatty acids between 1:1 and 1:4, whereas eggs from battery-raised hens have a ratio of omega-3 to omega-6 fatty acids of 1:20.

Studies show that omega-3 fatty acids are helpful against high blood pressure, heart disease, blood clotting, diabetes, colitis, and inflammatory diseases. So-called battery-raised hens are kept in coops where a light is always burning. This confuses the hens into thinking it is daytime, which makes them lay more eggs.

In addition to containing DHA, omega-3 eggs contain significant amounts of vitamin E and B_{12} as well as the antioxidants lutein and beta-carotene. By eating two high omega-3 eggs, you can get as much as 150 milligrams of DHA. Eggs are healthiest when they are poached, soft boiled, or consumed raw in smoothies. Frying and scrambling eggs can damage some of the nutrients contained in the yolk. Omega-3 eggs make a wonderful addition to any diet.

Extra Virgin Coconut Oil

I want to say a few things more about extra virgin coconut oil, which is an extremely healthy fat. This oil contains large amounts of lauric acid, one of the chief fatty acids in breast milk. According to scientific and clinical research, consuming extra virgin coconut oil can reduce the risk of deadly degenerative diseases such as cancer, heart disease, and diabetes. Extra virgin coconut oil supports the immune system and helps prevent bacterial, viral, and fungal infections.

Reportedly, coconut oil can reduce the symptoms of Crohn's disease, ulcerative colitis, diverticulosis, IBS, and constipation. Extra virgin coconut oil is one of the best oils to cook with because it can withstand heat without oxidation. People who suffer from digestive disorders often notice an improvement in symptoms after they substitute extra virgin coconut oil for whatever cooking oil they use.

Grass-Fed Red Meat

Grass-fed red meat, including beef, venison, buffalo, and lamb, is an excellent source of high-quality protein and B vitamins like B_3, B_6, and B_{12}. Grass-fed red meat provides protective nutrients such as CLA (conjugated linoleic acid) and carnitine and creatine. Grass-fed meat also has a much higher omega-3 fatty acid content than grain-fed meat.

Unheated Honey

Raw, unheated honey is Nature's only predigested food. Unheated honey supplies a rich array of nutrients, including amino acids and enzymes. The body uses pure honey for quick energy. Consumed in small amounts, honey does not contribute to blood sugar imbalances. Raw, unheated honey is the only sweetener we recommend. Nevertheless, you should consume it in moderation.

Fatty Fish

High-fat ocean fish such as salmon, sardines, mackerel, herring, and tuna are Nature's richest source of the omega-3 fatty acids eicosapentaenoic acid (EPA) and DHA. Dr. Weston Price found that cultures that relied on fish as their main source of protein were the healthiest among all the indigenous groups he studied.

Fish provides easily absorbable protein and minerals and is great for the heart. Eating fresh fish is best, but canned sardines and herring (with skin and bones) may be the exception to the rule. Canned sardines contain healthy levels of omega-3 fatty acids, are high in calcium, and are one of Nature's richest sources of nucleic acids.

Grass-Fed Organ Meats

Almost all of the ancient cultures that Dr. Weston Price studied prized organ meats for their ability to build strength and vitality. Organ meats are a rich source of fat-soluble vitamin A and D. They contain a great balance of B vitamins and are one of the best sources of minerals, including zinc. It is important to note that organ meats must come from organic or free-range animals. Toxins tend to concentrate in the organs of animals that are given growth hormones and pesticides. For that reason, eating organ meats from animals that were not properly raised can be harmful.

Cod Liver Oil

For those who can't stomach organ meats, and even those who can, cod liver oil is the next best thing. Cod liver oil contains large amounts of fat-soluble vitamin A and D, as well as the essential fatty acids EPA and DHA.

EPA and DHA are long-chain polyunsaturated fats known as omega-3 fatty acids, which are found in cold-water fish and eggs from chickens that run around and eat worms. But EPA and DHA are best found in cold-water fish, especially the golden oils extracted from the filleted livers of Icelandic cod.

This rich source of valuable nutrients began showing up in the fishing communities of Norway, Scotland, and Iceland in the middle of the 19th century as people discovered the health benefits of cod liver oil. They endured harsh winters with long periods of darkness in some of the most remote places in the world, so whenever someone came off the fishing boats sneezing up a storm from a winter cold, they couldn't run down to local pharmacy for a cold-and-flu medication.

Instead, they turned to cod liver oil because they had learned over the years that its medicinal properties were a natural, effective remedy to many of the infections that ailed them. Cod liver oil became popular in this country at the turn of the century, and I'm sure your parents or grandparents haven't forgotten the time when they held their noses while their parents administered a teaspoon of the fishy-smelling liquid. For a long time, however, cod liver oil had a reputation as a vile substance.

When improvements in the extraction and preparation in cod liver oil occurred, progress was made in how it smelled and tasted. These days, cod liver oil comes in lemon mint and other flavors that mask the "fishy" odor and taste. I'll admit that cod liver oil is an acquired taste, but after a week or two, you'll get used to swallowing a spoonful.

I added cod liver oil to my daily diet more than twenty years ago during my recovery from illness, and now I'm to the point where I can drink the stuff right out of the bottle. I recommend that you consume between one teaspoon and one tablespoon of this enduring, time-proven nutritional gem each day. Cod liver oil helps prevent bone deterioration in adults, improves cardiovascular function, and contributes to long life. Life insurance data and genetic research have shown that Iceland is now ahead of Japan for longevity, and the Icelandic people are medical marvels, displaying less heart disease and high blood pressure than most other cultures in the world.

As you can tell, I'm bullish on cod liver oil, and I could go on and on about the enduring, time-proven value of adding this inexpensive supplement to your diet. Sure, cod liver oil may be as old as the hills and not real fancy, but study after study shows that people who use cod liver oil are less likely to develop multiple sclerosis, arthritis, or coronary heart disease. That's why cod liver oil is one of the best-selling supplements in Europe, and it should be the same on this side of the Atlantic Ocean as well.

Organic Berries

Berries are some of Nature's richest sources of antioxidants. Organic blueberries, strawberries, raspberries, and blackberries contain powerful disease-fighting phytochemicals such as ellagic acid, quercetin, vitamin C, and anthocyanins. Berries are also high in fiber. A great way to enjoy the antioxidant power of berries is to incorporate them into smoothies, or top them with yogurt.

There is a test conducted at Tufts University called ORAC—short for Oxygen Radical Absorbance Capacity—that measures the ability of foods, blood plasma, and just about any substance to subdue oxygen-free radicals in the test tube. Studies at the Jean Mayer USDA Human Nutrition Research Center on Aging at Tufts University in Boston suggest that consuming fruits and vegetables with a high-ORAC value may help slow the aging process in both body and brain.

Consuming foods with a high-ORAC score are a great way to eat healthy. Here are the ORAC scores as ranked by USDA scientists at Tufts University:

- dried plums (5770)
- raisins (2830)
- blueberries (2700)
- blackberries (2036)
- strawberries (1546)
- raspberries (1220)
- plums (949)
- oranges (750)
- pink grapefruit (483)
- cantaloupe (252)
- apples (218)
- pears (134)

Cultured Vegetables

Raw, cultured vegetables are a great source of naturally occurring probiotics and enzymes. Cultured vegetables can aid in the digestion of meals that contain cooked animal protein. The daily consumption of raw, cultured vegetables, including sauerkraut, kimchi, or fermented beets, carrots, and ginger, can help keep the digestive tract healthy and even eliminate harmful microorganisms such as *C. albicansi.*

Vegetable Juice

Vegetable juice, especially green juices, is a potent source of enzymes, vitamins, and trace minerals. The body finds vegetable juices easy to assimilate. They supply many of the nutrients that are needed to rebuild health.

Cereal Grass Juice

Cereal grass juices from the young leaves of wheat, oat, and barley are nutrient powerhouses. Wheatgrass juice has been consumed around the world and taken as a primary therapy for digestive disorders such as IBS, ulcers, and inflammatory bowel disease for nearly a century.

Wheatgrass contains minerals, lightweight vegetable proteins, and chlorophyll and is Nature's richest source of trace minerals.

Stocks

Properly prepared soup stocks from meat, fish, and poultry contain many life-giving nutrients, including minerals, gelatin, and electrolytes from vegetables. Many people are unaware of the research that has been done on the naturally occurring gelatin found in stocks. Gelatin acts as a digestive aid and has been used successfully in the treatment of many intestinal disorders, including non-ulcerative dyspepsia (sour stomach), IBS, ulcers, and Crohn's disease.

Stocks also contain cartilage and collagen, both of which have been used to aid in the health of those suffering from arthritis and other inflammatory conditions. Consumption of stocks in chicken soup can help heal the digestive lining and reduce the inflammation that occurs in many severe digestive disorders.

Fiber

The consumption of dietary fiber from sources such as properly prepared seeds, legumes, and grains is extremely important. I mentioned Dr. Denis Burkitt, a missionary surgeon to Africa following World War II. He was the first individual to bring the importance of consuming adequate dietary fiber to the forefront. Like Dr. Weston A. Price, Dr. Burkitt traveled around the world and discovered that natives who consumed high amounts of fiber between 35 to 75 grams per day were free from many of today's common ailments including constipation, hemorrhoids, IBS, heart disease, inflammation, and more.

Fermented Beverages

Few people have heard of fermented beverages such as kefir, grape cooler, natural ginger ale, as well as kombucha and kvass, but they are worth checking out in well-stocked health food stores. They can even be made at home. These beverages contain lactic acid and supply beneficial probiotics, enzymes, and minerals to the digestive system. Fermented beverages relieve constipation problems, cleanse the colon and gall bladder, aid in the relief of arthritis, and promote overall well-being.

Kombucha (pronounced kom-BOO-cha) has become quite popular in the last decade. This fermented beverage made from black or green tea and a fungus culture may sound awful, but I've been known to drink several of these exotic beverages a week. Some people say kombucha is too tart and fizzy, but I don't think kombucha tastes that bad. While kombucha has a cidery flavor and a definite fizziness, I like the way the beverage boosts my energy and lightens my mood.

Kombucha is not a drink you guzzle down like a cold bottle of water after playing two sets of tennis. You probably don't want to drink more than four ounces at a time.

PART III

HEALTH AND HEALING

11

THE HEALING PROTOCOLS

This chapter presents protocols, or plans of treatment, for many of the common diseases, disorders, and health conditions that we face today. Keep in mind that taking care of your gastrointestinal health is key to getting your health back on track.

Over the years, I've heard from and met many people who told me that following these healing protocols dramatically enhanced their absorption and assimilation of foods and nutrients. They also improved their elimination of toxins, experienced greater clarity of mind, felt more vitality, and saw improvements in their immune function. In short, they dramatically improved their overall health.

Many were able to overcome long-standing symptoms and remain free of disease by following these healing protocols. They were able to reduce or discontinue medications (after being in consultation with their physician, of course).

On the following pages, you will find under each disease description specific instructions and practical techniques to help you resolve the condition and alleviate the symptoms that are associated with it. As part of each protocol, you will find recommendations for:

- **Diet.** These foods will promote optimal health and initiate your body's healing response.
- **Therapeutic foods.** These are specific foods that should be consumed as often as possible and can positively contribute to the health of the immune system and digestive tract.

- **Supplements.** The health supplements I describe should help to alleviate symptoms and improve your overall health, as well as support various health issues.

The focus of this protocol section is to help you to enjoy super health and even regain your fitness if you have lost it. I believe that the health of the gastrointestinal tract and immune system, both interlinked themselves, are fundamental to your overall well-being. If you follow these protocols diligently, you should see improvement in the first month—perhaps even in the first few days if not hours. Your body is a wonderfully sensitive machine, and it will respond to beneficial changes in your dietary and lifestyle habits almost immediately.

What's more, you might experience other health benefits. You will have more energy, attain and maintain proper weight for your body type, experience increased lean muscle mass, and improve skin tone. Your memory and ability to concentrate will improve.

If you are suffering from a severe illness, however, you may not notice any significant improvement for as long as ninety days. If after that period you see little or no results and you can honestly say that you followed the Maker's Diet protocol diligently, this program may not be right for you. I would advise that you seek help elsewhere.

Lifestyle Therapies

Throughout this chapter, I outline therapeutic foods you can eat to improve your health. I understand that this may be a new way of eating for you, but don't forget that changing your lifestyle is an important part of an optimal health program. With that thought in mind, let me recommend the following lifestyle therapies that you should adopt.

- **Squatting for elimination:** Squatting aligns the colon properly for elimination and empties the colon more completely. Using an elimination bench to raise the legs during elimination can help to fully detoxify the colon. This is essential for those suffering from digestive problems including IBS, constipation, and hemorrhoids.
- **Exercise:** As well as toning and strengthening muscles, exercising encourages peristalsis, the wavelike expanding and contracting of

the digestive system that eliminates waste. Exercise also enhances the health of the lymphatic system, which is important for proper detoxification and immune system function. If your condition allows it, I recommend performing some form of moderate exercise daily, be that something as simple as walking briskly. In fact, for some conditions, such as weight problems, exercise has been shown to markedly synergize the benefits of your nutritional supplements.

- **Avoiding hormonal contraceptives (females):** Evidence shows that hormonal contraceptives, whether taken orally, implanted, or administered by injection, can lead to imbalanced intestinal flora and contribute to yeast overgrowth (candidiasis), as well as increase the risk for developing ulcerative colitis and breast and liver cancer.

- **Sunlight:** Most of the vitamin D you obtain comes from sunlight, so spend approximately twenty minutes each day in the sun. Many people with chronic diseases including digestive disorders have less than optimal levels of vitamin D. Getting proper levels of vitamin D is crucial for proper calcium absorption and utilization.

- **Breathing properly:** Performing five to fifteen minutes of deep breathing exercises can be very beneficial. Inhale through your nose for three to seven seconds and exhale quickly through your mouth. Deep breathing can enhance oxygen utilization and improve the functioning of the immune system.

- **Sauna/steam detoxification:** Spend at least twenty to thirty minutes daily in a sauna or steam bath, especially during periods of detoxification. Be sure to drink plenty of water and stay hydrated. I recommend low-heat saunas with temperatures ranging from 120 to 140 degrees Fahrenheit. Raising the temperature of your body helps it to detoxify and expel foreign substances such as bacteria and viruses, as well as heavy metals, pesticides, and industrial chemicals.

- **Detoxification baths:** Take baths with essential oils, clays, and other healing compounds. Doing so aids the body's ability to detoxify harmful chemicals. To make a clay bath, fill the tub with hot water (as hot as you can tolerate) and add one-half to one cup of powdered clay (available in the cosmetic section of most health food stores). Stay in the bath for five to thirty minutes. These baths may cause a temporary feeling of weakness and other detoxification symptoms, so you may have to stay in the bath for short periods of time at first. After the bath, consume 16 ounces of structured water, vegetable juice, or water.

- **Skin brushing:** Skin brushing removes dead skin, improves circulation, and aids in the detoxification of harmful chemicals.
- **Sleep:** Getting enough sleep is essential, especially if you have a digestive disorder. Nighttime is when the body detoxifies and regenerates. When you sleep matters as much as how much sleep you get. Try to get at least one to three hours of sleep before midnight. Groundbreaking research on health and regeneration has shown that sleep before midnight is much more beneficial than sleep after midnight.

    It's important to note that in biblical times and throughout ancient history, people would rise and retire with the rising and setting of the sun. I believe this to be the healthiest way for us to function today, resulting in improved digestion, immune system health, and mood. It's my experience that the amount and quality of your sleep, as well as the times you retire and rise, are as important to your health as diet, supplements, and exercise.

- **Chewing properly:** Chew each bite of food thirty to fifty times to ensure proper digestion and absorption. Eating slowly and chewing properly greatly decreases indigestion.
- **Eating smaller meals:** Eat small meals instead of overstuffing yourself. Many foods recommended in this program greatly enhance metabolism. When large portions are consumed, however, metabolism slows down, digestion is stressed, and feelings of weakness and lethargy ensue.
- **Avoid ice-cold foods and beverages:** Ice-cold foods and beverages may shock the digestive tract and shut down digestive function. The body must work hard to raise the temperature of the food or beverage to body temperature. People in Eastern cultures never consume ice-cold foods because they "weaken digestive fire." Even foods from the refrigerator can be left at room temperature for

ten minutes or so to help dispel the cold. Our ancestors rarely consumed cold food because refrigeration has only existed for the past hundred years or so.

∽

Important Notice

This book is not intended to provide medical advice or to take the place of medical advice and treatment from your personal physician. Readers are advised to consult their own doctors or other qualified health professionals regarding treatment of their medical problems. Neither the publisher nor the author takes any responsibility for any possible consequences from any treatment, action, or application of medicine, supplement, herb, or preparation to any person reading or following the information in this book. If readers are taking prescription medications, they should consult with their physicians before beginning any nutrition or supplementation program.

∽

THE A-Z GUIDE TO CONDITIONS

Acne…see Skin Health
Addiction…see Mental Disorders
Alzheimer's Disease…see Brain Health
Agoraphobia…see Mental Disorders
Angina…see Cardiovascular Health
Ankylosing Spondylitis…see Joint Disorders
Anxiety…see Mental Disorders
Asthma…see Upper Respiratory Health
Atherosclerosis/Arteriosclerosis…see Cardiovascular Health
Atopic Dermatitis (eczema)…see Skin Health
Attention Deficit Hyperactivity Disorder…see Children's Health
Autism…see Children's Health

Autoimmune Disease

- Type 1 Diabetes
- Myasthenia Gravis
- Grave's Disease
- Rheumatoid Arthritis
- Lupus
- Scleroderma
- Multiple Sclerosis

Overview

The word *auto* is the Greek word for self. The immune system is a complicated network of cells and cell components (called molecules) that normally work to defend the body and eliminate infections caused by bacteria, viruses, and other invading microbes.

When a person has an autoimmune disease, the immune system mistakenly attacks self, targeting the cells, tissues, and organs of a person's own body. A collection of immune system cells and molecules at a target site is broadly referred to as inflammation.

There are many different autoimmune diseases, and they can each affect the body in different ways. For example:

- In multiple sclerosis, the autoimmune reaction is directed against the myelin sheath of the nervous system.
- The joints are targeted in rheumatoid arthritis.
- The skin and internal organs are targeted in scleroderma.

In other autoimmune diseases such as systemic lupus erythematosus (lupus), affected tissues and organs may vary among individuals with the same disease. One person with lupus may have affected skin and joints whereas another may have affected skin, kidneys, and lungs. Ultimately, damage to certain tissues by the immune system may be permanent because of the destruction of insulin-producing cells inside the pancreas. That is what's known as type 1 diabetes mellitus.

Many of the autoimmune diseases, such as *Myasthenia gravis* (a chronic autoimmune neuromuscular disease characterized by varying degrees of weakness of the voluntary muscles of the body) are rare. As a group, however, autoimmune diseases afflict millions of Americans. Most autoimmune diseases strike women more often than men; in particular, they affect women of working age and during their childbearing years.

Some autoimmune diseases occur more frequently in certain minority populations. For example, lupus is more common in African-American and Hispanic women than in Caucasian women of European ancestry. Rheumatoid arthritis and scleroderma affect a higher percentage of residents in some Native American communities than in the general U.S. population. Multiple sclerosis seems to be more prevalent in the northern latitudes.

Diet

Follow the Maker's Diet as best you can for six to twelve months. If symptoms are completely gone for at least three months, you may gradually add foods from the "Average" or "Trouble" categories, if you desire. Because people with autoimmune diseases appear to have a predisposed weakness in their immune systems, however, I strongly recommend that they adhere to a diet of foods in the "Extraordinary" category for the rest of their lives.

Therapeutic Foods

These therapeutic foods will help you get well:

Cultured goat's milk dairy products: Consume 8 to 32 ounces of the highest quality cultured dairy products from goat's milk. Try to find yogurt that does not contain the organism *Streptococcus thermophilus*, a bacterial microbe that has been known to make immune system disorders worse.

Grass-fed red meat: Red meat from grass-fed cattle, buffalo, and lamb is very healthy and can be eaten a few times per week. This meat is a great source of protein, minerals, vitamin B_{12}, vitamins A and D, omega-3 fats, and CLA.

Organic, pasture-raised eggs: Consume as many as one to three organic eggs high in omega-3 fatty acids each day. These eggs contain DHA, vitamins E and B_{12}, and antioxidants including lutein.

Extra virgin coconut oil: This oil is perhaps the healthiest of the widely available oils. I recommend cooking almost exclusively with extra virgin coconut oil. Consume as much as two to four tablespoons per day of the oil in cooking, smoothies, or right off the spoon. Coconut oil contains large amounts of lauric acid, a potent antimicrobial and one of the chief fatty acids found in breast milk.

Ocean-caught fish: This type of fish is perhaps the healthiest of all protein sources. Salmon, sardines, mackerel, herring, and albacore tuna are high in the omega-3 fatty acids EPA and DHA. Ocean-caught fish can be consumed every day to enhance digestive and immune system health.

Cod liver oil: Take one to three teaspoons of an excellent cod liver oil each day, or caplets. The amount consumed should be based upon the amount of sunlight you receive. People in colder climates generally need to consume larger amounts. Cod liver oil is a fantastic source of the omega-3 fats DHA and EPA, as well as fat-soluble vitamins A and D.

Vegetable juice: Consume vegetable juices that are low in carbohydrates, such as celery and green juices mixed with a small amount of higher carbohydrate veggies such as carrot or beet. Mix in some form of healthy fat with each glass of the juice. One to three teaspoons of cultured goat's milk, extra virgin coconut oil, canned or fresh coconut milk and cream, or flaxseed oil enhance absorption of minerals and prevents spikes in blood sugar.

Fermented vegetables: Consume a few tablespoons of fermented vegetables such as sauerkraut with each meal to aid in digestion. Fermented vegetables are an excellent source of naturally occurring probiotics and enzymes.

Stocks: It is a great idea to consume stocks on a regular basis, especially when you have a cold or flu. Stocks made from the bones of chicken, fish, lamb, and beef contain minerals, gelatin, cartilage, collagen, and electrolytes from the vegetables. Stocks are an excellent source of proteins, especially collagen. They help to heal the gut lining and reduce inflammation.

Supplements

Consume the following dietary supplements, along with the recommended foods and beverages, to help overcome this condition:

A probiotic, enzyme, and herbs formulation designed to fight autoimmune disease.

A probiotic with SBOs. Take six to twelve capsules per day and stay on that amount for three to six months or when tests for your affliction are negative. Then begin to gradually decrease to a maintenance dosage of between three to six capsules per day. Probiotics with SBOs are best taken first thing in the morning and right before bedtime with eight ounces pure water. Probiotics with SBOs may be taken with other nutritional supplements, but should be taken one hour apart from medications. If you experience symptoms of detoxification (i.e., increased elimination, loose stools, constipation, excess gas, flu-like symptoms, or fever), reduce the dosage and work up slowly to twelve per day.

A green superfood powder. Take two tablespoons twice daily with eight ounces water or fresh vegetable juice. Best taken on an empty stomach away from food.

Digestive enzymes. Take one to three capsules with each meal or snack.

An organic fiber supplement with chia seed. Consume one serving twice per day, morning and evening, with eight or more ounces of purified water. (Consuming a fiber supplement is essential during the first two weeks of the program. Thereafter, consume fiber as needed.)

A protein powder from bone broth. Take one to three servings per day mixed in water, juice, smoothies, yogurt, or can be used in many recipes.

Additional Therapies

For people who have or may have imbalanced immune systems, avoiding contact with chlorinated water is of the utmost importance. That includes bathing water and drinking water. Chlorine kills bacteria, friendly and unfriendly, in the intestines and can be absorbed through the skin. I recommend installing a shower filter to remove chlorine. Avoid swimming in chlorinated water as well.

Benign Prostatic Hypertrophy…see Male Health

Blood Pressure (elevated)…see Cardiovascular Health

Blood Sugar Imbalances

- Type 2 Diabetes
- Syndrome X
- Hypoglycemia

Overview

There are two tragedies associated with adult-onset diabetes today. The first is that by the time patients have been diagnosed with this condition, they've likely had diabetes for several years or longer. Extensive damage to the nervous and circulatory systems and even their vision may have already occurred.

Currently, 9 percent of our population presently has diabetes. That's 30.3 million Americans, according to the American Diabetes Association. Many experts believe that percentage will increase even more as aging Baby Boomers enter their sixties and seventies. Seniors are most at risk because one-fourth of all Americans sixty-five years or older are either diagnosed or undiagnosed with diabetes.

With more than 1.5 million Americans being diagnosed with diabetes each year, this is not good news because diabetes remains the seventh leading cause of death in the United States.

Just as disconcerting are the statistics that up to a quarter of the adult population will experience a related condition called Syndrome X. This sinister-sounding term stands for a cluster of conditions that, when occurring together, indicate a predisposition to diabetes, hypertension, heart disease, and other common deadly diseases.

Syndrome X, also known as metabolic syndrome, was first coined by a group of researchers at Stanford University to describe a cluster of disease-causing symptoms that include high blood pressure, high triglycerides, decreased high-density lipoprotein (HDL, the "good" cholesterol), insulin resistance, and obesity. These indicators of poor health tend to appear together in some individuals and increase their risk for diabetes, heart disease, and possibly cancer as well as many other diseases.

Be aware that type 2 diabetes and Syndrome X have much in common. Both are complex conditions where insulin deficiency is not the problem.

Rather, the problem is the body's *resistance* to insulin. In other words, the body may be producing plenty of insulin, but the hormone isn't being metabolized for optimal use. This condition, known as peripheral insulin resistance, is difficult to treat, even with our best medical drugs.

Clearly, the underlying theme of effective diabetes treatment is that for most adult cases of diabetes, front-line therapy should consist of improved diet with a reduction in carbohydrates and an increase in healthy fats, followed up with exercise.

Diet

Follow the Maker's Diet as best you can for six to twelve months. People with blood sugar imbalances (either diabetes or hypoglycemia) should do very well following the Maker's Diet. One should choose more high protein and low carbohydrate foods until blood sugar levels are under control.

The consumption of healthy fats and proteins along with low glycemic carbohydrates should lead to tremendous improvements in health and far better insulin sensitivity. I recommend that people with a propensity to blood sugar imbalances choose most of their foods from the "Extraordinary" category. After symptoms are completely gone for at least three months, you may gradually add foods from the "Average" or "Trouble" categories, if you desire.

Therapeutic Foods

These therapeutic foods will help you get well:

Cultured goat's milk dairy products: Consume 8 to 32 ounces of the highest quality cultured dairy products from goat's milk. Try to find yogurt that does not contain the organism *Streptococcus thermophilus*, a bacterial microbe that has been known to make immune system disorders worse.

Grass-fed red meat: Red meat from grass-fed cattle, buffalo, and lamb is very healthy and can be eaten a few times per week. This meat is a great source of protein, minerals, vitamin B_{12}, vitamins A and D, omega-3 fats, and CLA.

Organic, pasture-raised eggs: Consume as many as one to three organic eggs high in omega-3 fatty acids each day. These eggs contain DHA, vitamins E and B_{12}, and antioxidants including lutein.

Extra virgin coconut oil: This oil is perhaps the healthiest of the widely available oils. I recommend cooking almost exclusively with extra virgin coconut oil. Consume as much as two to four tablespoons per day of the oil in cooking, smoothies, or right off the spoon. Coconut oil contains large amounts of lauric acid, a potent antimicrobial and one of the chief fatty acids found in breast milk.

Ocean-caught fish: This type of fish is perhaps the healthiest of all protein sources. Salmon, sardines, mackerel, herring, and albacore tuna are high in the omega-3 fatty acids EPA and DHA. Ocean-caught fish can be consumed every day to enhance digestive and immune system health.

Cod liver oil: Take one to three teaspoons of an excellent cod liver oil each day, or caplets. The amount consumed should be based upon the amount of sunlight you receive. People in colder climates generally need to consume larger amounts. Cod liver oil is a fantastic source of the omega-3 fats DHA and EPA, as well as fat-soluble vitamins A and D.

Vegetable juice: Consume vegetable juices that are low in carbohydrates, such as celery and green juices mixed with a small amount of higher carbohydrate veggies such as carrots or beets. Mix in some form of healthy fat with each glass of the juice. One to three teaspoons of cultured goat's milk, extra virgin coconut oil, canned or fresh coconut milk and cream, or flaxseed oil enhance absorption of minerals and prevents spikes in blood sugar.

Fermented vegetables: Consume a few tablespoons of fermented vegetables such as sauerkraut with each meal to aid in digestion. Fermented vegetables are an excellent source of naturally occurring probiotics and enzymes.

Stocks: It is a great idea to consume stocks on a regular basis, especially when you have a cold or flu. Stocks made from the bones of chicken, fish, lamb, and beef contain minerals, gelatin, cartilage, collagen, and electrolytes from the vegetables. Stocks are an excellent source of proteins, especially collagen. They help to heal the gut lining and reduce inflammation.

Supplements

Consume the following dietary supplements, along with the recommended foods and beverages, to help overcome this condition:

A probiotic, enzyme, and herbs formulation designed to fight blood sugar imbalances.

A probiotic with SBOs. Take six to twelve capsules per day and stay on that amount for three to six months or when tests for your affliction are negative. Then begin to gradually decrease to a maintenance dosage of between three to six capsules per day. Probiotics with SBOs are best taken first thing in the morning and right before bedtime with eight ounces pure water. Probiotics with SBOs may be taken with other nutritional supplements, but should be taken one hour apart from medications. If you experience symptoms of detoxification (i.e., increased elimination, loose stools, constipation, excess gas, flu-like symptoms, or fever), reduce the dosage and work up slowly to twelve per day.

A green superfood powder. Take two tablespoons twice daily with eight ounces water or fresh vegetable juice. Best taken on an empty stomach away from food.

Digestive enzymes. Take one to three capsules with each meal or snack.

An organic fiber supplement with chia seed. Consume one serving twice per day, morning and evening, with eight or more ounces of purified water. (Consuming a fiber supplement is essential during the first two weeks of the program. Thereafter, consume fiber as needed.)

A protein powder from bone broth. Take one to three servings per day mixed in water, juice, smoothies, yogurt, or can be used in many recipes.

Additional Therapies

For people who have or may have imbalanced intestinal flora or a weakened immune system, avoiding contact with chlorinated water is of the utmost importance. That includes bathing water and drinking water. Chlorine kills bacteria, friendly and unfriendly, in the intestines and can be absorbed through the skin. I recommend installing a shower filter to remove chlorine. Avoid swimming in chlorinated water as well.

Brain Health

- Alzheimer's Disease
- Memory Loss
- Dementia
- Parkinson's Disease

Overview

The ability to think creatively, react quickly to new intellectual challenges and circumstances, remember phone numbers, addresses, even where we parked our car are just some of the valuable functions of a brain operating at peak efficiency. In a very real sense, our intelligence is perhaps our greatest gift.

Yet the cells of the brain are under siege daily from both the inexorable and natural processes of aging, including exposure to cell-damaging free radicals, an age-related decrease in activity of important neuro-transmitters, and exposure to toxic chemicals found in a wide range of consumer products, especially petroleum-based household cleaners, paints, and home and garden pesticides.

It's not surprising that experts have found the brain measurably loses function starting as early as age forty-five. Many otherwise healthy adults will lose a full 50 percent of their brain function related to memory, learning, and concentration over the course of their lives. While the decline of memory function is a normal process of aging, it may be a result of a pathological condition like Alzheimer's disease.

A decline in mental function can have a significant impact on both our physical and emotional health. Psychologist John Barefoot, of Duke University Medical Center, reports that in a study that began in 1964 and followed people for several decades, people with the highest scores for despair, poor self-esteem, difficulty concentrating, and low motivation had a 70 percent higher risk of heart attack and 60 percent higher risk of overall death compared to men and women with the lowest scores.

"We are living in a graying world," noted Ursula Lehr, Ph.D., of the University of Heidelberg and former Secretary of Health in Germany.

"Never before in the world could so many people reach such an advanced age. Many studies have found that people who are mentally more active, have higher IQs, a wider range of interests, a farther-reaching perspective, and a greater number of social contacts, reach old age with greater feelings of psycho-physical well-being. It has been established that cognitive activity is essential for healthy aging."

Diet

Follow the Maker's Diet as best you can for six to twelve months. If symptoms are completely gone for at least three months, you may gradually add foods from the "Average" or "Trouble" categories, if you desire. Because people with brain disorders (Parkinson's, Alzheimer's, dementia) appear to have a predisposed weakness which presents itself as a brain disorder, however, I strongly recommend that they adhere to a diet of foods in the "Extraordinary" category for the rest of their lives.

Therapeutic Foods

These therapeutic foods will help you get well:

Cultured goat's milk dairy products: Consume 8 to 32 ounces of the highest quality cultured dairy products from goat's milk. Try to find yogurt that does not contain the organism *Streptococcus thermophilus*, a bacterial microbe that has been known to make immune system disorders worse.

Grass-fed red meat: Red meat from grass-fed cattle, buffalo, and lamb is very healthy and can be eaten a few times per week. This meat is a great source of protein, minerals, vitamin B_{12}, vitamins A and D, omega-3 fats, and CLA.

Organic, pasture-raised eggs: Consume as many as one to three organic eggs high in omega-3 fatty acids each day. These eggs contain DHA, vitamins E and B_{12}, and antioxidants including lutein.

Extra virgin coconut oil: This oil is perhaps the healthiest of the widely available oils. I recommend cooking almost exclusively with extra virgin coconut oil. Consume as much as two to four tablespoons per day of the oil in cooking, smoothies, or right off the spoon. Coconut oil contains large amounts of lauric acid, a potent antimicrobial and one of the chief fatty acids found in breast milk.

Ocean-caught fish: This type of fish is perhaps the healthiest of all protein sources. Salmon, sardines, mackerel, herring, and albacore tuna are high in the omega-3 fatty acids EPA and DHA. Ocean-caught fish can be consumed every day to enhance digestive and immune system health.

Cod liver oil: Take one to three teaspoons of an excellent cod liver oil each day, or caplets. The amount consumed should be based upon the amount of sunlight you receive. People in colder climates generally need to consume larger amounts. Cod liver oil is a fantastic source of the omega-3 fats DHA and EPA, as well as fat-soluble vitamins A and D.

Vegetable juice: Consume vegetable juices that are low in carbohydrates, such as celery and green juices mixed with a small amount of higher carbohydrate veggies such as carrots or beets. Mix in some form of healthy fat with each glass of the juice. One to three teaspoons of cultured goat's milk, extra virgin coconut oil, canned or fresh coconut milk and cream, or flaxseed oil enhance absorption of minerals and prevents spikes in blood sugar.

Berries: Berries such as blueberries, raspberries, blackberries, and strawberries are perhaps the greatest sources of dietary antioxidants available. Scientists at Tufts University have shown that blueberries serve as the premiere dietary source of antioxidants and may reduce the damaging effects of age-related memory loss.

Fermented vegetables: Consume a few tablespoons of fermented vegetables such as sauerkraut with each meal to aid in digestion. Fermented vegetables are an excellent source of naturally occurring probiotics and enzymes.

Stocks: It is a great idea to consume stocks on a regular basis, especially when you have a cold or flu. Stocks made from the bones of chicken, fish, lamb, and beef contain minerals, gelatin, cartilage, collagen, and electrolytes from the vegetables. Stocks are an excellent source of proteins, especially collagen. They help to heal the gut lining and reduce inflammation.

Supplements

Consume the following dietary supplements, along with the recommended foods and beverages, to help overcome this condition:

A probiotic, enzyme, and herbs formulation designed to support brain health.

A probiotic with SBOs. Take six to twelve capsules per day and stay on that amount for three to six months or when tests for your affliction are negative. Then begin to gradually decrease to a maintenance dosage of between three to six capsules per day. Probiotics with SBOs are best taken first thing in the morning and right before bedtime with eight ounces pure water. Probiotics with SBOs may be taken with other nutritional supplements, but should be taken one hour apart from medications. If you experience symptoms of detoxification (i.e., increased elimination, loose stools, constipation, excess gas, flu-like symptoms, or fever), reduce the dosage and work up slowly to twelve per day.

A green superfood powder. Take two tablespoons twice daily with eight ounces water or fresh vegetable juice. Best taken on an empty stomach away from food.

Digestive enzymes. Take one to three capsules with each meal or snack.

An organic fiber supplement with chia seed. Consume one serving twice per day, morning and evening, with eight or more ounces of purified water. (Consuming a fiber supplement is essential during the first two weeks of the program. Thereafter, consume fiber as needed.)

A protein powder from bone broth. Take one to three servings per day mixed in water, juice, smoothies, yogurt, or can be used in many recipes.

Additional Therapies

For people who have or may have unbalanced intestinal flora, avoiding contact with chlorinated water is of the utmost importance. That includes bathing water and drinking water. Chlorine kills bacteria, friendly and unfriendly, in the intestines, and can be absorbed through the skin. I recommend installing a shower filter to remove chlorine. Avoid swimming in chlorinated water as well.

Also consider limiting exposure to the following consumer products:

Food additives. Some food additives, such as artificial colors, contain lead that impairs mental function. Other types of food additives, known as excitotoxins, can actually kill brain cells. Examples of excitotoxins are monosodium glutamate (often found in hydrolyzed vegetable protein) and aspartame (also known as Nutrasweet).

Excess alcohol. While a single serving of alcohol daily appears to be protective against heart disease, excess alcohol intake can result in destruction of brain cells and cause long-term irreversible brain damage.

Hazardous chemicals. Household cleaning products, paints, auto products, and home and garden pesticides often contain toxic solvents and other chemicals that damage the nervous system. Shop for more environmentally friendly brands.

Bursitis…see Inflammatory Conditions

Cancer

- Bladder
- Lung
- Brain
- Lymphoma
- Breast
- Melanoma
- Colorectal
- Ovarian
- Endometrial
- Prostate
- Leukemia

Cancer is one of the leading killers in the world today. If you're a male, you have a one in two chance of being diagnosed with the Big C; if you're a woman, a one in three chance, according to the American Cancer Society.

Cancer is actually many diseases characterized by uncontrolled cell division, starting with a single cell that has begun to uncontrollably multiply. That's not how the body, which is made of many types of cells, is supposed to work.

Normally cells grow and divide to produce more cells when the body needs them. This orderly process helps keep the body healthy. Sometimes, however, cells keep dividing when new cells are not needed. These extra cells form a mass of tissue called a growth or tumor. Tumors can be benign or malignant.

Benign tumors are not cancerous. They can often be removed and, in most cases, they do not come back. Cells from benign tumors do not spread to other parts of the body. Most important, benign tumors are rarely a threat to life.

Malignant tumors, on the other hand, are cancerous and therefore dangerous. Cells in these tumors are abnormal and divide without control or order. They can invade and damage nearby tissues and organs. Also, cancer cells can break away from a malignant tumor and enter the bloodstream or the lymphatic system. That is how cancer spreads from the original cancer site to form new tumors in other organs. The spread of cancer is called metastasis.

Most cancers are named for the organ or type of cell in which they begin. For example, cancer that begins in the lung is lung cancer, and cancer that begins in cells in the skin known as melanocytes is called melanoma. Leukemia and lymphoma are cancers that arise in blood-forming cells. The abnormal cells circulate in the bloodstream and lymphatic system. They may also invade (infiltrate) body organs and form tumors.

When cancer spreads (metastasizes), cancer cells are often found in nearby or regional lymph nodes (sometimes called lymph glands). If the cancer has reached these nodes, it means that cancer cells may have spread to other organs, such as the liver, bones, or brain. When cancer spreads from its original location to another part of the body, the new tumor has the same kind of abnormal cells and the same name as the primary tumor. For example, if lung cancer spreads to the brain, the cancer cells in the brain are actually lung cancer cells. The disease is called metastatic lung cancer (it is not brain cancer).

Because cancer is a complicated and deadly disease, it is beyond the scope of this book to present a "plan" to defeat cancer. Until you do your research and speak with your oncologist, you can certainly take steps in the area of diet to boost your chances of beating cancer.

Diet

Follow the Maker's Diet diligently for six to twelve months, in conjunction with feedback from your doctor. This would be an important time to make "Extraordinary" foods the largest part of your diet.

Therapeutic Foods

These therapeutic foods will help you in your fight against cancer:

Cultured goat's milk dairy products: Consume 8 to 32 ounces of the highest quality cultured dairy products from goat's milk. Try to find yogurt that does not contain the organism *Streptococcus thermophilus*, a bacterial microbe that has been known to make immune system disorders worse.

Grass-fed red meat: Red meat from grass-fed cattle, buffalo, and lamb is very healthy and can be eaten a few times per week. This meat is a great source of protein, minerals, vitamin B$_{12}$, vitamins A and D, omega-3 fats, and CLA.

Organic, pasture-raised eggs: Consume as many as two organic eggs high in omega-3 fatty acids each day. These eggs contain DHA, vitamins E and B$_{12}$, and antioxidants including lutein.

Extra virgin coconut oil: This oil is perhaps the healthiest of the widely available oils. I recommend cooking almost exclusively with extra virgin coconut oil. Consume as much as two to four tablespoons per day of the oil in cooking, smoothies, or right off the spoon. Coconut oil contains large amounts of lauric acid, a potent antimicrobial and one of the chief fatty acids found in breast milk.

Ocean-caught fish: This type of fish is perhaps the healthiest of all protein sources. Salmon, sardines, mackerel, herring, and albacore tuna are high in the omega-3 fatty acids EPA and DHA. Ocean-caught fish can be consumed every day to enhance digestive and immune system health.

Cod liver oil: Take one to three teaspoons of an excellent cod liver oil each day, or caplets. The amount consumed should be based upon the amount of sunlight you receive. People in colder climates generally need to consume larger amounts. Cod liver oil is a fantastic source of the omega-3 fats DHA and EPA, as well as fat-soluble vitamins A and D.

Vegetable juice: Consume vegetable juices that are low in carbohydrates, such as celery and green juices mixed with a small amount of higher carbohydrate veggies such as carrot or beet. Mix in some form of healthy fat with each glass of the juice. One to three teaspoons of cultured goat's milk, extra virgin coconut oil, canned or fresh coconut milk and cream, or flaxseed oil enhance absorption of minerals and prevents spikes in blood sugar.

Fermented vegetables: Consume a few tablespoons of fermented vegetables such as sauerkraut with each meal to aid in digestion. Fermented vegetables are an excellent source of naturally occurring probiotics and enzymes.

Stocks: It is a great idea to consume stocks on a regular basis, especially when you are undergoing treatment. Stocks made from the bones of chicken, fish, lamb, and beef contain minerals, gelatin, cartilage, collagen, and electrolytes from the vegetables. Stocks are an excellent source of proteins, especially collagen. They help to heal the gut lining and reduce inflammation.

Supplements

Consume the following dietary supplements, along with the recommended foods and beverages, to help overcome this condition:

A probiotic, enzyme, and herbs formulation designed to support the fight against cancer.

A probiotic with SBOs. Take six to twelve capsules per day and stay on that amount for three to six months or when tests for your affliction are negative. Then begin to gradually decrease to a maintenance dosage of between three to six capsules per day. Probiotics with SBOs are best taken first thing in the morning and right before bedtime with eight ounces pure water. Probiotics with SBOs may be taken with other nutritional supplements, but should be taken one hour apart from medications. If you experience symptoms of detoxification (i.e., increased elimination, loose stools, constipation, excess gas, flu-like symptoms, or fever), reduce the dosage and work up slowly to twelve per day.

A green superfood powder. Take two tablespoons twice daily with eight ounces water or fresh vegetable juice. Best taken on an empty stomach away from food.

Digestive enzymes. Take one to three capsules with each meal or snack.

An organic fiber supplement with chia seed. Consume one serving twice per day, morning and evening, with eight or more ounces of purified water. (Consuming a fiber supplement is essential during the first two weeks of the program. Thereafter, consume fiber as needed.)

A protein powder from bone broth. Take one to three servings per day mixed in water, juice, smoothies, yogurt, or can be used in many recipes.

Additional Therapies

For people who have or may have a weakened immune system, avoiding contact with chlorinated water is of the utmost importance. That includes bathing water and drinking water. Chlorine kills bacteria, friendly and unfriendly, in the intestines and can be absorbed through the skin. I recommend installing a shower filter to remove chlorine. Avoid swimming in chlorinated water as well.

Candidiasis

C. albicans, a common yeast, is part of the regular flora (bacteria) in the digestive tract. In a healthy state, they live in a ratio of about one candida cell to one million other microorganisms. Due to our modern lifestyles, however, women who take birth control pills and men or women who consume large amounts of carbohydrates, especially refined carbohydrates (e.g., refined sugars and fruit juices), or have used antibiotics or corticosteroids might experience candida overgrowth. Women might also experience yeast overgrowth premenstrually or during pregnancy because progesterone levels seem to enhance yeast growth. Stress is also a cause of yeast overgrowth.

When this happens, yeast overgrowth-related disorders may develop—yeast infections, rectal itch, constipation, bloating and weight gain, skin problems, brain fog, and many others.

With long-term infestation, candida shifts into a fungal form that develops roots called rhizoids. These can grow right into the intestinal wall and cause the intestine to become porous, allowing toxins and undigested proteins and carbohydrates to flow through the bowel wall and be absorbed into the body and the bloodstream. This condition is called leaky gut syndrome. So many seemingly untreatable health problems start with candida overgrowth, which can evolve into leaky gut syndrome.

The next step in this vicious cycle is that the immune system of the individual makes antibodies (which are proteins) that attempt to neutralize the candida overgrowth. These antibodies can cause the body to become hypersensitive to certain foods and molds, and they can create a wide variety of food allergies. They can also interfere with hormonal activity and cause nutritional deficiencies.

The yeast syndrome is characterized by patients saying they "feel sick all over." Major symptoms include fatigue or lethargy; feeling "drained"; poor memory; feeling "spacey" or "unreal"; depression; numbness; burning or tingling; muscle aches and weakness; pain and/or swelling in the joints; abdominal pain and bloating; constipation and/or diarrhea; persistent vaginal itch or burning; endometriosis; cramps and other menstrual irregularities including premenstrual tension; erratic vision including spots in front of eyes; allergies; immune system malfunction; chemical sensitivities; and digestive disturbances.

The best method for diagnosing chronic candidiasis is clinical evaluation by a physician knowledgeable about yeast-related illness. The manner in which the doctor will diagnose the yeast syndrome will probably be based on clinical judgment from a detailed medical history and patient questionnaire. The doctor may also employ laboratory techniques such as stool cultures for candida and measurement of antibody levels to candida or candida antigens in the blood.

Once diagnosed, most physicians prescribe drugs such as nystatin, ketoconazole, and diflucan as well as various natural anti-candida agents, but these rarely produce significant long-term results because they fail to address the underlying factors that promote candida overgrowth.

Therefore, a holistic and integrative approach involving diet, lifestyle, and whole-food nutritional supplements is essential for long-term improvement and prevention.

Diet

Follow the Maker's Diet as best you can for six to twelve months. For the first thirty days, it's best to limit or even restrict fruit and honey consumption. Make sure that if you do consume fruit, then choose the less sweet, high-nutrient, high-fiber fruits such as berries, apples, or grapefruit.

After symptoms are completely gone for at least six months, you may gradually add foods from the "Average" or "Trouble" categories, if you desire. I recommend that people with a propensity to blood sugar imbalances choose most of their foods from the "Extraordinary" category.

Bear in mind that many people suffering from systemic yeast overgrowth will need to eliminate almost all grains and fruit for the first three months of the program. Because people with fungal and parasitic over-growth appear to have a predisposed weakness in their intestinal tracts, I strongly recommend that they adhere to a diet of "Extraordinary" foods for the rest of their lives.

Therapeutic Foods

These therapeutic foods will help you get well:

Cultured goat's milk dairy products: Consume 8 to 32 ounces of the highest quality cultured dairy products from goat's milk. Try to find yogurt that does not contain the organism *Streptococcus thermophilus*, a bacterial microbe that has been known to make immune system disorders worse.

Grass-fed red meat: Red meat from grass-fed cattle, buffalo, and lamb is very healthy and can be eaten a few times per week. This meat is a great source of protein, minerals, vitamin B$_{12}$, vitamins A and D, omega-3 fats, and CLA.

Organic, pasture-raised eggs: Consume as many as one to three organic eggs high in omega-3 fatty acids each day. These eggs contain DHA, vitamins E and B$_{12}$, and antioxidants including lutein.

Extra virgin coconut oil: This oil is perhaps the healthiest of the widely available oils. I recommend cooking almost exclusively with extra virgin coconut oil. Consume as much as two to four tablespoons per day of the oil in cooking, smoothies, or right off the spoon. Coconut oil contains large amounts of lauric acid, a potent antimicrobial and one of the chief fatty acids found in breast milk.

Ocean-caught fish: This type of fish is perhaps the healthiest of all protein sources. Salmon, sardines, mackerel, herring, and albacore tuna are high in the omega-3 fatty acids EPA and DHA. Ocean-caught fish can be consumed every day to enhance digestive and immune system health.

Cod liver oil: Take one to three teaspoons of an excellent cod liver oil each day, or caplets. The amount consumed should be based upon the amount of sunlight you receive. People in colder climates generally need to consume larger amounts. Cod liver oil is a fantastic source of the omega-3 fats DHA and EPA, as well as fat-soluble vitamins A and D.

Vegetable juice: Consume vegetable juices that are low in carbohy-drates, such as celery and green juices mixed with a small amount of higher carbohydrate veggies such as carrot or beet. Mix in some form of healthy fat with each glass of the juice. One to three teaspoons of cultured goat's milk, extra virgin coconut oil, canned or fresh coconut milk and cream, or flaxseed oil enhance absorption of minerals and prevents spikes in blood sugar.

Fermented vegetables: Consume a few tablespoons of fermented vegetables such as sauerkraut with each meal to aid in digestion. Fermented vegetables are an excellent source of naturally occurring probiotics and enzymes.

Stocks: It is a great idea to consume stocks on a regular basis, especially when you have a cold or flu. Stocks made from the bones of chicken, fish, lamb, and beef contain minerals, gelatin, cartilage, collagen, and electrolytes from the vegetables. Stocks are an excellent source of proteins, especially collagen. They help to heal the gut lining and reduce inflammation.

Supplements

Consume the following dietary supplements, along with the recommended foods and beverages, to help overcome this condition:

A probiotic, enzyme, and herbs formulation designed to support candidiasis.

A probiotic with SBOs. Take six to twelve capsules per day and stay on that amount for three to six months or when tests for your affliction are negative. Then begin to gradually decrease to a maintenance dosage of between three to six capsules per day. Probiotics with SBOs are best taken first thing in the morning and right before bedtime with eight ounces pure water. Probiotics with SBOs may be taken with other nutritional supplements, but should be taken one hour apart from medications. If you experience symptoms of detoxification (i.e., increased elimination, loose stools, constipation, excess gas, flu-like symptoms, or fever), reduce the dosage and work up slowly to twelve per day.

A green superfood powder. Take two tablespoons twice daily with eight ounces water or fresh vegetable juice. Best taken on an empty stomach away from food.

Digestive enzymes. Take one to three capsules with each meal or snack.

An organic fiber supplement with chia seed. Consume one serving twice per day, morning and evening, with eight or more ounces of purified water. (Consuming a fiber supplement is essential during the first two weeks of the program. Thereafter, consume fiber as needed.)

A protein powder from bone broth. Take one to three servings per day mixed in water, juice, smoothies, yogurt, or can be used in many recipes.

Additional Therapies

For people who have or may have imbalanced intestinal flora, avoiding contact with chlorinated water is of the utmost importance. That includes bathing water and drinking water. Chlorine kills bacteria, friendly and unfriendly, in the intestines and can be absorbed through the skin. I recommend installing a shower filter to remove chlorine. Avoid swimming in chlorinated water as well.

In treating chronic candidiasis, a comprehensive approach is more effective than simply trying to kill the candida with a drug or a natural anti-candida agent. For example, most physicians fail to recognize that a number of dietary factors appear to promote the overgrowth of candida. It is also important to increase digestive secretions; enhance immunity; promote detoxification and elimination; and use a comprehensive nutritional supplement program, including the use of the natural anti-yeast herbal extracts. Follow these guidelines.

Limit sugar. Sugar is the chief nutrient for *C. albicans*. Restriction of sugar intake is an absolute necessity in the treatment of chronic candidiasis. Most people do well by simply avoiding grains, flours, pasta, refined sugar, and large amounts of honey, maple syrup, and fruit juice and limiting overall consumption of carbohydrates to less than 100 grams per day.

Limit milk and dairy products. There are several reasons to restrict or eliminate the intake of milk in chronic candidiasis. Milk's high lactose content promotes the overgrowth of candida. Milk is also one of the most common food allergens and may even contain trace levels of antibiotics, which can further disrupt the gastrointestinal bacterial flora and promote candida overgrowth. The consumption of a cultured goat's milk yogurt is beneficial to those suffering from candidiasis.

Avoid mold- and yeast-containing foods. It is generally recommended by many experts that individuals with chronic candidiasis avoid foods with a high content of yeast or mold, including alcoholic beverages, grains, cheeses, dried fruits, and peanuts.

Increase digestive secretions. In many cases, an important step in treating chronic candidiasis is improving digestive secretions. Gastric hydrochloric acid, pancreatic enzymes, and bile all inhibit the overgrowth of candida and prevent its penetration into the absorptive surfaces of the small intestine. Decreased production of any of these important digestive components can lead to overgrowth of *C. albicans* in the gastrointestinal tract. Therefore, restoration of normal digestive secretions through the use of digestive enzymes is critical in the treatment of chronic candidiasis.

Restoring immune function. Restoring proper immune function is one of the key goals in the treatment of chronic candidiasis. Consuming immune-enhancing supplements can greatly aid in the body's fight against candida overgrowth.

Promoting detoxification. Candida patients usually exhibit multiple chemical sensitivities and allergies, an indication that detoxification reactions are stressed. Therefore, the liver function of the candida patient needs to be supported. In fact, improving the health of the liver and promoting detoxification may be one of the most critical factors in the successful treatment of candidiasis.

Damage to the liver is often an underlying factor in chronic candidiasis as well as chronic fatigue. When the liver is even slightly damaged by a toxic chemical, immune function is severely compromised. Liver injury is also linked to candida overgrowth, as evident in studies of mice demonstrating that when the liver is even slightly damaged, candida runs rampant through the body. Consuming a high-quality green food supplement can greatly enhance the liver's ability to properly detoxify the body.

Promoting elimination. In addition to directly supporting liver function, proper detoxification involves proper elimination. A diet that focuses on high-fiber plant foods should be sufficient to promote proper elimination by supplying an ample amount of dietary fiber. If additional support is needed, fiber formulas can be taken. These formulas are composed of natural plant fibers derived from seeds, vegetables, and grains.

Natural anti-yeast compounds. There are a number of natural agents with proven activity against *C. albicans*. Among natural agents recommended to treat *C. albicans* are garlic and wild oregano.

Garlic has demonstrated significant antifungal activity. In fact, its inhibition of *C. albicans* in both animal and test tube studies has shown it to be more potent than nystatin, gentian violet, and six other reputed antifungal agents.

There is no doubt that candida overgrowth is a major health problem today among men and especially women. It is also equally clear that conventional treatments fail to address the underlying condition that allowed the overgrowth to occur. By following the steps in this natural program, you can overcome candida and start feeling great all over.

Cardiovascular Health

- Angina
- Cholesterol (elevated)
- Arteriosclerosis/Atherosclerosis
- Homocysteine levels (elevated)
- Blood pressure (elevated)
- Triglycerides (elevated)

Overview

Cardiovascular disease, principally heart disease and stroke, is the nation's leading killer for both men and women among all racial and ethnic groups. More than 800,000 Americans die of cardiovascular disease each year, accounting for one in three deaths, according to the American Heart Association and National Institutes of Health. About 92 million Americans (around 30 percent of the nation's population) live with some form of cardiovascular disease or the after-effects of a stroke.

Heart disease and stroke are the leading causes of premature, permanent disability among working adults. Stroke kills nearly 133,000 people a year and ranks fifth among all causes of death in the United States.

Angina

Angina pectoris (angina) is a recurring pain or discomfort in the chest that happens when some part of the heart does not receive enough blood. It is a common symptom of coronary heart disease, which occurs when vessels that carry blood to the heart become narrowed and blocked due to atherosclerosis. Angina is usually precipitated by exertion.

Arteriosclerosis/Atherosclerosis

Arteriosclerosis is a group of diseases characterized by the thickening of the artery wall—the hardening and calcification of the arteries—and in the narrowing of its lumen. Hardening of the arterial wall is due to various depositions within the plaque including lipids, cholesterol crystals, and calcium salts. These depositions make the arteries bone-like rigid tubes. They are most prominently found in the disease known as atherosclerosis.

Atherosclerosis is a specific type of arteriosclerosis involving fatty deposits that affect large arteries, and it is the underlying pathologic condition in most cases of coronary heart disease, aortic aneurysm, peripheral vascular disease, and stroke.

Blood Pressure (Elevated)

Blood pressure is the force of blood against the walls of arteries. Blood pressure rises and falls during the day. When blood pressure stays elevated over time, it is called high blood pressure or hypertension.

Blood pressure is typically recorded as two numbers—the systolic pressure (as the heart beats) over the diastolic pressure (as the heart relaxes between beats). A consistent blood pressure reading of 140/90 mm Hg or higher is considered high blood pressure.

Systolic pressure is the force of blood in the arteries as the heart beats. It is shown as the top number in a blood pressure reading. High blood pressure is 140 mm Hg and higher for systolic pressure. Diastolic pressure does not need to be nearly as high (usually over 80 mm Hg) for you to have high blood pressure.

If left uncontrolled, high blood pressure can lead to stroke, heart attack, congestive heart failure, kidney damage, blindness, or other conditions. Yet, most Americans do not have their systolic pressure under control.

Cholesterol (Elevated)

We can all agree on the American Heart Association's description of cholesterol as a soft, waxy substance found among the lipids (fats) in the bloodstream and in all your body's cells. We can even all agree that it's normal to have cholesterol. After all, cholesterol is an important part of a healthy body because it's used to form cell membranes, some hormones, and serve other needed bodily functions.

With this in mind, it's disturbing that cholesterol has been given such a terrible beating by the medical establishment over the last couple of decades. Cholesterol doesn't deserve its evil reputation. Keep in mind the following points so eloquently summarized by Danish physician Uffe Ravnskov, M.D., Ph.D.:

- A high cholesterol is not dangerous by itself, but may reflect an unhealthy condition, or it may be totally innocent.
- High blood cholesterol is said to promote atherosclerosis and thus also coronary heart disease. But many studies have shown that people whose blood cholesterol is low become just as atherosclerotic as people whose cholesterol is high.
- The body produces three to four times more cholesterol than you eat. The production of cholesterol increases when you eat little cholesterol and decreases when you eat much. This explains why a "prudent" diet or a "low cholesterol" diet cannot lower cholesterol more than, on average, a few percent.
- There is no evidence that too much animal fat and cholesterol in the diet promotes atherosclerosis or heart attacks. For instance, more than twenty studies have shown that people who have had a heart attack haven't eaten more fat of any kind than other people, and degree of atherosclerosis at autopsy is unrelated with the diet.
- Cholesterol-lowering drugs like statins prevent cardiovascular disease, but this is due to other mechanisms than the lowering of cholesterol.
- Many of these facts have been presented in scientific journals and books for decades but are rarely told to the public because drug

companies press the media to report on the use of cholesterol-lowering drugs since these drugs represent major profits to corporate interests.

- The reason why laymen, doctors, and most scientists have been misled about the benefits of cholesterol in the body is because opposing and disagreeing results are systematically ignored or misquoted in the scientific press.

Homocysteine (Elevated)

A more likely culprit in heart disease is elevated homocysteine. In the optimally functioning body, homocysteine is an intermediate point in a metabolic pathway that starts with consumption of foods rich in the essential amino acid methionine. At the end of this pathway, methionine generally is metabolized to cysteine.

For this conversion to be completed, however, the body requires the help of an enzyme called cystathionine synthetase, and the coenzyme pyridoxal phosphate. If this metabolic pathway is stymied, homocysteine accumulates in the blood and exerts a toxic effect on the inner linings of the body's vessels, causing low-density lipoprotein cholesterol to accumulate.

There are several causes of elevated homocysteine levels. The most dramatic elevation, which leads to life-threatening vascular abnormalities at a young age, is due to rare genetic enzymatic defects at various points in the metabolic pathway. A far more common cause of elevated levels is diet. In particular, three members of the vitamin B complex family—folate (also known as folic acid), vitamin B_6, and vitamin B_{12}—enable this full conversion to take place.

Foods rich in folate include deep green leafy vegetables, carrots, liver, egg yolk, cantaloupe, apricots, pumpkins, avocados, beans, and whole dark rye flour. Vitamin B_6-rich foods are brewer's yeast, wheat germ, liver, fermented soy foods, cantaloupe, cabbage, blackstrap molasses, brown rice, eggs, oats, peanuts, and walnuts; those rich in vitamin B_{12} include animal foods such as liver, beef, eggs, milk, and cheese. A study published in the *Netherland Journal of Medicine* reports that vegetarians and vegans have higher levels of homocysteine compared to people who have high fat and meat intakes.

It is also quite clear that the homocysteine theory of heart disease might someday displace the fat/cholesterol theory. What makes the homocysteine theory even more appealing is that Kilmer McCully M.D., the doctor and a scientist who must be credited with its founding, is also a pathologist. He found the smoking gun—signs of homocysteine toxicity—even in arteries of people with normal to low cholesterol levels who had been felled by heart disease.

Triglycerides (Elevated)

Triglycerides are the form in which fat exists in meats, cheese, fish, nuts, vegetable oils, and the greasy layer on the surface of soup stocks or in a pan used to fry bacon. In a healthy person, triglycerides and other fatty substances are normally moved into the liver and into adipose cells to provide energy for later use. Triglycerides are the chemical form in which most fat exists in the body.

The current conventional wisdom is that high levels of triglycerides create a high risk for a heart attack or stroke. No less a publication than *Circulation* from the American Heart Association has been in the forefront of exposing the triglyceride–heart disease link. There is merit to this work. But I see high triglycerides as symptomatic of a diet that is too high in carbohydrates and refined foods and low in protein and the good fats. I think this truly is the key issue.

Epidemiological studies from Harvard University make it clear that the good fats are not only benign when it comes to heart disease but actually reduce risk. Therefore, the Maker's Diet, with adequate protein and fats from the proper foods, is beneficial in healing heart disease. The real culprit in heart disease is our overly processed, carbohydrate-rich food supply. The promoters of low-protein, low-fat diets remain oblivious to many factors, but most important is that no amount of supplementation can substitute for the proper balance of fat and protein that is obtained from eating healthy foods, the way our Maker intended.

Diet

Follow the Maker's Diet as best you can for six to twelve months. After symptoms are completely gone for at least three months, you may gradually add foods from the "Average" or "Trouble" categories, if you desire.

Because people with cardiovascular disorders appear to have a predisposed weakness that manifests as a cardiovascular condition, I strongly recommend that you adhere to a diet of foods in the "Extraordinary" category for the rest of your life.

Therapeutic Foods

These therapeutic foods will help you get well:

Cultured goat's milk dairy products: Consume 8 to 32 ounces of the highest quality cultured dairy products from goat's milk. Try to find yogurt that does not contain the organism *Streptococcus thermophilus*, a bacterial microbe that has been known to make immune system disorders worse.

Grass-fed red meat: Red meat from grass-fed cattle, buffalo, and lamb is very healthy and can be eaten a few times per week. This meat is a great source of protein, minerals, vitamin B_{12}, vitamins A and D, omega-3 fats, and CLA.

Organic, pasture-raised eggs: Consume as many as one to three organic eggs high in omega-3 fatty acids each day. These eggs contain DHA, vitamins E and B_{12}, and antioxidants including lutein.

Extra virgin coconut oil: This oil is perhaps the healthiest of the widely available oils. I recommend cooking almost exclusively with extra virgin coconut oil. Consume as much as two to four tablespoons per day of the oil in cooking, smoothies, or right off the spoon. Coconut oil contains large amounts of lauric acid, a potent antimicrobial and one of the chief fatty acids found in breast milk.

Ocean-caught fish: This type of fish is perhaps the healthiest of all protein sources. Salmon, sardines, mackerel, herring, and albacore tuna are high in the omega-3 fatty acids EPA and DHA. Ocean-caught fish can be consumed every day to enhance digestive and immune system health.

Cod liver oil: Take one to three teaspoons of an excellent cod liver oil each day, or caplets. The amount consumed should be based upon the amount of sunlight you receive. People in colder climates generally need to consume larger amounts. Cod liver oil is a fantastic source of the omega-3 fats DHA and EPA, as well as fat-soluble vitamins A and D.

Vegetable juice: Consume vegetable juices that are low in carbohydrates, such as celery and green juices mixed with a small amount of higher carbohydrate veggies such as carrot or beet. Mix in some form of healthy fat with each glass of the juice. One to three teaspoons of cultured goat's milk, extra virgin coconut oil, canned or fresh coconut milk and cream, or flaxseed oil enhance absorption of minerals and prevents spikes in blood sugar.

Fermented vegetables: Consume a few tablespoons of fermented vegetables such as sauerkraut with each meal to aid in digestion. Fermented vegetables are an excellent source of naturally occurring probiotics and enzymes.

Stocks: It is a great idea to consume stocks on a regular basis, especially when you have a cold or flu. Stocks made from the bones of chicken, fish, lamb, and beef contain minerals, gelatin, cartilage, collagen, and electrolytes from the vegetables. Stocks are an excellent source of proteins, especially collagen. They help to heal the gut lining and reduce inflammation.

Supplements

Consume the following dietary supplements, along with the recommended foods and beverages, to help overcome this condition:

A probiotic, enzyme, and herbs formulation designed to support cardiovascular health.

A probiotic with SBOs. Take six to twelve capsules per day and stay on that amount for three to six months or when tests for your affliction are negative. Then begin to gradually decrease to a maintenance dosage of between three to six capsules per day. Probiotics with SBOs are best taken first thing in the morning and right before bedtime with eight ounces pure water. Probiotics with SBOs may be taken with other nutritional supplements, but should be taken one hour apart from medications. If you experience symptoms of detoxification (i.e., increased elimination, loose stools, constipation, excess gas, flu-like symptoms, or fever), reduce the dosage and work up slowly to twelve per day.

A green superfood powder. Take two tablespoons twice daily with eight ounces water or fresh vegetable juice. Best taken on an empty stomach away from food.

Digestive enzymes. Take one to three capsules with each meal or snack.

An organic fiber supplement with chia seed. Consume one serving twice per day, morning and evening, with eight or more ounces of purified water. (Consuming a fiber supplement is essential during the first two weeks of the program. Thereafter, consume fiber as needed.)

A protein powder from bone broth. Take one to three servings per day mixed in water, juice, smoothies, yogurt, or can be used in many recipes.

Additional Therapies

In order to maintain a healthy balance of intestinal flora, avoiding contact with chlorinated water is of the utmost importance. That includes bathing water and drinking water. Chlorine kills bacteria, friendly and unfriendly, in the intestines and can be absorbed through the skin. I recommend installing a shower filter to remove chlorine. Avoid swimming in chlorinated water as well.

Many researchers now believe that heart disease can be caused by infections that originate in the oral cavity. While the diet outlined in this book is sure to improve dental health, I recommend that you find and use a toothbrush, mouthwash, and dental floss that contains antimicrobial essential oils. It may be helpful to use a tongue cleaner. Natural toothpaste, mouthwash, dental floss, and tongue cleaners are available at your local health food store.

Celiac Disease...see Chronic Digestive Disease

Children's Health

- Attention Deficit Disorder (ADD)
- Autism
- Attention Deficit/Hyperactivity Disorder (ADHD)
- Pervasive Developmental Disorders (PDD)

Attention Deficit Disorder and Attention Deficit/Hyperactivity Disorder

ADHD and ADD are characterized by developmentally inappropriate inattention and impulsivity, with or without hyperactivity. ADHD is implicated in learning disorders and is diagnosed two or three times more frequently in boys than girls, according to Mayo Clinic researchers. Boys are also up to nine times more likely than girls to be referred for treatment and evaluation. Despite the frequent references to ADHD as a neurobiological disorder, the cause of ADHD remains unknown.

The primary signs of ADD with or without hyperactivity are the display of inattention and impulsivity. ADHD with hyperactivity is diagnosed when signs of overactivity are obvious. Inattention is described as a failure to finish tasks started, easy distractibility, seeming lack of attention, and difficulty concentrating on tasks requiring sustained attention. Impulsivity is described as acting before thinking, difficulty taking turns, problems organizing work, and constant shifting from one activity to another. Hyperactivity is described as difficulty staying seated and sitting still, and running or climbing excessively.

Autism

Autism symptoms usually manifest within the first two to four years of life. Once considered a rare disorder with an incidence of only one case per 10,000 births thirty years ago, autism is now reaching epidemic proportions with an incidence of more than *fifty* cases per 10,000 children, according to the Centers for Disease Control. Autism now ranks third among childhood developmental disorders, making it more common than Down's syndrome, multiple sclerosis, and cystic fibrosis.

Why the huge increase? Scientists aren't sure if this is due to a broadening of the disorder's definition or an actual increase in the number of individuals who have autism. A subject of controversy is whether childhood vaccinations play a role in the stratospheric rise of autism. The traditional medical community says there's no link between autism—or GMOs and pesticides that contains glyphosates—to autism.

At the moment, I think it's fair to say that the jury is out on why so many children are being diagnosed with autism, a neurological disorder characterized by impairments in language, cognitive, and social development.

Pervasive Developmental Disorder

Autism and PDD are developmental disabilities that share many of the same characteristics. Usually evident by age three, autism and PDD are neurological disorders that affect a child's ability to communicate, understand language, play, and relate to others.

Diet

Have your children follow the Maker's Diet as best they can for six to twelve months. Many children have poor health or even illness due to poor nutrition and improper detoxification. The improvement in diet and the addition of key nutrients can improve your children's health and may even aid in the reversal of many childhood health problems, especially as we find that these disorders are exacerbated or, in some cases, caused by gastrointestinal imbalances.

When your children follow the Maker's Diet, I believe each child will have excellent health, improved learning ability, and the potential to grow into a healthy adult.

Therapeutic Foods

These therapeutic foods will help you get well:

Cultured goat's milk dairy products: Consume 8 to 32 ounces of the highest quality cultured dairy products from goat's milk. Try to find yogurt that does not contain the organism *Streptococcus thermophilus*, a bacterial microbe that has been known to make immune system disorders worse.

Grass-fed red meat: Red meat from grass-fed cattle, buffalo, and lamb is very healthy and can be eaten a few times per week. This meat is a great source of protein, minerals, vitamin B12, vitamins A and D, omega-3 fats, and CLA.

Organic, pasture-raised eggs: Consume as many as one to three organic eggs high in omega-3 fatty acids each day. These eggs contain DHA, vitamins E and B12, and antioxidants including lutein.

Extra virgin coconut oil: This oil is perhaps the healthiest of the widely available oils. I recommend cooking almost exclusively with extra virgin coconut oil. Consume as much as two to four tablespoons per day of the oil in cooking, smoothies, or right off the spoon. Coconut oil contains large amounts of lauric acid, a potent antimicrobial and one of the chief fatty acids found in breast milk.

Ocean-caught fish: This type of fish is perhaps the healthiest of all protein sources. Salmon, sardines, mackerel, herring, and albacore tuna are high in the omega-3 fatty acids EPA and DHA. Ocean-caught fish can be consumed every day to enhance digestive and immune system health.

Cod liver oil: Take one to three teaspoons of an excellent cod liver oil each day, or caplets. The amount consumed should be based upon the amount of sunlight you receive. People in colder climates generally need to consume larger amounts. Cod liver oil is a fantastic source of the omega-3 fats DHA and EPA, as well as fat-soluble vitamins A and D.

Vegetable juice: Consume vegetable juices that are low in carbohydrates, such as celery and green juices mixed with a small amount of higher carbohydrate veggies such as carrot or beet. Mix in some form of healthy fat with each glass of the juice. One to three teaspoons of cultured goat's milk, extra virgin coconut oil, canned or fresh coconut milk and cream, or flaxseed oil enhance absorption of minerals and prevents spikes in blood sugar.

Fermented vegetables: Consume a few tablespoons of fermented vegetables such as sauerkraut with each meal to aid in digestion. Fermented vegetables are an excellent source of naturally occurring probiotics and enzymes.

Stocks: It is a great idea to consume stocks on a regular basis, especially when you have a cold or flu. Stocks made from the bones of chicken, fish, lamb, and beef contain minerals, gelatin, cartilage, collagen, and electrolytes from the vegetables. Stocks are an excellent source of proteins, especially collagen. They help to heal the gut lining and reduce inflammation.

Supplements

Consume the following dietary supplements, along with the recommended foods and beverages, to help overcome this condition:

A probiotic, enzyme, and herbs formulation designed to support children's health.

A probiotic with SBOs. Take six to twelve capsules per day and stay on that amount for three to six months or when tests for your affliction are negative. Then begin to gradually decrease to a maintenance dosage of between three to six capsules per day. Probiotics with SBOs are best taken first thing in the morning and right before bedtime with eight ounces pure water. Probiotics with SBOs may be taken with other nutritional supplements, but should be taken one hour apart from medications. If you experience symptoms of detoxification (i.e., increased elimination, loose stools, constipation, excess gas, flu-like symptoms, or fever), reduce the dosage and work up slowly to twelve per day.

A green superfood powder. Take two tablespoons twice daily with eight ounces water or fresh vegetable juice. Best taken on an empty stomach away from food.

Digestive enzymes. Take one to three capsules with each meal or snack.

An organic fiber supplement with chia seed. Consume one serving twice per day, morning and evening, with eight or more ounces of purified water. (Consuming a fiber supplement is essential during the first two weeks of the program. Thereafter, consume fiber as needed.)

A protein powder from bone broth. Take one to three servings per day mixed in water, juice, smoothies, yogurt, or can be used in many recipes.

Additional Therapies

For children who are rapidly developing a strong immune system, avoiding contact with chlorinated water is of the utmost importance. That includes bathing water and drinking water. Chlorine kills bacteria, friendly and unfriendly, in the intestines, and can be absorbed through the skin. I recommend installing a shower filter to remove chlorine. Avoid swimming in chlorinated water as well.

Cholesterol (Elevated)…Cardiovascular Health

Chronic Constipation…see Functional Bowel Disorders

Chronic Diarrhea…see Functional Bowel Disorders

Chronic Digestive Disease

- Celiac Disease
- Ulcerative Colitis
- Crohn's Disease
- Ulcers
- Diverticulitis

Overview

Chronic digestive diseases usually involve an intestinal condition characterized by a combination of:

- abdominal pain
- constipation
- diarrhea
- increased secretion of colon-related mucus
- dyspeptic symptoms such as flatulence, nausea, and anorexia.

Each condition has specific causes and symptoms as well as varying degrees of anxiety or depression:

- Celiac disease is characterized by gluten intolerance and severe wasting.
- Crohn's disease is a condition in which the intestinal wall thickens and causes narrowing of the bowel channel, blocking the intestinal tract.
- Diverticulitis is inflammation of an abnormal pouch or sac opening from a hollow organ (as the intestine or bladder).
- Ulcerative colitis is a nonspecific inflammatory disease of the colon of unknown cause characterized by diarrhea with discharge of mucus and blood, cramping abdominal pain, and inflammation and edema of the mucous membrane with patches of ulceration.
- An ulcer involves a break in the gastrointestinal mucous membrane with loss of surface tissue, disintegration, and necrosis of epithelial tissue.

The onset for chronic digestive diseases peak during young adulthood, although gastrointestinal ulcers afflict persons of all ages. Restoration of the balance of friendly bacteria to the gastrointestinal tract is essential to recovery. The complete avoidance of disaccharide-containing foods such as grains, most beans, sugar, maple syrup, non-cultured fluid dairy products (milk and ice cream), potatoes, and corn is a must in order to heal the digestive tract and improve the microbial balance.

Diet

Follow the Maker's Diet as best you can for six to twelve months. It is imperative to avoid all grains, even those in the "Extraordinary" category, which include soaked sprouted or sour leavened grains for the first six months.

While the aforementioned properly prepared grains are healthy for most people, those suffering from chronic digestive disease often have problems digesting grains in any form. After symptoms are completely gone for at least three months, you may gradually add foods from the "Average" or "Trouble" categories, if you desire. Because people with chronic digestive diseases (Crohn's, IBS, celiac disease, and ulcerative colitis) appear to have a predisposed weakness in their intestinal tracts, I strongly recommend that you adhere to a diet of foods in the "Extraordinary" category for the rest of your life.

Therapeutic Foods

These therapeutic foods will help you get well:

Cultured goat's milk dairy products: Consume 8 to 32 ounces of the highest quality cultured dairy products from goat's milk. Try to find yogurt that does not contain the organism *Streptococcus thermophilus*, a bacterial microbe that has been known to make immune system disorders worse.

Grass-fed red meat: Red meat from grass-fed cattle, buffalo, and lamb is very healthy and can be eaten a few times per week. This meat is a great source of protein, minerals, vitamin B_{12}, vitamins A and D, omega-3 fats, and CLA.

Organic, pasture-raised eggs: Consume as many as one to three organic eggs high in omega-3 fatty acids each day. These eggs contain DHA, vitamins E and B_{12}, and antioxidants including lutein.

Extra virgin coconut oil: This oil is perhaps the healthiest of the widely available oils. I recommend cooking almost exclusively with extra virgin coconut oil. Consume as much as two to four tablespoons per day of the oil in cooking, smoothies, or right off the spoon. Coconut oil contains large amounts of lauric acid, a potent antimicrobial and one of the chief fatty acids found in breast milk.

Ocean-caught fish: This type of fish is perhaps the healthiest of all protein sources. Salmon, sardines, mackerel, herring, and albacore tuna are high in the omega-3 fatty acids EPA and DHA. Ocean-caught fish can be consumed every day to enhance digestive and immune system health.

Cod liver oil: Take one to three teaspoons of an excellent cod liver oil each day, or caplets. The amount consumed should be based upon the amount of sunlight you receive. People in colder climates generally need to consume larger amounts. Cod liver oil is a fantastic source of the omega-3 fats DHA and EPA, as well as fat-soluble vitamins A and D.

Vegetable juice: As long as diarrhea is not active, consume vegetable juices that are low in carbohydrates, such as celery and green juices mixed with a small amount of higher carbohydrate veggies, such as carrot or beet. Mix in some form of healthy fat with each glass of the juice. One to three teaspoons of cultured goat's milk, extra virgin coconut oil, canned or fresh coconut milk and cream, or flaxseed oil enhance absorption of minerals and prevents spikes in blood sugar.

Fermented vegetables: Consume a few tablespoons of fermented vegetables such as sauerkraut with each meal to aid in digestion. Fermented vegetables are an excellent source of naturally occurring probiotics and enzymes.

Berries: Berries, particularly blueberries and raspberries, can be very beneficial for those suffering from chronic digestive diseases. These berries are high in antioxidant nutrients and are great sources of fiber.

Stocks: It is a great idea to consume stocks on a regular basis, especially when you have a cold or flu. Stocks made from the bones of chicken, fish, lamb, and beef contain minerals, gelatin, cartilage, collagen, and electrolytes from the vegetables. Stocks are an excellent source of proteins, especially collagen. They help to heal the gut lining and reduce inflammation.

Supplements

Consume the following dietary supplements, along with the recommended foods and beverages, to help overcome this condition:

A probiotic, enzyme, and herbs formulation designed to support digestive health.

A probiotic with SBOs. Take six to twelve capsules per day and stay on that amount for three to six months or when tests for your affliction are negative. Then begin to gradually decrease to a maintenance dosage of between three to six capsules per day. Probiotics with SBOs are best taken first thing in the morning and right before bedtime with eight ounces pure water. Probiotics with SBOs may be taken with other nutritional supplements, but should be taken one hour apart from medications. If you experience symptoms of detoxification (i.e., increased elimination, loose stools, constipation, excess gas, flu-like symptoms, or fever), reduce the dosage and work up slowly to twelve per day.

A green superfood powder. Take two tablespoons twice daily with eight ounces water or fresh vegetable juice. Best taken on an empty stomach away from food.

Digestive enzymes. Take one to three capsules with each meal or snack.

An organic fiber supplement with chia seed. Consume one serving twice per day, morning and evening, with eight or more ounces of purified water. (Consuming a fiber supplement is essential during the first two weeks of the program. Thereafter, consume fiber as needed.)

A protein powder from bone broth. Take one to three servings per day mixed in water, juice, smoothies, yogurt, or can be used in many recipes.

Additional Therapies

For people who have or may have unbalanced intestinal flora, avoiding contact with chlorinated water is of the utmost importance. That includes bathing water and drinking water. Chlorine kills bacteria, friendly and unfriendly, in the intestines, and can be absorbed through the skin. I recommend installing a shower filter to remove chlorine. Avoid swimming in chlorinated water as well.

Chronic Fatigue/Fibromyalgia

Overview

Chronic fatigue syndrome and fibromyalgia are complex and debilitating chronic illnesses that affect the brain and multiple body systems. Chronic pain and fatigue are common symptoms, but the difference is that in fibromyalgia, fatigue takes a back seat to debilitating muscle pain.

Chronic fatigue syndrome is characterized by incapacitating fatigue (experienced as profound exhaustion and extremely poor stamina) and problems with concentration and short-term memory. It is also accompanied by flu-like symptoms such as pain in the joints and muscles, unrefreshing sleep, tender lymph nodes, sore throat, and headache.

Persons with chronic fatigue syndrome or fibromyalgia have symptoms that vary from person to person and fluctuate in severity. Specific symptoms may come and go, complicating treatment and the person's ability to cope with the illness. Many symptoms are invisible to the doctor's eye, which makes it difficult for others to understand the vast array of debilitating symptoms with which such people contend.

Diet

Follow the Maker's Diet as best you can for six to twelve months. After symptoms are completely gone for at least three months, you may gradually add foods from the "Average" or "Trouble" categories, if you desire. Because people suffering from chronic fatigue or fibromyalgia appear to have a predisposed weakness in their immune systems and intestinal tracts, I strongly recommend that you adhere to a diet of foods in the "Extraordinary" category for the rest of your life.

Therapeutic Foods

These therapeutic foods will help you get well:

Cultured goat's milk dairy products: Consume 8 to 32 ounces of the highest quality cultured dairy products from goat's milk. Try to find yogurt that does not contain the organism *Streptococcus thermophilus*, a bacterial microbe that has been known to make immune system disorders worse.

Grass-fed red meat: Red meat from grass-fed cattle, buffalo, and lamb is very healthy and can be eaten a few times per week. This meat is a great source of protein, minerals, vitamin B12, vitamins A and D, omega-3 fats, and CLA.

Organic, pasture-raised eggs: Consume as many as one to three organic eggs high in omega-3 fatty acids each day. These eggs contain DHA, vitamins E and B12, and antioxidants including lutein.

Extra virgin coconut oil: This oil is perhaps the healthiest of the widely available oils. I recommend cooking almost exclusively with extra virgin coconut oil. Consume as much as two to four tablespoons per day of the oil in cooking, smoothies, or right off the spoon. Coconut oil contains large amounts of lauric acid, a potent antimicrobial and one of the chief fatty acids found in breast milk.

Ocean-caught fish: This type of fish is perhaps the healthiest of all protein sources. Salmon, sardines, mackerel, herring, and albacore tuna are high in the omega-3 fatty acids EPA and DHA. Ocean-caught fish can be consumed every day to enhance digestive and immune system health.

Cod liver oil: Take one to three teaspoons of an excellent cod liver oil each day, or caplets. The amount consumed should be based upon the amount of sunlight you receive. People in colder climates generally need to consume larger amounts. Cod liver oil is a fantastic source of the omega-3 fats DHA and EPA, as well as fat-soluble vitamins A and D.

Vegetable juice: Consume vegetable juices that are low in carbohydrates, such as celery and green juices mixed with a small amount of higher carbohydrate veggies such as carrot or beet. Mix in some form of healthy fat with each glass of the juice. One to three teaspoons of cultured goat's milk, extra virgin coconut oil, canned or fresh coconut milk and cream, or flaxseed oil enhance absorption of minerals and prevents spikes in blood sugar.

Fermented vegetables: Consume a few tablespoons of fermented vegetables such as sauerkraut with each meal to aid in digestion. Fermented vegetables are an excellent source of naturally occurring probiotics and enzymes.

Stocks: It is a great idea to consume stocks on a regular basis, especially when you have a cold or flu. Stocks made from the bones of chicken, fish, lamb, and beef contain minerals, gelatin, cartilage, collagen, and electrolytes from the vegetables. Stocks are an excellent source of proteins, especially collagen. They help to heal the gut lining and reduce inflammation.

Supplements

Consume the following dietary supplements, along with the recommended foods and beverages, to support chronic fatigue:

A probiotic with SBOs. When it comes to chronic fatigue, be sure to use a supplement with SBOs because human herpes virus-6 (HHV-6) is one of numerous causes of chronic fatigue syndrome.

HHV-6 is a nasty virus that infects a wide range of the body's cells, including brain, immune, and endothelial cells. The virus comes in two variants (A and B) with the A variant attracting most of the attention. Not surprisingly, HHV-6 is closely related to herpes simplex virus-1—that herpes virus most of us have heard about, which causes genital and oral herpes—but it's potentially far more devastating and might cause many different kinds of autoimmune disorders as well.

SBOs can help because they produce bio-surfactants that destroy lipid-enveloped viruses such as HHV-6. The addition of SBOs ensures that the immune system is brought back into balance by normalizing overproduction of compounds such as interleukins and tumor necrosis factor-alpha.

Take six to twelve capsules of a probiotic with SBOs per day and stay on that amount for three to six months or when tests for your affliction are negative. Then begin to gradually decrease to a maintenance dosage of between three to six capsules per day. Probiotics with SBOs are best taken first thing in the morning and right before bedtime with eight ounces pure water. Probiotics with SBOs may be taken with other nutritional supplements, but should be taken one hour apart from medications. If you experience symptoms of detoxification (i.e., increased elimination, loose stools, constipation, excess gas, flu-like symptoms, or fever), reduce the dosage and work up slowly to twelve per day.

A green superfood powder. Take two tablespoons twice daily with eight ounces water or fresh vegetable juice. Best taken on an empty stomach away from food.

Digestive enzymes. Take one to three capsules with each meal or snack.

An organic fiber supplement with chia seed. Consume one serving twice per day, morning and evening, with eight or more ounces of purified water. (Consuming a fiber supplement is essential during the first two weeks of the program. Thereafter, consume fiber as needed.)

A protein powder from bone broth. Take one to three servings per day mixed in water, juice, smoothies, yogurt, or can be used in many recipes.

Additional Therapies

For people who have or may have an imbalanced immune system, avoiding contact with chlorinated water is of the utmost importance. That includes bathing water and drinking water. Chlorine kills bacteria, friendly and unfriendly, in the intestines and can be absorbed through the skin. I recommend installing a shower filter to remove chlorine. Avoid swimming in chlorinated water as well.

Cold and Flu (also see Viral Diseases)

Overview

Seasonal colds and flus can be inconvenient to one's lifestyle. The best course of action is to use natural means and allow the seasonal bug to run its course. I believe that every time one is able to overcome a cold or flu without medication, he or she will be healthier for it.

Occasionally, we need a good cold or flu to stimulate the body's cleansing processes. Maybe there is a good reason for us to get a cold or flu every once in a while. While we admit it is no fun to be laid up in bed, aching, feverish, and nauseous, your body might actually be doing something terrific for your long-term health.

One line of thought posits that when we become feverish, our bodies actually do much more than simply vanquish a single pathogen but actually cleanse the tissues of many pathogens and even cancerous cells. Thus, an occasional cold or flu is your body's natural cleansing and detoxifying response.

When we take antibiotics or prevent this process altogether, however, we may be weakening our health by not allowing the body to go through this cleansing.

Diet

During a bout of cold or flu, it's important to only eat when hungry, which gives the body ample opportunity to heal itself. Consuming the foods mentioned below can insure a healthy and speedy recovery.

Therapeutic Foods

These therapeutic foods will help you get well:

Extra virgin coconut oil: This oil is perhaps the healthiest of the widely available oils. I recommend cooking almost exclusively with extra virgin coconut oil. Consume as much as two to four tablespoons per day during a bout of cold or flu. Extra virgin coconut oil can be used in cooking, in smoothies, or consumed right off the spoon. Extra virgin coconut oil contains large amounts of lauric, capric, and caprylic acids, which are potent antiviral and antifungal compounds.

Ocean-caught fish: This type of fish is perhaps the healthiest of all protein sources. It's important to consume a high-quality source of protein during a cold or flu bout, and fish is a great source. Salmon, sardines, mackerel, herring, and albacore tuna are high in the omega-3 fatty acids EPA and DHA. Ocean-caught fish can be consumed every day to enhance digestive and immune system health.

Cod liver oil: Take three teaspoons of an excellent cod liver for the duration of a cold or flu. The amount consumed should be based upon the amount of sunlight you receive. People in colder climates generally need to consume larger amounts. Cod liver oil is a fantastic source of the omega-3 fats DHA and EPA, as well as fat-soluble vitamins A and D.

Vegetable juice: Consume vegetable juices that are low in carbohydrates, such as celery and green juices mixed with a small amount of higher carbohydrate veggies such as carrot or beet. Mix in some form of healthy fat with each glass of the juice. One to three teaspoons of cultured goat's milk, extra virgin coconut oil, canned or fresh coconut milk and cream, or flaxseed oil enhance absorption of minerals and prevents spikes in blood sugar.

Chicken Soup: It's a great idea to consume chicken soup (or stocks) on a regular basis, especially when you have a cold or flu. Going on a one- to three-day chicken soup fast can be extremely helpful to eliminate even the toughest cold or flu. Even if you don't go on an exclusively chicken soup diet, consuming some chicken soup daily will be very helpful.

Supplements

Consume the following dietary supplements, along with the recommended foods and beverages, to overcome a flu or cold:

A probiotic with SBOs. Probiotics with SBOs are best taken first thing in the morning and right before bedtime with eight ounces pure water. Probiotics with SBOs may be taken with other nutritional supplements, but should be taken one hour apart from medications. If you experience symptoms of detoxification (i.e., increased elimination, loose stools, constipation, excess gas, flu-like symptoms, or fever), reduce the dosage and work up slowly to twelve per day.

A green superfood powder. Take two tablespoons twice daily with eight ounces water or fresh vegetable juice. Best taken on an empty stomach away from food.

An organic fiber supplement with chia seed. Consume one serving twice per day, morning and evening, with eight or more ounces of purified water. (Consuming a fiber supplement is essential during the first two weeks of the program. Thereafter, consume fiber as needed.)

A protein powder from bone broth. Take one to three servings per day mixed in water, juice, smoothies, yogurt, or can be used in many recipes.

Additional Therapies

For people who have or may have imbalanced intestinal flora, avoiding contact with chlorinated water is of the utmost importance. That includes bathing water and drinking water. Chlorine kills bacteria, friendly and unfriendly, in the intestines and can be absorbed through the skin. I recommend installing a shower filter to remove chlorine. Avoid swimming in chlorinated water as well.

Colon Cleansing

I discussed the relationship of intestinal toxemia to poor health in Chapter 3, so it should be clear that colon cleansing is not only important but essential in order to regain your health and maintain it. With daily colon cleansing, you will avoid buildup of harmful bacteria and mucus. Our colon should be cleansed daily through the consumption of foods rich in probiotics and enzymes.

Diet

Follow the Maker's Diet as best you can for six to twelve months. For those who want to thoroughly cleanse the colon, consume large amounts of vegetables as well as cleansing fruits such as figs, grapes, watermelon, stone fruits (plums, apricots, and peaches) and small berries such as blueberries and raspberries. Be sure to consume cleansing beverages such as cultured goat's milk yogurt, fermented vegetables, vegetable juices, and lacto-fermented beverages daily.

Therapeutic Foods

These therapeutic foods will help you get well:

Cultured goat's milk dairy products: Consume 8 to 32 ounces of the highest quality cultured dairy products from goat's milk.

Grass-fed red meat: Red meat from grass-fed cattle, buffalo, and lamb is very healthy and can be eaten a few times per week. This meat is a great source of protein, minerals, vitamin B_{12}, vitamins A and D, omega-3 fats, and CLA.

Organic, pasture-raised eggs: Consume as many as two organic eggs high in omega-3 fatty acids each day. These eggs contain DHA, vitamins E and B_{12}, and antioxidants including lutein.

Extra virgin coconut oil: This oil is perhaps the healthiest of the widely available oils. I recommend cooking almost exclusively with extra virgin coconut oil. Consume as much as two to four tablespoons per day of the oil in cooking, smoothies, or right off the spoon. Coconut oil contains large amounts of lauric acid, a potent antimicrobial and one of the chief fatty acids found in breast milk.

Ocean-caught fish: This type of fish is perhaps the healthiest of all protein sources. Salmon, sardines, mackerel, herring, and albacore tuna are high in the omega-3 fatty acids EPA and DHA. Ocean-caught fish can be consumed every day to enhance digestive and immune system health.

Cod liver oil: Take one to three teaspoons of an excellent cod liver oil each day, or caplets. The amount consumed should be based upon the amount of sunlight you receive. People in colder climates generally need to consume larger amounts. Cod liver oil is a fantastic source of the omega-3 fats DHA and EPA, as well as fat-soluble vitamins A and D.

Vegetable juice: Consume vegetable juices that are low in carbohydrates, such as celery and green juices mixed with a small amount of higher carbohydrate veggies such as carrot or beet. Mix in some form of healthy fat with each glass of the juice. One to three teaspoons of cultured goat's milk, extra virgin coconut oil, canned or fresh coconut milk and cream, or flaxseed oil enhance absorption of minerals and prevents spikes in blood sugar.

Fermented vegetables: Consume a few tablespoons of fermented vegetables such as sauerkraut with each meal to aid in digestion. Fermented vegetables are an excellent source of naturally occurring probiotics and enzymes.

Berries: Consuming high-fiber berries such as blueberries and raspberries can lead to effective daily colon cleansing as well as provide the body with antioxidants.

Stocks: It is a great idea to consume stocks on a regular basis, especially when you have a cold or flu. Stocks made from the bones of chicken, fish, lamb, and beef contain minerals, gelatin, cartilage, collagen, and electrolytes from the vegetables. Stocks are an excellent source of proteins, especially collagen. They help to heal the gut lining and reduce inflammation.

Supplements

Take these health supplements to alleviate symptoms and get well:

A probiotic with SBOs. Start with one caplet per day on an empty stomach, thirty minutes before or one hour after meals. Increase usage by adding one additional caplet per day (i.e., one caplet the first day, two the second day, three the third day, and so on). Once your dosage is up to twelve caplets per day, stay on that amount for a minimum of three months and then begin to gradually decrease to a maintenance dosage of between three to six caplets per day. A probiotic with SBOs is best taken first thing in the morning and right before bedtime with eight ounces pure water. If you experience symptoms of detoxification (i.e., increased elimination, loose stools, constipation, excess gas, flu-like symptoms, or fever), reduce the dosage and work up slowly to twelve per day.

A green superfood powder. Take two tablespoons twice daily with eight ounces water or fresh vegetable juice. Best taken on an empty stomach away from food.

Digestive enzymes. Take one to three capsules with each meal or snack.

An organic fiber supplement with chia seed. Consume one serving twice per day, morning and evening, with eight or more ounces of purified water. (Consuming a fiber supplement is essential during the first two weeks of the program. Thereafter, consume fiber as needed.)

A protein powder from bone broth. Take one to three servings per day mixed in water, juice, smoothies, yogurt, or can be used in many recipes.

Additional Therapies

For people who have or may have imbalanced intestinal flora, avoiding contact with chlorinated water is of the utmost importance. That includes bathing water and drinking water. Chlorine kills bacteria, friendly and unfriendly, in the intestines, and can be absorbed through the skin. I recommend installing a shower filter to remove chlorine. Avoid swimming in chlorinated water as well.

Be sure to read the Lifestyle Therapies section at the start of this chapter.

Crohn's Disease...see Chronic Digestive Disease

Dementia...see Brain Health

Depression...see Mental Disorders

Dermatitis...see Skin Health

Detoxification

Detoxification in our modern vernacular is usually thought of as unburdening the human body of chemical toxins such as pesticides, heavy metals, industrial chemicals, radiation, and other toxins. This is an essential process to relieve each individual's growing burden of toxicity, which can lead to cancer, heart disease, premature aging, and many other maladies.

Diet

Follow the Maker's Diet as best you can for six to twelve months. After the body has been properly detoxified, I strongly recommend that you adhere to a diet of foods in the "Extraordinary" category for the rest of your life.

Therapeutic Foods

These therapeutic foods will help you get well:

Cultured goat's milk dairy products: Consume 8 to 32 ounces of the highest quality cultured dairy products from goat's milk. Try to find yogurt that does not contain the organism *Streptococcus thermophilus*, a bacterial microbe that has been known to make immune system disorders worse.

Grass-fed red meat: Red meat from grass-fed cattle, buffalo, and lamb is very healthy and can be eaten a few times per week. This meat is a great source of protein, minerals, vitamin B_{12}, vitamins A and D, omega-3 fats, and CLA.

Organic, pasture-raised eggs: Consume as many as one to three organic eggs high in omega-3 fatty acids each day. These eggs contain DHA, vitamins E and B_{12}, and antioxidants including lutein.

Extra virgin coconut oil: This oil is perhaps the healthiest of the widely available oils. I recommend cooking almost exclusively with extra virgin coconut oil. Consume as much as two to four tablespoons per day of the oil in cooking, smoothies, or right off the spoon. Coconut oil contains large amounts of lauric acid, a potent antimicrobial and one of the chief fatty acids found in breast milk.

Ocean-caught fish: This type of fish is perhaps the healthiest of all protein sources. Salmon, sardines, mackerel, herring, and albacore tuna are high in the omega-3 fatty acids EPA and DHA. Ocean-caught fish can be consumed every day to enhance digestive and immune system health.

Cod liver oil: Take one to three teaspoons of an excellent cod liver oil each day, or caplets. The amount consumed should be based upon the amount of sunlight you receive. People in colder climates generally need to consume larger amounts. Cod liver oil is a fantastic source of the omega-3 fats DHA and EPA, as well as fat-soluble vitamins A and D.

Berries: The daily consumption of berries, including blueberries, strawberries, blackberries, and raspberries, can provide the body with antioxidants that can neutralize harmful toxins damaging to the body. Berries supply rich sources of dietary fiber.

Vegetable juice: Consume vegetable juices that are low in carbohydrates, such as celery and green juices mixed with a small amount of higher carbohydrate veggies such as carrot or beet. Mix in some form of healthy fat with each glass of the juice. One to three teaspoons of cultured goat's milk, extra virgin coconut oil, canned or fresh coconut milk and cream, or flaxseed oil enhance absorption of minerals and prevents spikes in blood sugar.

Fermented vegetables: Consume a few tablespoons of fermented vegetables such as sauerkraut with each meal to aid in digestion. Fermented vegetables are an excellent source of naturally occurring probiotics and enzymes.

Stocks: It is a great idea to consume stocks on a regular basis, especially when you have a cold or flu. Stocks made from the bones of chicken, fish, lamb, and beef contain minerals, gelatin, cartilage, collagen, and electrolytes from the vegetables. Stocks are an excellent source of proteins, especially collagen. They help to heal the gut lining and reduce inflammation.

Supplements

Consume the following dietary supplements, along with the recommended foods and beverages, to help overcome this condition:

A probiotic, enzyme, and herbs formulation designed to support detoxification.

A probiotic with SBOs. Take six to twelve capsules per day and stay on that amount for three to six months or when tests for your affliction are negative. Then begin to gradually decrease to a maintenance dosage of between three to six capsules per day. Probiotics with SBOs are best taken first thing in the morning and right before bedtime with eight ounces pure water. Probiotics with SBOs may be taken with other nutritional supplements, but should be taken one hour apart from medications. If you experience symptoms of detoxification (i.e., increased elimination, loose stools, constipation, excess gas, flu-like symptoms, or fever), reduce the dosage and work up slowly to twelve per day.

A green superfood powder. Take two tablespoons twice daily with eight ounces water or fresh vegetable juice. Best taken on an empty stomach away from food.

Digestive enzymes. Take one to three capsules with each meal or snack.

An organic fiber supplement with chia seed. Consume one serving twice per day, morning and evening, with eight or more ounces of purified water. (Consuming a fiber supplement is essential during the first two weeks of the program. Thereafter, consume fiber as needed.)

A protein powder from bone broth. Take one to three servings per day mixed in water, juice, smoothies, yogurt, or can be used in many recipes.

Additional Therapies

In order to properly detoxify the body, avoiding contact with chlorinated water is of the utmost importance. That includes bathing water and drinking water. Chlorine kills bacteria, friendly and unfriendly, in the intestines, and can be absorbed through the skin. I recommend installing a shower filter to remove chlorine. Avoid swimming in chlorinated water as well.

I especially recommend regular use of low-heat saunas.

Diabetes Type 1…see Autoimmune Disease

Diabetes Type 2…see Blood Sugar Imbalances

Diverticulitis…see Chronic Digestive Disease

Dyspepsia...see Functional Bowel Disorders

Eczema...see Skin Health

Endometriosis...see Female Health

Epstein–Barr Virus...see Viral Diseases

Erectile Dysfunction...see Male Health

Female Health

- Endometriosis
- Ovarian Cysts
- Fibrocystic Breast Disease
- Premenstrual Syndrome (PMS)
- Menopause
- Uterine Fibroids
- Osteoporosis

Overview

One of the key issues for women's health is to maintain balanced estrogen levels. By improving their estrogen profile, women can markedly reduce their risk of breast cancer, one of the major causes of death for women. This can be done by following dietary measures and avoiding exposure to environmental xenoestrogens.

Most of us know that estrogen is the hormone responsible for stimulating development of female characteristics as well as the hormone that changes girls into women. There is nothing evil or bad about estrogen—as long as the estrogen to which your body is exposed is derived from the healthy functioning of your organs and glands.

The key here is the body's balance of estrogen. Different aspects of your diet, lifestyle, medications prescribed by your doctor, the cosmetics you use, and consumption of alcohol all influence estrogen balance in your body.

The body produces different types of estrogen—estradiol, estrone, and estriol. Estrone and estriol are much weaker estrogens than estradiol.

The body converts estradiol, the most potent estrogen, either to "good" estrogen (2-hydroxyestrone), which is weakly anti-estrogenic and reduces risk of breast cancer, or "bad" estrogen (16-alpha-hydroxyestrone), which is more long-lived and potent, stimulates breast cell proliferation, and is carcinogenic. High levels of this bad estrogen are a "risk marker" or an indication of increased risk of breast cancer.

Phytoestrogens and lignans are a group of naturally occurring chemicals derived from plants; they have a structure similar to estrogen and form part of our diet. They also have potentially anticarcinogenic biological activity.

Thus, they appear to be an effective dietary means for reducing cancer risk by improving estrogen metabolism. Many studies associate higher levels of circulating phytoestrogens and lignans with overall improved women's health and improved estrogen profiles.

And just how should women go about raising their blood levels of the lignans? That answer comes to us from a report published in the *European Journal of Clinical Nutrition*.

The purpose of this study was to investigate the effects of flaxseed supplementation as a part of daily diet on serum lipids, fatty acids, and plasma enterolactone. Eighty volunteers participated in this clinical nutrition study, which was carried out in a controlled, double-blind manner. There was a significant increase in serum alpha-linolenic acid, eicosapentaenoic acid, and DHA, the major omega-3 fatty acids found in flaxseed. Serum enterolactone concentration was doubled during flaxseed supplementation.

"In this study we were able to show that by adding ground flaxseed and flaxseed oil to one or two daily meals, it was possible to obtain significant effects on serum levels of enterolactone and alpha-linolenic acid," the researchers said.

This leads to the next dramatic finding—that by raising levels of alpha-linolenic, eicosapentaenoic, and DHA, women are further protecting themselves against breast cancer (as well as heart disease and arthritis).

Experimental studies have indicated that omega-3 fatty acids, including alpha-linolenic, eicosapentaenoic, and DHA, inhibit mammary tumor growth and metastasis. To clinically evaluate whether omega-3 fatty acids protect against breast cancer, researchers in a study published in the *International Journal of Cancer* examined the fatty acid composition in adipose tissue from 241 patients with invasive, non-metastatic breast carcinoma and from 88 patients with benign breast disease, in a case-control study in Tours, central France.

Women with the highest levels of alpha-linolenic acid had a 61 percent reduced risk of breast cancer compared to women with the lowest levels. In a similar way, women with the highest levels of DHA had a reduced risk of 69 percent, compared to women with the lowest levels. "In conclusion, our data based on fatty acids levels in breast adipose tissue suggest a protective effect of n-3 fatty acids on breast cancer risk and support the hypothesis that the balance between n-3 and n-6 fatty acids plays a role in breast cancer," the researchers said.

It is clear that by reducing levels of "bad" estrogen a women's risk of breast cancer is reduced. The most effective and safe way of doing so is with diet—including more flaxseeds, fish, high omega-3 eggs, and fermented foods.

Diet

Choose mainly foods from the "Extraordinary" category until optimal health is achieved for at least three months (or if experiencing symptoms such as painful PMS, hot flashes, bone loss, low libido, or low energy). Once symptoms are greatly improved, you may gradually add foods from the "Average" or "Trouble" categories if desired.

Therapeutic Foods

These therapeutic foods will help you feel better:

Cultured goat's milk dairy products: Consume 8 to 32 ounces of the highest quality cultured dairy products from goat's milk. Try to find yogurt that does not contain the organism *Streptococcus thermophilus*, a bacterial microbe that has been known to make immune system disorders worse.

Grass-fed red meat: Red meat from grass-fed cattle, buffalo, and lamb is very healthy and can be eaten a few times per week. This meat is a great source of protein, minerals, vitamin B_{12}, vitamins A and D, omega-3 fats, and CLA.

Organic, pasture-raised eggs: Consume as many as two organic eggs high in omega-3 fatty acids each day. These eggs contain DHA, vitamins E and B$_{12}$, and antioxidants including lutein.

Extra virgin coconut oil: This oil is perhaps the healthiest of the widely available oils. I recommend cooking almost exclusively with extra virgin coconut oil. Consume as much as two to four tablespoons per day of the oil in cooking, smoothies, or right off the spoon. Coconut oil contains large amounts of lauric acid, a potent antimicrobial and one of the chief fatty acids found in breast milk.

Ocean-caught fish: This type of fish is perhaps the healthiest of all protein sources. Salmon, sardines, mackerel, herring, and albacore tuna are high in the omega-3 fatty acids EPA and DHA. Ocean-caught fish can be consumed every day to enhance digestive and immune system health.

Cod liver oil: Take one to three teaspoons of an excellent cod liver oil each day, or caplets. The amount consumed should be based upon the amount of sunlight you receive. People in colder climates generally need to consume larger amounts. Cod liver oil is a fantastic source of the omega-3 fats DHA and EPA, as well as fat-soluble vitamins A and D.

Vegetable juice: Consume vegetable juices that are low in carbohydrates, such as celery and green juices mixed with a small amount of higher carbohydrate veggies such as carrot or beet. Mix in some form of healthy fat with each glass of the juice. One to three teaspoons of cultured goat's milk, extra virgin coconut oil, canned or fresh coconut milk and cream, or flaxseed oil enhance absorption of minerals and prevents spikes in blood sugar.

Fermented vegetables: Consume a few tablespoons of fermented vegetables such as sauerkraut with each meal to aid in digestion. Fermented vegetables are an excellent source of naturally occurring probiotics and enzymes.

Stocks: It is a great idea to consume stocks on a regular basis, especially when you are undergoing treatment. Stocks made from the bones of chicken, fish, lamb, and beef contain minerals, gelatin, cartilage, collagen, and electrolytes from the vegetables. Stocks are an excellent source of proteins, especially collagen. They help to heal the gut lining and reduce inflammation.

Supplements

Take these health supplements to alleviate symptoms and get well:

A probiotic, enzyme, and herbs formulation designed to support women's health.

A probiotic with SBOs. Take six to twelve capsules per day and stay on that amount for three to six months or when tests for your affliction are negative. Then begin to gradually decrease to a maintenance dosage of between three to six capsules per day. Probiotics with SBOs are best taken first thing in the morning and right before bedtime with eight ounces pure water. Probiotics with SBOs may be taken with other nutritional supplements, but should be taken one hour apart from medications. If you experience symptoms of detoxification (i.e., increased elimination, loose stools, constipation, excess gas, flu-like symptoms, or fever), reduce the dosage and work up slowly to twelve per day.

A green superfood powder. Take two tablespoons twice daily with eight ounces water or fresh vegetable juice. Best taken on an empty stomach away from food.

Digestive enzymes. Take one to three capsules with each meal or snack.

An organic fiber supplement with chia seed. Consume one serving twice per day, morning and evening, with eight or more ounces of purified water. (Consuming a fiber supplement is essential during the first two weeks of the program. Thereafter, consume fiber as needed.)

A protein powder from bone broth. Take one to three servings per day mixed in water, juice, smoothies, yogurt, or can be used in many recipes.

Additional Therapies

For those who have or may have imbalanced intestinal flora or a weak immune system, avoiding contact with chlorinated water is of the utmost importance. That includes bathing water and drinking water. Chlorine kills bacteria, friendly and unfriendly, in the intestines and can be absorbed through the skin. I recommend installing a shower filter to remove chlorine. Avoid swimming in chlorinated water as well.

Fibrocystic Breast Disease…see Female Health

Flu…see Cold and Flu and Viral Diseases

Food Allergies/Chemical Sensitivities

Overview

Food allergies and chemical sensitivities are conditions marked by our modern lifestyles. Food allergies may be life-threatening and debilitating or simply result in uncomfortable symptoms ranging from intestinal distress to faintness and rapid heartbeat (as in the case of persons sensitive to MSG).

It's not uncommon to find chronic diseases linked with long-standing food allergies. In many cases, helping to restore proper digestion and a healthy intestinal lining are key to improving food allergies and intolerances.

Diet

Choose mainly foods from the "Extraordinary" category until optimal health is achieved for at least three months. If you have known allergies to certain foods, it's best to limit those for at least the first few months on the program. You can often return to eating foods that you were previously allergic to once the gastrointestinal and immune systems are functioning properly.

Once symptoms are greatly improved, you may gradually add foods from the "Average" and "Trouble" categories if desired. Because people with food allergies and/or chemical sensitivities appear to have a predisposed weakness in their gastrointestinal tract, I strongly recommend that they adhere to a diet of foods in the "Extraordinary" category for the rest of their lives.

Therapeutic Foods

These therapeutic foods will help you get well:

Cultured goat's milk dairy products: Consume 8 to 32 ounces of the highest quality cultured dairy products from goat's milk. Try to find yogurt that does not contain the organism *Streptococcus thermophilus*, a bacterial microbe that has been known to make immune system disorders worse.

Grass-fed red meat: Red meat from grass-fed cattle, buffalo, and lamb is very healthy and can be eaten a few times per week. This meat is a great source of protein, minerals, vitamin B_{12}, vitamins A and D, omega-3 fats, and CLA.

Organic, pasture-raised eggs: Consume as many as two organic eggs high in omega-3 fatty acids each day. These eggs contain DHA, vitamins E and B$_{12}$, and antioxidants including lutein.

Extra virgin coconut oil: This oil is perhaps the healthiest of the widely available oils. I recommend cooking almost exclusively with extra virgin coconut oil. Consume as much as two to four tablespoons per day of the oil in cooking, smoothies, or right off the spoon. Coconut oil contains large amounts of lauric acid, a potent antimicrobial and one of the chief fatty acids found in breast milk.

Ocean-caught fish: This type of fish is perhaps the healthiest of all protein sources. Salmon, sardines, mackerel, herring, and albacore tuna are high in the omega-3 fatty acids EPA and DHA. Ocean-caught fish can be consumed every day to enhance digestive and immune system health.

Cod liver oil: Take one to three teaspoons of an excellent cod liver oil each day, or caplets. The amount consumed should be based upon the amount of sunlight you receive. People in colder climates generally need to consume larger amounts. Cod liver oil is a fantastic source of the omega-3 fats DHA and EPA, as well as fat-soluble vitamins A and D.

Vegetable juice: Consume vegetable juices that are low in carbohydrates, such as celery and green juices mixed with a small amount of higher carbohydrate veggies such as carrot or beet. Mix in some form of healthy fat with each glass of the juice. One to three teaspoons of cultured goat's milk, extra virgin coconut oil, canned or fresh coconut milk and cream, or flaxseed oil enhance absorption of minerals and prevents spikes in blood sugar.

Fermented vegetables: Consume a few tablespoons of fermented vegetables such as sauerkraut with each meal to aid in digestion. Fermented vegetables are an excellent source of naturally occurring probiotics and enzymes.

Stocks: It is a great idea to consume stocks on a regular basis, especially when you are undergoing treatment. Stocks made from the bones of chicken, fish, lamb, and beef contain minerals, gelatin, cartilage, collagen, and electrolytes from the vegetables. Stocks are an excellent source of proteins, especially collagen. They help to heal the gut lining and reduce inflammation.

Supplements

Take these health supplements to alleviate symptoms and get well:

A probiotic, enzyme, and herbs formulation designed to support food allergies and chemical sensitivities.

A probiotic with SBOs. Take six to twelve capsules per day and stay on that amount for three to six months or when tests for your affliction are negative. Then begin to gradually decrease to a maintenance dosage of between three to six capsules per day. Probiotics with SBOs are best taken first thing in the morning and right before bedtime with eight ounces pure water. Probiotics with SBOs may be taken with other nutritional supplements, but should be taken one hour apart from medications. If you experience symptoms of detoxification (i.e., increased elimination, loose stools, constipation, excess gas, flu-like symptoms, or fever), reduce the dosage and work up slowly to twelve per day.

A green superfood powder. Take two tablespoons twice daily with eight ounces water or fresh vegetable juice. Best taken on an empty stomach away from food.

Digestive enzymes. Take one to three capsules with each meal or snack.

An organic fiber supplement with chia seed. Consume one serving twice per day, morning and evening, with eight or more ounces of purified water. (Consuming a fiber supplement is essential during the first two weeks of the program. Thereafter, consume fiber as needed.)

A protein powder from bone broth. Take one to three servings per day mixed in water, juice, smoothies, yogurt, or can be used in many recipes.

Additional Therapies

For people who have or may have imbalanced intestinal flora or a weak immune system, avoiding contact with chlorinated water is of the utmost importance. That includes bathing water and drinking water. Chlorine kills bacteria, friendly and unfriendly, in the intestines and can be absorbed through the skin. I recommend installing a shower filter to remove chlorine. Avoid swimming in chlorinated water as well.

Functional Bowel Disorders

- Chronic Constipation
- IBS
- Chronic Diarrhea
- Lactose Intolerance
- Dyspepsia
- Leaky Gut Syndrome

Overview

Gastrointestinal disorders affect millions of people of all ages—men, women, and children. They are the most commonly presented gastrointestinal illnesses seen by physicians in primary care or gastroenterology. IBS and dyspepsia are the most common, notes the International Foundation for Functional Gastrointestinal Disorders.

As the international foundation further notes, "A functional disorder does not show any evidence of an organic or physical disease, and the cause of a functional GI disorder doesn't show up in a blood test or an X-ray. The disorders are diagnosed based on symptoms and often require tests to rule out the likelihood of another disease."

It's apparent that functional disorders increase morbidity and diminish a patient's quality of life. For sure, the social and economic costs of gastrointestinal disorders are enormous. The symptoms of these disorders cause discomfort that ranges from inconvenience to deep personal distress. For those with severe symptoms, the disorders can be debilitating, leaving them unable to fully participate in life and work.

Diet

Choose mainly foods from the "Extraordinary" category until optimal health is achieved for at least three months. If you have known allergies to certain foods, it's best to limit those for at least the first few months on the program. You can often return to eating foods that you were previously allergic to once the gastrointestinal and immune systems are functioning properly.

Once symptoms are greatly improved, you may gradually add foods from the "Average" and "Trouble" categories if desired. Because people with functional bowel disorders appear to have a predisposed weakness in their immune systems, I strongly recommend that they adhere to a diet of foods in the "Extraordinary" category for the rest of their lives.

Therapeutic Foods

These therapeutic foods will help you get well:

Cultured goat's milk dairy products: Consume 8 to 32 ounces of the highest quality cultured dairy products from goat's milk. Try to find yogurt that does not contain the organism *Streptococcus thermophilus*, a bacterial microbe that has been known to make immune system disorders worse.

Grass-fed red meat: Red meat from grass-fed cattle, buffalo, and lamb is very healthy and can be eaten a few times per week. This meat is a great source of protein, minerals, vitamin B_{12}, vitamins A and D, omega-3 fats, and CLA.

Organic, pasture-raised eggs: Consume as many as two organic eggs high in omega-3 fatty acids each day. These eggs contain DHA, vitamins E and B_{12}, and antioxidants including lutein.

Extra virgin coconut oil: This oil is perhaps the healthiest of the widely available oils. I recommend cooking almost exclusively with extra virgin coconut oil. Consume as much as two to four tablespoons per day of the oil in cooking, smoothies, or right off the spoon. Coconut oil contains large amounts of lauric acid, a potent antimicrobial and one of the chief fatty acids found in breast milk.

Ocean-caught fish: This type of fish is perhaps the healthiest of all protein sources. Salmon, sardines, mackerel, herring, and albacore tuna are high in the omega-3 fatty acids EPA and DHA. Ocean-caught fish can be consumed every day to enhance digestive and immune system health.

Cod liver oil: Take one to three teaspoons of an excellent cod liver oil each day, or caplets. The amount consumed should be based upon the amount of sunlight you receive. People in colder climates generally need to consume larger amounts. Cod liver oil is a fantastic source of the omega-3 fats DHA and EPA, as well as fat-soluble vitamins A and D.

Vegetable juice: Consume vegetable juices that are low in carbohydrates, such as celery and green juices mixed with a small amount of higher carbohydrate veggies such as carrot or beet. Mix in some form of healthy fat with each glass of the juice. One to three teaspoons of cultured goat's milk, extra virgin coconut oil, canned or fresh coconut milk and cream, or flaxseed oil enhance absorption of minerals and prevents spikes in blood sugar.

Fermented vegetables: Consume a few tablespoons of fermented vegetables such as sauerkraut with each meal to aid in digestion. Fermented vegetables are an excellent source of naturally occurring probiotics and enzymes.

Stocks: It is a great idea to consume stocks on a regular basis, especially when you are undergoing treatment. Stocks made from the bones of chicken, fish, lamb, and beef contain minerals, gelatin, cartilage, collagen, and electrolytes from the vegetables. Stocks are an excellent source of proteins, especially collagen. They help to heal the gut lining and reduce inflammation.

Supplements

Take these health supplements to alleviate symptoms and get well:

A probiotic, enzyme, and herbs formulation designed to support gastrointestinal health.

A probiotic with SBOs. Start with one caplet per day on an empty stomach, thirty minutes before or one hour after meals. Increase usage by adding one additional caplet per day (i.e., one caplet the first day, two the second day, three the third day, and so on). Once your dosage is up to twelve caplets per day, stay on that amount for a minimum of three months and then begin to gradually decrease to a maintenance dosage of between three to six caplets per day.

Probiotics with SBOs are best taken first thing in the morning and right before bedtime with eight ounces pure water. Probiotics with SBOs may be taken with other nutritional supplements, but should be taken one hour apart from medications. If you experience symptoms of detoxification (i.e., increased elimination, loose stools, constipation, excess gas, flu-like symptoms, or fever), reduce the dosage and work up slowly to twelve per day.

A green superfood powder. Take two tablespoons twice daily with eight ounces water or fresh vegetable juice. Best taken on an empty stomach away from food.

Digestive enzymes. Take one to three capsules with each meal or snack.

An organic fiber supplement with chia seed. Consume one serving twice per day, morning and evening, with eight or more ounces of purified water. (Consuming a fiber supplement is essential during the first two weeks of the program. Thereafter, consume fiber as needed.)

A protein powder from bone broth. Take one to three servings per day mixed in water, juice, smoothies, yogurt, or can be used in many recipes.

Additional Therapies

For people who have or may have imbalanced intestinal flora or a weak immune system, avoiding contact with chlorinated water is of the utmost importance. That includes bathing water and drinking water. Chlorine kills bacteria, friendly and unfriendly, in the intestines and can be absorbed through the skin. I recommend installing a shower filter to remove chlorine. Avoid swimming in chlorinated water as well.

General Health Maintenance

In today's world, it's crucial to prevent disease before it starts. By following the principals outlined in *Patient Heal Thyself,* you can improve your health and make great strides in preventing future diseases.

Diet

Follow the Maker's Diet as best you can for ninety days. I strongly recommend that you adhere to a diet of foods in the "Extraordinary" category for the rest of your life.

Therapeutic Foods

These therapeutic foods will help you maintain a feeling of wellness:

Cultured goat's milk dairy products: Consume 8 to 32 ounces of the highest quality cultured dairy products from goat's milk. Try to find yogurt that does not contain the organism *Streptococcus thermophilus*, a bacterial microbe that has been known to make immune system disorders worse.

Grass-fed red meat: Red meat from grass-fed cattle, buffalo, and lamb is very healthy and can be eaten a few times per week. This meat is a great source of protein, minerals, vitamin B$_{12}$, vitamins A and D, omega-3 fats, and CLA.

Organic, pasture-raised eggs: Consume as many as one to three organic eggs high in omega-3 fatty acids each day. These eggs contain DHA, vitamins E and B$_{12}$, and antioxidants including lutein.

Extra virgin coconut oil: This oil is perhaps the healthiest of the widely available oils. I recommend cooking almost exclusively with extra virgin coconut oil. Consume as much as two to four tablespoons per day of the oil in cooking, smoothies, or right off the spoon. Coconut oil contains large amounts of lauric acid, a potent antimicrobial and one of the chief fatty acids found in breast milk.

Ocean-caught fish: This type of fish is perhaps the healthiest of all protein sources. Salmon, sardines, mackerel, herring, and albacore tuna are high in the omega-3 fatty acids EPA and DHA. Ocean-caught fish can be consumed every day to enhance digestive and immune system health.

Cod liver oil: Take one to three teaspoons of an excellent cod liver oil each day, or caplets. The amount consumed should be based upon the amount of sunlight you receive. People in colder climates generally need to consume larger amounts. Cod liver oil is a fantastic source of the omega-3 fats DHA and EPA, as well as fat-soluble vitamins A and D.

Vegetable juice: Consume vegetable juices that are low in carbohydrates, such as celery and green juices mixed with a small amount of higher carbohydrate veggies such as carrot or beet. Mix in some form of healthy fat with each glass of the juice. One to three teaspoons of cultured goat's milk, extra virgin coconut oil, canned or fresh coconut milk and cream, or flaxseed oil enhance absorption of minerals and prevents spikes in blood sugar.

Berries: The daily consumption of berries, including blueberries, strawberries, blackberries, and raspberries, can provide the body with antioxidants that neutralize harmful toxins damaging to the body. Berries supply rich sources of dietary fiber to enhance elimination.

Fermented vegetables: Consume a few tablespoons of fermented vegetables such as sauerkraut with each meal to aid in digestion. Fermented vegetables are an excellent source of naturally occurring probiotics and enzymes.

Stocks: It is a great idea to consume stocks on a regular basis, especially when you have a cold or flu. Stocks made from the bones of chicken, fish, lamb, and beef contain minerals, gelatin, cartilage, collagen, and electrolytes from the vegetables. Stocks are an excellent source of proteins, especially collagen. They help to heal the gut lining and reduce inflammation.

Supplements

Consume the following dietary supplements, along with the recommended foods and beverages, to help overcome this condition:

A probiotic, enzyme, and herbs formulation designed to support general health.

A probiotic with SBOs. Start with one caplet per day on an empty stomach, thirty minutes before or one hour after meals. Increase usage by adding one additional caplet per day (i.e., one caplet the first day, two the second day, three the third day, and so on). Once your dosage is up to twelve caplets per day, stay on that amount for a minimum of three months and then begin to gradually decrease to a maintenance dosage of between three to six caplets per day.

Probiotics with SBOs are best taken first thing in the morning and right before bedtime with eight ounces pure water. Probiotics with SBOs may be taken with other nutritional supplements, but should be taken one hour apart from medications. If you experience symptoms of detoxification (i.e., increased elimination, loose stools, constipation, excess gas, flu-like symptoms, or fever), reduce the dosage and work up slowly to twelve per day.

A green superfood powder. Take two tablespoons twice daily with eight ounces water or fresh vegetable juice. Best taken on an empty stomach away from food.

Digestive enzymes. Take one to three capsules with each meal or snack.

An organic fiber supplement with chia seed. Consume one serving twice per day, morning and evening, with eight or more ounces of purified water. (Consuming a fiber supplement is essential during the first two weeks of the program. Thereafter, consume fiber as needed.)

A protein powder from bone broth. Take one to three servings per day mixed in water, juice, smoothies, yogurt, or can be used in many recipes.

Additional Therapies

In order to maintain health and prevent disease, avoiding contact with chlorinated water is of the utmost importance. That includes bathing water and drinking water. Chlorine kills bacteria, friendly and unfriendly, in the intestines and can be absorbed through the skin. I recommend installing a shower filter to remove chlorine. Avoid swimming in chlorinated water as well.

Gastroesophageal Reflux Disease (GERD)

Overview

When the acidic juices of the stomach splash upward into the esophagus, the result is heartburn. Normally, a ring of muscles called the esophageal sphincter prevents stomach acid from entering the esophagus. But if the muscles relax or open under pressure from acidic juices in the stomach, heartburn may result.

Everyone gets heartburn from time to time, but severe, persistent heartburn that occurs two or more times per week is called gastroesophageal reflux disease, or GERD. Chronic GERD has the potential to scar and damage the lining of the esophagus. The condition can also lead to a condition called Barrett's esophagus, which carries the risk of developing esophageal cancer.

Heartburn has many different causes. Heartburn may be caused by overeating, stress, lying down soon after eating, or even wearing clothes that fit too tightly. In addition, alcohol, nicotine, and caffeine relax the esophageal sphincter and allow stomach acid to enter the esophagus. Certain kinds of spicy food can also cause heartburn in some people. Poor digestion is another major contributor to GERD.

Diet

Choose mainly foods from the "Extraordinary" category until optimal health is achieved for at least three months. Once symptoms are greatly improved, you may gradually add foods from the "Average" or "Trouble" categories if desired. Because people with GERD appear to have a predisposed weakness in their gastrointestinal tract, I strongly recommend that they adhere to a diet of foods in the "Extraordinary" category for the rest of their lives.

Therapeutic Foods

These therapeutic foods will help you get well:

Cultured goat's milk dairy products: Consume 8 to 32 ounces of the highest quality cultured dairy products from goat's milk. Try to find yogurt that does not contain the organism *Streptococcus thermophilus*, a bacterial microbe that has been known to make immune system disorders worse.

Grass-fed red meat: Red meat from grass-fed cattle, buffalo, and lamb is very healthy and can be eaten a few times per week. This meat is a great source of protein, minerals, vitamin B_{12}, vitamins A and D, omega-3 fats, and CLA.

Organic, pasture-raised eggs: Consume as many as two organic eggs high in omega-3 fatty acids each day. These eggs contain DHA, vitamins E and B_{12}, and antioxidants including lutein.

Extra virgin coconut oil: This oil is perhaps the healthiest of the widely available oils. I recommend cooking almost exclusively with extra virgin coconut oil. Consume as much as two to four tablespoons per day of the oil in cooking, smoothies, or right off the spoon. Coconut oil contains large amounts of lauric acid, a potent antimicrobial and one of the chief fatty acids found in breast milk.

Ocean-caught fish: This type of fish is perhaps the healthiest of all protein sources. Salmon, sardines, mackerel, herring, and albacore tuna are high in the omega-3 fatty acids EPA and DHA. Ocean-caught fish can be consumed every day to enhance digestive and immune system health.

Cod liver oil: Take one to three teaspoons of an excellent cod liver oil each day, or caplets. The amount consumed should be based upon the amount of sunlight you receive. People in colder climates generally need to consume larger amounts. Cod liver oil is a fantastic source of the omega-3 fats DHA and EPA, as well as fat-soluble vitamins A and D.

Vegetable juice: Consume vegetable juices that are low in carbohydrates, such as celery and green juices mixed with a small amount of higher carbohydrate veggies such as carrot or beet. Mix in some form of healthy fat with each glass of the juice. One to three teaspoons of cultured goat's milk, extra virgin coconut oil, canned or fresh coconut milk and cream, or flaxseed oil enhance absorption of minerals and prevents spikes in blood sugar.

Fermented vegetables: Consume a few tablespoons of fermented vegetables such as sauerkraut with each meal to aid in digestion. Fermented vegetables are an excellent source of naturally occurring probiotics and enzymes.

Stocks: It is a great idea to consume stocks on a regular basis, especially when you are undergoing treatment. Stocks made from the bones of chicken, fish, lamb, and beef contain minerals, gelatin, cartilage, collagen, and electrolytes from the vegetables. Stocks are an excellent source of proteins, especially collagen. They help to heal the gut lining and reduce inflammation.

Supplements

Take these health supplements to alleviate symptoms and get well:

A probiotic, enzyme, and herbs formulation designed to support gastrointestinal health.

A probiotic with SBOs. Start with one caplet per day on an empty stomach, thirty minutes before or one hour after meals. Increase usage by adding one additional caplet per day (i.e., one caplet the first day, two the second day, three the third day, and so on). Once your dosage is up to twelve caplets per day, stay on that amount for a minimum of three months and then begin to gradually decrease to a maintenance dosage of between three to six caplets per day.

Probiotics with SBOs are best taken first thing in the morning and right before bedtime with eight ounces pure water. Probiotics with SBOs may be taken with other nutritional supplements, but should be taken one hour apart from medications. If you experience symptoms of detoxification (i.e., increased elimination, loose stools, constipation, excess gas, flu-like symptoms, or fever), reduce the dosage and work up slowly to twelve per day.

A green superfood powder. Take two tablespoons twice daily with eight ounces water or fresh vegetable juice. Best taken on an empty stomach away from food.

Digestive enzymes. Take one to three capsules with each meal or snack.

An organic fiber supplement with chia seed. Consume one serving twice per day, morning and evening, with eight or more ounces of purified water. (Consuming a fiber supplement is essential during the first two weeks of the program. Thereafter, consume fiber as needed.)

A protein powder from bone broth. Take one to three servings per day mixed in water, juice, smoothies, yogurt, or can be used in many recipes.

Additional Therapies

For people who have or may have imbalanced intestinal flora or a weak immune system, avoiding contact with chlorinated water is of the utmost importance. That includes bathing water and drinking water. Chlorine kills bacteria, friendly and unfriendly, in the intestines and can be absorbed through the skin. I recommend installing a shower filter to remove chlorine. Avoid swimming in chlorinated water as well.

Gout…see Joint Disorders

Grave's Disease…see Autoimmune Disease

Heartburn…see Gastroesophageal Reflux Disease (GERD)

Heavy Metal Poisoning…Detoxification

Hepatitis…see Viral Diseases

Herpes…see Viral Diseases

Hypoglycemia…see Blood Sugar Imbalances

Immune Health (Optional)

By now readers are certainly aware of my strongly held belief that immune health and gastrointestinal health are inexorably intertwined. Whether we are presently enjoying super health or suffering from illness, our immune system is of paramount importance to our well-being.

If you are healthy, your immune system is charged with the important mission of maintaining your equilibrium. If you are ill, your immune system is charged with helping you to become well. No matter what your level of health, your immune system will play a role. That is why taking care of your immune health is so important to your overall health.

Diet

For general health, it's best to consume a majority of your diet from the "Extraordinary" category.

Therapeutic Foods

These therapeutic foods will help you stay well:

Cultured goat's milk dairy products: Consume 8 to 32 ounces of the highest quality cultured dairy products from goat's milk. Try to find yogurt that does not contain the organism *Streptococcus thermophilus*, a bacterial microbe that has been known to make immune system disorders worse.

Grass-fed red meat: Red meat from grass-fed cattle, buffalo, and lamb is very healthy and can be eaten a few times per week. This meat is a great source of protein, minerals, vitamin B_{12}, vitamins A and D, omega-3 fats, and CLA.

Organic, pasture-raised eggs: Consume as many as one to three organic eggs high in omega-3 fatty acids each day. These eggs contain DHA, vitamins E and B_{12}, and antioxidants including lutein.

Extra virgin coconut oil: This oil is perhaps the healthiest of the widely available oils. I recommend cooking almost exclusively with extra virgin coconut oil. Consume as much as two to four tablespoons per day of the oil in cooking, smoothies, or right off the spoon. Coconut oil contains large amounts of lauric acid, a potent antimicrobial and one of the chief fatty acids found in breast milk.

Ocean-caught fish: This type of fish is perhaps the healthiest of all protein sources. Salmon, sardines, mackerel, herring, and albacore tuna are high in the omega-3 fatty acids EPA and DHA. Ocean-caught fish can be consumed every day to enhance digestive and immune system health.

Cod liver oil: Take one to three teaspoons of an excellent cod liver oil each day, or caplets. The amount consumed should be based upon the amount of sunlight you receive. People in colder climates generally need to consume larger amounts. Cod liver oil is a fantastic source of the omega-3 fats DHA and EPA, as well as fat-soluble vitamins A and D.

Berries: The daily consumption of berries, including blueberries, strawberries, blackberries, and raspberries, can provide the body with antioxidants that can neutralize harmful toxins damaging to the body. Berries supply rich sources of dietary fiber.

Vegetable juice: Consume vegetable juices that are low in carbohydrates, such as celery and green juices mixed with a small amount of higher carbohydrate veggies such as carrot or beet. Mix in some form of healthy fat with each glass of the juice. One to three teaspoons of cultured goat's milk, extra virgin coconut oil, canned or fresh coconut milk and cream, or flaxseed oil enhance absorption of minerals and prevents spikes in blood sugar.

Fermented vegetables: Consume a few tablespoons of fermented vegetables such as sauerkraut with each meal to aid in digestion. Fermented vegetables are an excellent source of naturally occurring probiotics and enzymes.

Stocks: It is a great idea to consume stocks on a regular basis, especially when you have a cold or flu. Stocks made from the bones of chicken, fish, lamb, and beef contain minerals, gelatin, cartilage, collagen, and electrolytes from the vegetables. Stocks are an excellent source of proteins, especially collagen. They help to heal the gut lining and reduce inflammation.

Supplements

Take these health supplements to maintain immune health:

A probiotic with SBOs. Take three to six capsules per day. Probiotics with SBOs are best taken first thing in the morning and right before bedtime with eight ounces pure water.

A green superfood powder. Take two tablespoons twice daily with eight ounces water or fresh vegetable juice. Best taken on an empty stomach away from food.

Digestive enzymes. Take one to three capsules with each meal or snack.

An organic fiber supplement with chia seed. Consume one serving twice per day, morning and evening, with eight or more ounces of purified water. (Consuming a fiber supplement is essential during the first two weeks of the program. Thereafter, consume fiber as needed.)

A protein powder from bone broth. Take one to three servings per day mixed in water, juice, smoothies, yogurt, or can be used in many recipes.

Additional Therapies

For people who want to maintain balanced intestinal flora and a strong immune system, avoiding contact with chlorinated water is of the utmost importance. That includes bathing water and drinking water. Chlorine kills bacteria, friendly and unfriendly, in the intestines, and can be absorbed through the skin. I recommend installing a shower filter to remove chlorine. Avoid swimming in chlorinated water as well.

I especially recommend regular use of low-heat saunas.

Inflammatory Conditions

Inflammation is an underlying cause of many illnesses, including heart disease and stroke, as well as cancer and autoimmune conditions such as rheumatoid arthritis and asthma, to name but a few. The entire program detailed in this book will help to maintain normal levels of inflammation. To determine inflammatory levels, ask your doctor to perform a relatively inexpensive and noninvasive high-sensitivity C-reactive protein test.

Diet

Follow the Maker's Diet diligently for six to twelve months. After symptoms are completely gone for at least three months, you may gradually add foods from the "Average" or "Trouble" categories if desired.

Because people suffering from chronic inflammation appear to have a predisposed weakness in their immune systems, I strongly recommend that they adhere to a diet of foods in the "Extraordinary" category for the rest of their lives.

Therapeutic Foods

Appendix A lists sources where you can obtain these foods. These therapeutic foods will help you feel better:

Cultured goat's milk dairy products: Consume 8 to 32 ounces of the highest quality cultured dairy products from goat's milk. Try to find yogurt that does not contain the organism *Streptococcus thermophilus*, a bacterial microbe that has been known to make immune system disorders worse.

Grass-fed red meat: Red meat from grass-fed cattle, buffalo, and lamb is very healthy and can be eaten a few times per week. This meat is a great source of protein, minerals, vitamin B_{12}, vitamins A and D, omega-3 fats, and CLA.

Organic, pasture-raised eggs: Consume as many as two organic eggs high in omega-3 fatty acids each day. These eggs contain DHA, vitamins E and B_{12}, and antioxidants including lutein.

Extra virgin coconut oil: This oil is perhaps the healthiest of the widely available oils. I recommend cooking almost exclusively with extra virgin coconut oil. Consume as much as two to four tablespoons per day of the oil in cooking, smoothies, or right off the spoon. Coconut oil contains large amounts of lauric acid, a potent antimicrobial and one of the chief fatty acids found in breast milk.

Ocean-caught fish: This type of fish is perhaps the healthiest of all protein sources. Salmon, sardines, mackerel, herring, and albacore tuna are high in the omega-3 fatty acids EPA and DHA. Ocean-caught fish can be consumed every day to enhance digestive and immune system health.

Cod liver oil: Take one to three teaspoons of an excellent cod liver oil each day, or caplets. The amount consumed should be based upon the amount of sunlight you receive. People in colder climates generally need to consume larger amounts. Cod liver oil is a fantastic source of the omega-3 fats DHA and EPA, as well as fat-soluble vitamins A and D.

Vegetable juice: Consume vegetable juices that are low in carbohydrates, such as celery and green juices mixed with a small amount of higher carbohydrate veggies such as carrot or beet. Mix in some form of healthy fat with each glass of the juice. One to three teaspoons of cultured goat's milk, extra virgin coconut oil, canned or fresh coconut milk and cream, or flaxseed oil enhance absorption of minerals and prevents spikes in blood sugar.

Fermented vegetables: Consume a few tablespoons of fermented vegetables such as sauerkraut with each meal to aid in digestion. Fermented vegetables are an excellent source of naturally occurring probiotics and enzymes.

Stocks: It is a great idea to consume stocks on a regular basis, especially when you are undergoing treatment. Stocks made from the bones of chicken, fish, lamb, and beef contain minerals, gelatin, cartilage, collagen, and electrolytes from the vegetables. Stocks are an excellent source of proteins, especially collagen. They help to heal the gut lining and reduce inflammation.

Supplements

Take these health supplements to alleviate symptoms and get well:

A probiotic, enzyme, and herbs formulation designed to support immune health.

A probiotic with SBOs. Start with one caplet per day on an empty stomach, thirty minutes before or one hour after meals. Increase usage by adding one additional caplet per day (i.e., one caplet the first day, two the second day, three the third day, and so on). Once your dosage is up to twelve caplets per day, stay on that amount for a minimum of three months and then begin to gradually decrease to a maintenance dosage of between three to six caplets per day.

Probiotics with SBOs are best taken first thing in the morning and right before bedtime with eight ounces pure water. Probiotics with SBOs may be taken with other nutritional supplements, but should be taken one hour apart from medications. If you experience symptoms of detoxification (i.e., increased elimination, loose stools, constipation, excess gas, flu-like symptoms, or fever), reduce the dosage and work up slowly to twelve per day.

A green superfood powder. Take two tablespoons twice daily with eight ounces water or fresh vegetable juice. Best taken on an empty stomach away from food.

Digestive enzymes. Take one to three capsules with each meal or snack.

An organic fiber supplement with chia seed. Consume one serving twice per day, morning and evening, with eight or more ounces of purified water. (Consuming a fiber supplement is essential during the first two weeks of the program. Thereafter, consume fiber as needed.)

A protein powder from bone broth. Take one to three servings per day mixed in water, juice, smoothies, yogurt, or can be used in many recipes.

Additional Therapies

For people who have or may have an imbalanced immune system, avoiding contact with chlorinated water is of the utmost importance. That includes bathing water and drinking water. Chlorine kills bacteria, friendly and unfriendly, in the intestines and can be absorbed through the skin. I recommend installing a shower filter to remove chlorine. Avoid swimming in chlorinated water as well.

Joint Disorders

- Ankylosing Spondylitis
- Osteoarthritis
- Gout
- Rheumatoid Arthritis

Overview

Arthritis is a general medical term that refers to inflammation of the joints. The word *arthritis* is a blend of the Greek words *arthron* for joint and *itis* for inflammation. Frequent cracking of the joints and early morning stiffness are common symptoms of osteoarthritis, even during pain-free periods. Some will joke that they can tell a weather change is ahead when their knees act up, but that's because painful joints can be sensitive to a falling of barometric pressure, which signals rain in the forecast.

Arthritis and related conditions affect more than 50 million Americans, or about one of every seven people, making it one of the most prevalent diseases in the United States. By 2020, as the Baby Boom generation solidly hits their senior years, an estimated 60 million Americans will be affected by arthritis.

Arthritis is the leading cause of disability in the United States, and although cost-effective interventions are available to reduce the burden of arthritis, they are currently underused.

Ankylosing Spondylitis

Ankylosing spondylitis (spinal arthritis) causes immobility of the back and often the shoulders and neck. The affliction impacts more than 300,000 people—usually young men, often white, between the ages of sixteen and thirty-five.

Gout

Gout, usually associated with lifestyle and diet, affects some one million persons—usually men. Gout is caused by the buildup of acidic crystals that lodge in the joints. Painful gout attacks often are first felt in the big toe.

Osteoarthritis

The most common form of arthritis is osteoarthritis, which is a mechanical disease that results from cartilage deterioration and trauma. Under the age of forty-five, osteoarthritis is more common in men. After age forty-five, however, it's ten times more common in women than men.

Forty million Americans have some form of osteoarthritis from mild to severe, including 80 percent of people over age fifty. Some 30 million Americans suffer from disabling osteoarthritis. This number is likely to increase by three or four times over the next several decades.

Rheumatoid Arthritis

Rheumatoid arthritis is an inflammatory- and immune-mediated disease. Rheumatoid arthritis, also known simply as RA, affects about 1.3 million people—and the majority are women by a two to one margin.

Rheumatoid arthritis is a chronic disease of the joints characterized by alternating periods of active inflammation and absence of symptoms, both of variable duration. Some of the symptoms include a sense of utter fatigue and weakness while running a slight fever. The joints may become just a little stiff at first, but a few weeks later, they become much stiffer and swollen.

The stiffness and swelling may start in the small joints like the fingers and wrists but progress to larger joints and afflict both the joints and bodily organs. This is a systemic disease that affects the body inside and outside. Interestingly, symmetrical joints such as the hands, wrists, and ankles are often hit first with an attack. The joints may even be "hot" to the touch. About one-third of rheumatoid arthritis patients get luckier than most, meaning only a single joint area or two are affected. For most people, though, the pain will be spread throughout the entire body.

The usual age at which rheumatoid arthritis strikes is in the twenty to forty age group. In terms of gender differentiation, rheumatoid arthritis is most likely to strike women aged thirty to fifty, according to the Arthritis Foundation. The next major target is men forty-five to sixty. Some children and teenagers suffer various forms of rheumatoid arthritis.

Diet

Follow the Maker's Diet as best you can for six to twelve months. Once symptoms are completely gone for three months, you may gradually add foods from the "Average" or "Trouble" categories if desired.

Because people with chronic joint disorders appear to have a predisposed weakness in their immune systems, I strongly recommend that they adhere to a diet of foods in the "Extraordinary" category for the rest of their lives.

Therapeutic Foods

These therapeutic foods will help you feel better:

Cultured goat's milk dairy products: Consume 8 to 32 ounces of the highest quality cultured dairy products from goat's milk. Try to find yogurt that does not contain the organism *Streptococcus thermophilus*, a bacterial microbe that has been known to make immune system disorders worse.

Grass-fed red meat: Red meat from grass-fed cattle, buffalo, and lamb is very healthy and can be eaten a few times per week. This meat is a great source of protein, minerals, vitamin B_{12}, vitamins A and D, omega-3 fats, and CLA.

Organic, pasture-raised eggs: Consume as many as two organic eggs high in omega-3 fatty acids each day. These eggs contain DHA, vitamins E and B_{12}, and antioxidants including lutein.

Extra virgin coconut oil: This oil is perhaps the healthiest of the widely available oils. I recommend cooking almost exclusively with extra virgin coconut oil. Consume as much as two to four tablespoons per day of the oil in cooking, smoothies, or right off the spoon. Coconut oil contains large amounts of lauric acid, a potent antimicrobial and one of the chief fatty acids found in breast milk.

Ocean-caught fish: This type of fish is perhaps the healthiest of all protein sources. Salmon, sardines, mackerel, herring, and albacore tuna are high in the omega-3 fatty acids EPA and DHA. Ocean-caught fish can be consumed every day to enhance digestive and immune system health.

We've known for hundreds of years that fish oils play a role in fighting arthritis. British doctors used to give their patients cod liver oil to alleviate rheumatism. In particular, seafood rich in omega-3 fatty acids may prove to be extremely beneficial for anyone suffering inflammatory types of arthritis, especially rheumatoid arthritis. Three or more servings weekly of select seafood dishes could do more for your arthritis than any medical drug or surgery.

Salmon, tuna, sardines, herring, anchovies, and mackerel are rich sources of omega-3 fatty acids. These fatty acids, found in such limited amounts in most people's diet, suppress production of substances such as cytokines and leukotrienes that are produced by white blood cells and are responsible for the inflammation accompanying arthritis. Eating these fats is likely to reduce the body's overall inflammation levels, thin the blood, and reduce your risk for heart attack and stroke, as well as arthritis.

Cod liver oil: Take one to three teaspoons of an excellent cod liver oil each day, or caplets. The amount consumed should be based upon the amount of sunlight you receive. People in colder climates generally need to consume larger amounts. Cod liver oil is a fantastic source of the omega-3 fats DHA and EPA, as well as fat-soluble vitamins A and D.

Vegetable juice: Consume vegetable juices that are low in carbohydrates, such as celery and green juices mixed with a small amount of higher carbohydrate veggies such as carrot or beet. Mix in some form of healthy fat with each glass of the juice. One to three teaspoons of cultured goat's milk, extra virgin coconut oil, canned or fresh coconut milk and cream, or flaxseed oil enhance absorption of minerals and prevents spikes in blood sugar.

Fermented vegetables: Consume a few tablespoons of fermented vegetables such as sauerkraut with each meal to aid in digestion. Fermented vegetables are an excellent source of naturally occurring probiotics and enzymes.

Stocks: It is a great idea to consume stocks on a regular basis, especially when you are undergoing treatment. Stocks made from the bones of chicken, fish, lamb, and beef contain minerals, gelatin, cartilage, collagen, and electrolytes from the vegetables. Stocks are an excellent source of proteins, especially collagen. They help to heal the gut lining and reduce inflammation.

Supplements

Take these health supplements to alleviate symptoms and get well:

A probiotic, enzyme, and herbs formulation designed to support joint and tissue health.

A probiotic with SBOs. Start with one caplet per day on an empty stomach, thirty minutes before or one hour after meals. Increase usage by adding one additional caplet per day (i.e., one caplet the first day, two the second day, three the third day, and so on). Once your dosage is up to twelve caplets per day, stay on that amount for a minimum of three months and then begin to gradually decrease to a maintenance dosage of between three to six caplets per day.

Probiotics with SBOs are best taken first thing in the morning and right before bedtime with eight ounces pure water. Probiotics with SBOs may be taken with other nutritional supplements, but should be taken one hour apart from medications. If you experience symptoms of detoxification (i.e., increased elimination, loose stools, constipation, excess gas, flu-like symptoms, or fever), reduce the dosage and work up slowly to twelve per day.

A green superfood powder. Take two tablespoons twice daily with eight ounces water or fresh vegetable juice. Best taken on an empty stomach away from food.

Digestive enzymes. Take one to three capsules with each meal or snack.

An organic fiber supplement with chia seed. Consume one serving twice per day, morning and evening, with eight or more ounces of purified water. (Consuming a fiber supplement is essential during the first two weeks of the program. Thereafter, consume fiber as needed.)

A protein powder from bone broth. Take one to three servings per day mixed in water, juice, smoothies, yogurt, or can be used in many recipes.

Additional Therapies

For people who have or may have imbalanced intestinal flora or a weak immune system, avoiding contact with chlorinated water is of the utmost importance. That includes bathing water and drinking water. Chlorine kills bacteria, friendly and unfriendly, in the intestines and can be absorbed through the skin. I recommend installing a shower filter to remove chlorine. Avoid swimming in chlorinated water as well.

Lactose Intolerance…see Functional Bowel Disorders

Leaky Gut Syndrome…see Functional Bowel Disorders

Low Back Pain…see Inflammatory Conditions

Lupus…see Autoimmune Disease

Male Health

- Benign Prostatic Hypertrophy
- Prostatitis
- Erectile Dysfunction

Benign Prostatic Hypertrophy (BPH)

A combination of connective tissue, gland, and muscle, the prostate provides the power that propels the semen through the urethra and out the penis. The prostate plays a key role in men's sexuality, providing more than 90 percent of his ejaculate, including the enzyme-filled fluid called semen required for fertilization of the ovum. So you can see why the health of the prostate is key for maintaining lifetime potency and virility.

The prostate needs male hormones to function. The main male hormone is testosterone, which is made mainly by the testes.

Yet as men age, the prostate can become enlarged. This enlargement, in turn, can be the source of much suffering and embarrassment. Indeed, prostate enlargement, which your doctor may call benign prostatic hypertrophy (BPH) or hyperplasia, is the most common prostate disorder.

Men who have an enlarged prostate commonly begin producing a toxic form of testosterone called dihydrotestosterone (DHT). Interestingly, DHT is also linked to hair loss. In the case of the prostate, excess production of DHT is closely linked with enlarged prostate tissue.

Symptoms include difficulty starting and stopping urination, frequent nighttime trips to the bathroom, and the unsettling feeling that, although you've tried, voiding simply isn't complete. These all result when the prostate squeezes and pinches off the urethra, and the bladder outlet becomes obstructed.

By age sixty, at least half of all men are suffering from symptoms of an enlarged prostate; by age eighty-five, the number climbs to 90 percent, according to the American Urological Association. For some men, there may be only a minor discomfort, and the symptoms can be stoically shrugged off as simply a condition of aging. Other men, for whom the symptoms are more severe, however, require medical help.

Erectile Dysfunction

Impotence is a consistent inability to sustain an erection sufficient for sexual intercourse. Medical professionals often use the term *erectile dysfunction* or ED to describe this disorder and to differentiate it from other problems that interfere with sexual intercourse such as lack of sexual desire and problems with ejaculation and orgasm.

Impotence can be a total inability to achieve erection, an inconsistent ability to do so, or a tendency to sustain only brief erections. These variations make defining impotence and estimating its incidence difficult. Experts believe impotence affects more than 30 million American men, including 30 to 50 percent of men between the ages of forty and seventy. Many men are too embarrassed to seek help.

What is the truth about men's impotency? Some experts suggest 90 percent of cases of erectile dysfunction in men over age fifty are due to physical factors such as a health condition like diabetes or heart and circulatory disease, injury, or drug side effects. Any disorder that impairs blood flow in the penis has the potential to cause impotence. This is buttressed by a Massachusetts Male Aging Study that found that both psychological and organic factors affect the burdensome problems of aging, particularly men's potency.

As men age, their sexual function is impaired by the same types of atherosclerotic processes that cause heart disease. That is why for so many men erectile dysfunction should be taken seriously because it's often an early warning sign of heart disease. Like the arteries to the heart, when the vessels leading to the sexual organs clog up with plaque, blood flow is impaired. This makes achieving an erection difficult and also leads to poor sensation.

Natural remedies may require a longer time to bring a result, but they also offer many of the same therapeutic benefits as drug therapies without the sometime severe side effects.

Prostatitis

The prostate gland and seminal vesicle (the male appendages) form a unit anatomically and functionally. The prostate, an organ which is well supplied with blood and normally undergoes periods of congestion, is the central point of this organ system and is liable to be afflicted with acute or chronic infections.

Aside from the typical complex of complaints, acute prostatitis is often accompanied by fever and chills. In addition to analgesics, therapy includes high-dosed chemotherapy with antibiotics. Should the inflammation not be brought under control, a prostatic abscess or other condition may develop. In spite of specific chemotherapy, acute prostatitis regardless of the causative agent may develop into a chronic inflammation.

Chronic prostatitis, on the other hand, proceeds blandly and without fever. It is often the residual condition following acute prostatitis, although it may also ascend along the ducts or spread via the blood.

Diet

Choose mainly foods from the "Extraordinary" category until optimal health is achieved for at least three months, or if you're experiencing symptoms such as BPH, low libido, and low energy, until symptoms are gone for at least three months.

Once symptoms are greatly improved, you may gradually add foods from the "Average" and "Trouble" categories if desired. To attain and maintain vibrant health, I recommend consuming foods from the "Extraordinary" category as the main part of a healthy diet.

Therapeutic Foods

These therapeutic foods will help you stay well:

Cultured goat's milk dairy products: Consume 8 to 32 ounces of the highest quality cultured dairy products from goat's milk. Try to find yogurt that does not contain the organism *Streptococcus thermophilus*, a bacterial microbe that has been known to make immune system disorders worse.

Grass-fed red meat: Red meat from grass-fed cattle, buffalo, and lamb is very healthy and can be eaten a few times per week. This meat is a great source of protein, minerals, vitamin B$_{12}$, vitamins A and D, omega-3 fats, and CLA.

Organic, pasture-raised eggs: Consume as many as one to three organic eggs high in omega-3 fatty acids each day. These eggs contain DHA, vitamins E and B$_{12}$, and antioxidants including lutein.

Extra virgin coconut oil: This oil is perhaps the healthiest of the widely available oils. I recommend cooking almost exclusively with extra virgin coconut oil. Consume as much as two to four tablespoons per day of the oil in cooking, smoothies, or right off the spoon. Coconut oil contains large amounts of lauric acid, a potent antimicrobial and one of the chief fatty acids found in breast milk.

Ocean-caught fish: This type of fish is perhaps the healthiest of all protein sources. Salmon, sardines, mackerel, herring, and albacore tuna are high in the omega-3 fatty acids EPA and DHA. Ocean-caught fish can be consumed every day to enhance digestive and immune system health.

Cod liver oil: Take one to three teaspoons of an excellent cod liver oil each day, or caplets. The amount consumed should be based upon the amount of sunlight you receive. People in colder climates generally need to consume larger amounts. Cod liver oil is a fantastic source of the omega-3 fats DHA and EPA, as well as fat-soluble vitamins A and D.

Berries: The daily consumption of berries, including blueberries, strawberries, blackberries, and raspberries, can provide the body with antioxidants that can neutralize harmful toxins damaging to the body. Berries supply rich sources of dietary fiber.

Vegetable juice: Consume vegetable juices that are low in carbohydrates, such as celery and green juices mixed with a small amount of higher carbohydrate veggies such as carrot or beet. Mix in some form of healthy fat with each glass of the juice. One to three teaspoons of cultured goat's milk, extra virgin coconut oil, canned or fresh coconut milk and cream, or flaxseed oil enhance absorption of minerals and prevents spikes in blood sugar.

Fermented vegetables: Consume a few tablespoons of fermented vegetables such as sauerkraut with each meal to aid in digestion. Fermented vegetables are an excellent source of naturally occurring probiotics and enzymes.

Stocks: It is a great idea to consume stocks on a regular basis, especially when you have a cold or flu. Stocks made from the bones of chicken, fish, lamb, and beef contain minerals, gelatin, cartilage, collagen, and electrolytes from the vegetables. Stocks are an excellent source of proteins, especially collagen. They help to heal the gut lining and reduce inflammation.

Supplements

Take these health supplements to support potency:

Natural remedies. Do your online research to determine whether supplements like l-Arginine and Ginkgo Biloba could help.

A probiotic with SBOs. Take three to six capsules per day. Probiotics with SBOs are best taken first thing in the morning and right before bedtime with eight ounces pure water.

A green superfood powder. Take two tablespoons twice daily with eight ounces water or fresh vegetable juice. Best taken on an empty stomach away from food.

Digestive enzymes. Take one to three capsules with each meal or snack.

An organic fiber supplement with chia seed. Consume one serving twice per day, morning and evening, with eight or more ounces of purified water. (Consuming a fiber supplement is essential during the first two weeks of the program. Thereafter, consume fiber as needed.)

A protein powder from bone broth. Take one to three servings per day mixed in water, juice, smoothies, yogurt, or can be used in many recipes.

Memory Loss…see Brain Health

Menopause…see Female Health

Mental Disorders

- Addiction
- Violent, Impulsive Behavior
- Agoraphobia
- Postpartum Depression
- Anxiety
- Schizophrenia
- Depression Disorders

Overview

Mental disorders are common in the United States and internationally. An estimated 18 percent of Americans ages eighteen and older—a little less one in five adults—suffer from a diagnosable mental disorder in a given year, noted the National Institute for Mental Health.

When applied to the 2010 U.S. Census residential population estimate, this figure translates to 43.4 million people. In addition, four of the ten leading causes of disability in the United States and other developed countries are the following mental disorders: major depression, bipolar disorder, schizophrenia, and obsessive-compulsive disorder. Many people suffer from more than one mental disorder at a given time.

Addiction

Many view drug abuse and addiction as strictly a social problem. Parents, teens, older adults, and other members of the community tend to characterize people who take drugs as morally weak or as having criminal tendencies. They believe that drug abusers and addicts should be able to stop taking drugs if they are willing to change their behavior.

These myths have not only stereotyped those with drug-related problems, but also their families, their communities, and the health care professionals who work with them. Drug abuse and addiction comprise a public health problem that affects many people and has wide-ranging social consequences.

Addiction does begin with drug abuse when an individual makes a conscious choice to use drugs, but addiction is not just "a lot of drug use." Recent scientific research provides overwhelming evidence that not only do drugs interfere with normal brain functioning creating powerful feelings of pleasure, but they also have long-term effects on brain metabolism and activity. At some point, changes occur in the brain that can turn drug abuse into addiction or a chronic, relapsing illness. Those addicted to drugs suffer from a compulsive drug craving and usage and cannot quit by themselves.

Holistic treatment can have a profound effect not only on drug abusers, but on society as a whole by significantly improving social and psychological functioning, decreasing related criminality and violence, and reducing the spread of the HIV virus. A holistic approach to treatment can also dramatically reduce the costs to society of drug abuse.

Anxiety

Anxiety disorders include panic disorder, obsessive-compulsive disorder, posttraumatic stress disorder, generalized anxiety disorder, and phobias such as social phobia or agoraphobia, a fear of places or situations that lead to panic attacks or feelings of being trapped, helpless, or embarrassed. Consider these statistics:

- Anxiety disorders are the most common mental illness in the United States, affecting 40 million adults in the United States eighteen and older, or 18 percent of the population each year according to the statistics collected by the Anxiety and Depression Association of America.
- Anxiety disorders frequently co-occur with depressive disorders, eating disorders, or substance abuse.
- Many people have more than one anxiety disorder.
- Women are more likely than men to have an anxiety disorder. Approximately twice as many women as men suffer from panic disorder, posttraumatic stress disorder, generalized anxiety

disorder, agoraphobia, and specific phobia, though about equal numbers of women and men have obsessive-compulsive disorder and social phobia.

Agoraphobia

Agoraphobia involves intense fear and avoidance of any place or situation where escape might be difficult or help unavailable in the event of developing sudden panic-like symptoms. Approximately 1.8 million American adults ages eighteen and over have agoraphobia with a history of panic disorder. The median age of onset of agoraphobia is twenty years of age.

Depression

Depressive disorders encompass major depressive disorder, dysthymic disorder, and bipolar disorder. Bipolar disorder is included because people with this illness have depressive episodes as well as manic episodes.

- Approximately 16 million American adults, or around 7 percent of the U.S. population age eighteen and older, had a major depressive episode in the last year.
- Women are twice as likely to have depression or symptoms of depression. In addition, 12 percent of all women in the United States will experience symptoms of clinical depression some time during their lives.
- Depressive disorders may be appearing earlier in life in people born in recent decades compared to the past.
- Depressive disorders often co-occur with anxiety disorders and substance abuse.

Postpartum Depression

Having a baby is a joyous time for most women. After childbirth, though, many mothers feel sad, afraid, angry, or anxious. Most new mothers have these feelings in a mild form called postpartum blues, or otherwise known as "baby blues." Postpartum blues almost always go away in a few days.

Between 11 percent and 20 percent of new mothers, however, have a greater problem called postpartum depression, which lasts longer and is more intense, according to the Centers for Disease Control. Postpartum depression often requires counseling and treatment and can occur after any birth, not just the first.

Schizophrenia

Approximately 2.4 million American adults, or about 1.1 percent of the population age eighteen and older in a given year, have schizophrenia.

Schizophrenia, which affects men and women with equal frequency, often first appears earlier in men, usually in their late teens or early twenties, than in women, who are generally affected in their twenties or early thirties.

Violent, Impulsive Behavior

Spousal abuse, criminal activity, and other examples of violent, impulsive behavior can be linked to alcohol abuse, environmental pollution (especially industrial chemicals such as some pesticides and heavy metals), and genetics.

A Word About Omega-3s and Mental Health

I strongly urge persons with mental disorders to increase their intake of flaxseed and flax oil as well as omega-3 fatty acid-rich seafood.

Dr. Donald O. Rudin, the former director of the Department of Molecular Biology at the Eastern Pennsylvania Psychiatric Institute, was one of the first to conduct research into the impact of omega-3 fatty acids on mental health during the 1980s. He found the results to be astounding, even to the point where he observed that his patients' moods and depression lifted within two hours of receiving flax oil.

As a researcher with thirty-five years of experience, Dr. Rudin suspected that many modern diseases were signs of malnutrition and the key role that omega-3 fatty acids play in maintaining optimal mental health. At the same, he was aware that omega-3 fatty acids had declined to only 20 percent of the level found in diets a century ago.

We now know that omega-3 fatty acids can help the most common mood disorders, including depression, postpartum depression, bipolar disorder, and impulsive, violent behavior.

Diet

Follow the Maker's Diet diligently for six to twelve months. After symptoms are completely gone for at least three months, you may gradually add foods from the "Average" or "Trouble" categories if desired.

Because people with mental disorders appear to have derangements of the neuro-gastro immunomodulatory network, I strongly recommend that they adhere to a diet of foods in the "Extraordinary" category for the rest of their lives.

Therapeutic Foods

These therapeutic foods will help you feel better:

Cultured goat's milk dairy products: Consume 8 to 32 ounces of the highest quality cultured dairy products from goat's milk. Try to find yogurt that does not contain the organism *Streptococcus thermophilus*, a bacterial microbe that has been known to make immune system disorders worse.

Grass-fed red meat: Red meat from grass-fed cattle, buffalo, and lamb is very healthy and can be eaten a few times per week. This meat is a great source of protein, minerals, vitamin B_{12}, vitamins A and D, omega-3 fats, and CLA.

Organic, pasture-raised eggs: Consume as many as two organic eggs high in omega-3 fatty acids each day. These eggs contain DHA, vitamins E and B_{12}, and antioxidants including lutein.

Extra virgin coconut oil: This oil is perhaps the healthiest of the widely available oils. I recommend cooking almost exclusively with extra virgin coconut oil. Consume as much as two to four tablespoons per day of the oil in cooking, smoothies, or right off the spoon. Coconut oil contains large amounts of lauric acid, a potent antimicrobial and one of the chief fatty acids found in breast milk.

Ocean-caught fish: This type of fish is perhaps the healthiest of all protein sources. Salmon, sardines, mackerel, herring, and albacore tuna are high in the omega-3 fatty acids EPA and DHA. Ocean-caught fish can be consumed every day to enhance digestive and immune system health.

Cod liver oil: Take one to three teaspoons of an excellent cod liver oil each day, or caplets. The amount consumed should be based upon the amount of sunlight you receive. People in colder climates generally need to consume larger amounts. Cod liver oil is a fantastic source of the omega-3 fats DHA and EPA, as well as fat-soluble vitamins A and D.

Vegetable juice: Consume vegetable juices that are low in carbohydrates, such as celery and green juices mixed with a small amount of higher carbohydrate veggies such as carrot or beet. Mix in some form of healthy fat with each glass of the juice. One to three teaspoons of cultured goat's milk, extra virgin coconut oil, canned or fresh coconut milk and cream, or flaxseed oil enhance absorption of minerals and prevents spikes in blood sugar.

Fermented vegetables: Consume a few tablespoons of fermented vegetables such as sauerkraut with each meal to aid in digestion. Fermented vegetables are an excellent source of naturally occurring probiotics and enzymes.

Stocks: It is a great idea to consume stocks on a regular basis, especially when you are undergoing treatment. Stocks made from the bones of chicken, fish, lamb, and beef contain minerals, gelatin, cartilage, collagen, and electrolytes from the vegetables. Stocks are an excellent source of proteins, especially collagen. They help to heal the gut lining and reduce inflammation.

Supplements

Take these health supplements to alleviate symptoms and get well:

A probiotic with SBOs. Start with one caplet per day on an empty stomach, thirty minutes before or one hour after meals. Increase usage by adding one additional caplet per day (i.e., one caplet the first day, two the second day, three the third day, and so on). Once your dosage is up to twelve caplets per day, stay on that amount for a minimum of three months and then begin to gradually decrease to a maintenance dosage of between three to six caplets per day.

Probiotics with SBOs are best taken first thing in the morning and right before bedtime with eight ounces pure water. Probiotics with SBOs may be taken with other nutritional supplements, but should be taken one hour apart from medications. If you experience symptoms of detoxification (i.e., increased elimination, loose stools, constipation, excess gas,

flu-like symptoms, or fever), reduce the dosage and work up slowly to twelve per day.

A green superfood powder. Take two tablespoons twice daily with eight ounces water or fresh vegetable juice. Best taken on an empty stomach away from food.

Digestive enzymes. Take one to three capsules with each meal or snack.

An organic fiber supplement with chia seed. Consume one serving twice per day, morning and evening, with eight or more ounces of purified water. (Consuming a fiber supplement is essential during the first two weeks of the program. Thereafter, consume fiber as needed.)

A protein powder from bone broth. Take one to three servings per day mixed in water, juice, smoothies, yogurt, or can be used in many recipes.

Additional Therapies

For people who have or may have an imbalanced immune system, avoiding contact with chlorinated water is of the utmost importance. That includes bathing water and drinking water. Chlorine kills bacteria, friendly and unfriendly, in the intestines and can be absorbed through the skin. I recommend installing a shower filter to remove chlorine. Avoid swimming in chlorinated water as well.

Multiple Sclerosis…see Autoimmune Disease

Myasthenia Gravis…see Autoimmune Disease

Mycoplasma Infections

Overview

Human mycoplasma infection, a respiratory illness caused by a microscopic organism related to bacteria, is not new, but recognition by medical scientists and doctors has come relatively late. What researchers are understanding is that mycoplasma is spread through contact with droplets from the nose and throat of infected people, especially when they cough or sneeze.

Mycoplasmas are small microorganisms without cell walls. The word *mycoplasma* itself is derived from the ancient Greek *mykes,* which is a combined linguistic form for mushroom, fungus, and plasma, the non-cellular fluid portion of the blood. Thus, mycoplasmas are blood fungi. They are also *pleomorphic,* meaning they have the ability to change shape and form during their life cycle and under varying conditions. This gives them a highly unique ability to evade even healthily functioning immune systems (more on this later).

Unfortunately, diagnosis of mycoplasma infections is difficult, even though typical symptoms include fever, cough, bronchitis, sore throat, headache, and tiredness. Culturing mycoplasmas is difficult and may take months to obtain results. Until properly diagnosed, a common result of mycoplasma infection is "walking pneumonia" because it's usually mild and doesn't require hospitalization.

Even though you have probably never heard of mycoplasmas or their role with "walking pneumonia," their parasitic existence in the human body may be key to prolongation of disabling chronic diseases.

Among the most intractable medical conditions linked to myco-plasma infections are:

- chronic fatigue syndrome
- fibromyalgia
- rheumatoid arthritis
- respiratory maladies, including chronic asthma
- inflammatory bowel disease
- heart disease
- neurological disorders such as Parkinson's and amyotrophic lateral sclerosis, otherwise known as Lou Gehrig's disease

Diet

Follow the Maker's Diet as best you can for six to twelve months. For the first thirty days, it's best to limit or even restrict fruit and honey consumption. Make sure that if you do have some fruit that it's a less sweet, high-nutrient, high-fiber fruit such as berries, apples, or grapefruit.

Once symptoms are completely gone for at least six months, you may gradually add foods from the "Average" or "Trouble" categories if desired.

Because people with fungal and parasitic overgrowth appear to have a predisposed weakness in their intestinal tracts, I strongly recommend that they adhere to a diet of foods in the "Extraordinary" category for the rest of their lives.

Therapeutic Foods

These therapeutic foods will help you get well:

Cultured goat's milk dairy products: Consume 8 to 32 ounces of the highest quality cultured dairy products from goat's milk. Try to find yogurt that does not contain the organism *Streptococcus thermophilus*, a bacterial microbe that has been known to make immune system disorders worse.

Grass-fed red meat: Red meat from grass-fed cattle, buffalo, and lamb is very healthy and can be eaten a few times per week. This meat is a great source of protein, minerals, vitamin B_{12}, vitamins A and D, omega-3 fats, and CLA.

Organic, pasture-raised eggs: Consume as many as two organic eggs high in omega-3 fatty acids each day. These eggs contain DHA, vitamins E and B_{12}, and antioxidants including lutein.

Extra virgin coconut oil: This oil is perhaps the healthiest of the widely available oils. I recommend cooking almost exclusively with extra virgin coconut oil. Consume as much as two to four tablespoons per day of the oil in cooking, smoothies, or right off the spoon. Coconut oil contains large amounts of lauric acid, a potent antimicrobial and one of the chief fatty acids found in breast milk.

Ocean-caught fish: This type of fish is perhaps the healthiest of all protein sources. Salmon, sardines, mackerel, herring, and albacore tuna are high in the omega-3 fatty acids EPA and DHA. Ocean-caught fish can be consumed every day to enhance digestive and immune system health.

Cod liver oil: Take one to three teaspoons of an excellent cod liver oil each day, or caplets. The amount consumed should be based upon the amount of sunlight you receive. People in colder climates generally need to consume larger amounts. Cod liver oil is a fantastic source of the omega-3 fats DHA and EPA, as well as fat-soluble vitamins A and D.

Vegetable juice: Consume vegetable juices that are low in carbohydrates, such as celery and green juices mixed with a small amount of higher carbohydrate veggies such as carrot or beet. Mix in some form of healthy fat with each glass of the juice. One to three teaspoons of cultured goat's milk, extra virgin coconut oil, canned or fresh coconut milk and cream, or flaxseed oil enhance absorption of minerals and prevents spikes in blood sugar.

Fermented vegetables: Consume a few tablespoons of fermented vegetables such as sauerkraut with each meal to aid in digestion. Fermented vegetables are an excellent source of naturally occurring probiotics and enzymes.

Stocks: It is a great idea to consume stocks on a regular basis, especially when you are feeling under the weather. Stocks made from the bones of chicken, fish, lamb, and beef contain minerals, gelatin, cartilage, collagen, and electrolytes from the vegetables. Stocks are an excellent source of proteins, especially collagen. They help to heal the gut lining and reduce inflammation.

Supplements

Take these health supplements to alleviate symptoms and get well:

A probiotic, enzyme, and herbs formulation designed to support respiratory illnesses.

A probiotic with SBOs. Start with one caplet per day on an empty stomach, thirty minutes before or one hour after meals. Increase usage by adding one additional caplet per day (i.e., one caplet the first day, two the second day, three the third day, and so on). Once your dosage is up to twelve caplets per day, stay on that amount for a minimum of three months and then begin to gradually decrease to a maintenance dosage of between three to six caplets per day.

Probiotics with SBOs are best taken first thing in the morning and right before bedtime with eight ounces pure water. Probiotics with SBOs may be taken with other nutritional supplements, but should be taken one hour apart from medications. If you experience symptoms of detoxification (i.e., increased elimination, loose stools, constipation, excess gas,

flu-like symptoms, or fever), reduce the dosage and work up slowly to twelve per day.

A green superfood powder. Take two tablespoons twice daily with eight ounces water or fresh vegetable juice. Best taken on an empty stomach away from food.

Digestive enzymes. Take one to three capsules with each meal or snack.

An organic fiber supplement with chia seed. Consume one serving twice per day, morning and evening, with eight or more ounces of purified water. (Consuming a fiber supplement is essential during the first two weeks of the program. Thereafter, consume fiber as needed.)

A protein powder from bone broth. Take one to three servings per day mixed in water, juice, smoothies, yogurt, or can be used in many recipes.

Additional Therapies

For people who have or may have imbalanced intestinal flora or a weak immune system, avoiding contact with chlorinated water is of the utmost importance. That includes bathing water and drinking water. Chlorine kills bacteria, friendly and unfriendly, in the intestines and can be absorbed through the skin. I recommend installing a shower filter to remove chlorine. Avoid swimming in chlorinated water as well.

Osteoarthritis…see Joint Disorders

Osteoporosis…see Joint Disorders

Ovarian Cysts…see Female Health

Parkinson's Disease…see Brain Health

Pervasive Development Disorders…see Children's Health

Postpartum Depression…see Mental Disorders

Premenstrual Syndrome…see Female Health

Prostatitis…see Male Health

Psoriasis…see Skin Health

Rheumatoid Arthritis…see Joint Disorders and Autoimmune Disease

Schizophrenia…see Mental Disorders

Scleroderma…see Autoimmune Disease

Seasonal Allergies…see Upper Respiratory Health

Shingles…see Vital Diseases

Sinusitis…see Upper Respiratory Health

Skin Health

- Acne
- Atopic Dermatitis (Dermatitis, Eczema)
- Psoriasis

Overview

It's my experience that people suffering from acne, dermatitis, and psoriasis frequently suffer from imbalanced immune system and intestinal flora. Once these imbalances are corrected by eating the proper foods and rebalancing the digestive tract with SBOs, the symptoms of even the most serious skin disorders will greatly improve.

Acne

Acne is a disorder resulting from the action of hormones on the skin's oil glands (sebaceous glands), which leads to plugged pores and outbreaks of lesions commonly called pimples or zits. Acne lesions usually occur on the face, neck, back, chest, and shoulders.

Approximately 85 percent of people between the ages of twelve and twenty-four experience at least minor acne, which is why is acne the most common skin disease in this country. Although acne is not a serious health threat, severe acne can lead to disfiguring, permanent scarring, which can be upsetting to those affected by the disorder.

The exact cause of acne is unknown, but doctors believe it results from several related factors. One important factor is an increase in hormones called androgens, which increase in both boys and girls during puberty and cause the sebaceous glands to enlarge and make more sebum, an oily, waxy substance. Hormonal changes related to pregnancy or starting or stopping birth control pills can also cause acne.

Another factor is heredity or genetics. Researchers believe that the tendency to develop acne can be inherited from parents. For example, studies have shown that many school-age boys with acne have a family history of the disorder. Certain drugs, like those prescribed to treat epilepsy, bipolar disorder, and the thyroid, are known to cause acne. Greasy cosmetics may alter the cells of the follicles and make them stick together, producing a plug.

Many nutrition researchers believe that the outer appearance of the skin is directly related to the health of the digestive tract and immune system. An imbalance in intestinal flora and increased gut permeability (leaky gut syndrome) are almost always found in those suffering from acne. By following the diet and supplement recommendations in this book, the symptoms of acne should greatly improve.

Atopic Dermatitis (Eczema)

Atopic dermatitis is a chronic, long-lasting disease that affects the skin. The word *dermatitis* means inflammation of the skin. *Atopic* refers to a group of diseases that are hereditary (i.e., an affliction that runs in families) and often occur together, including asthma, allergies such as hay fever, and atopic dermatitis.

In atopic dermatitis, the skin becomes extremely itchy and inflamed, causing redness, swelling, cracking, weeping, crusting, and scaling. Atopic dermatitis most often affects infants and young children, but it can continue into adulthood or even show up later in life.

In most cases, there are periods of time when the disease is worse, called exacerbations or flares, followed by periods when the skin improves or clears up entirely, called remissions. Many children with atopic dermatitis will experience a permanent remission of the disease when they get older, although their skin often remains dry and easily irritated. Environmental factors can bring on symptoms of atopic dermatitis at any time in the lives of individuals who have inherited the atopic disease trait.

Atopic dermatitis is often referred to as *eczema,* which is a general term for the many types of dermatitis. Atopic dermatitis is the most common of the many types of eczema.

Psoriasis

Psoriasis is a chronic, long-lasting skin disease characterized by scaling and inflammation. Scaling occurs when cells in the outer layer of the skin reproduce faster than normal and pile up on the skin's surface.

Psoriasis affects around 2 percent of the United States population, or about 7.5 million people. Although the disease occurs in all age groups and about equally in men and women, adults have a brunt of the cases. People with psoriasis often suffer discomfort, including pain and itching, restricted motion in their joints, and emotional distress.

In its most typical form, psoriasis results in patches of thick, red skin covered with silvery scales. These patches, which are sometimes referred to as plaques, usually itch and burn. The skin at the joints may crack. Psoriasis most often occurs on the elbows, knees, scalp, lower back, face, palms, and soles of the feet, but it can affect any skin site. The disease may also affect the fingernails, the toenails, and the soft tissues inside the mouth and genitalia. A small percentage of people with psoriasis have joint inflammation that produces arthritis symptoms. This condition is called psoriatic arthritis.

Recent research indicates that psoriasis is likely a disorder of the immune system. This system includes a type of white blood cell, called a T cell, that normally helps protect the body against infection and disease. Scientists now think that, in psoriasis, an abnormal immune system causes activity by T cells in the skin. These T cells trigger inflammation and excessive skin cell reproduction seen in people with psoriasis.

In about one-third of the cases, psoriasis is inherited. Researchers are studying large families affected by psoriasis to identify a gene or genes that cause the disease. (Genes govern every bodily function and determine the inherited traits passed from parent to child.)

People with psoriasis may notice that there are times when their skin worsens, then improves. Conditions that may cause flare-ups include changes in climate, infections, stress, and dry skin. Also, certain medicines, most notably beta-blockers used to treat high blood pressure and lithium or drugs used to treat depression, may trigger an outbreak or worsen the disease.

Diet

Choose mainly foods from the "Extraordinary" category until optimal health is achieved for at least three months. Once symptoms are greatly improved, you may gradually add foods from the "Average" and "Trouble" categories if desired.

Because people with chronic skin problems appear to have a predisposed immune-gastrointestinal weaknesses that present skin problems, I strongly recommend that they adhere to a diet of foods in the "Extraordinary" category for the rest of their lives.

Therapeutic Foods

These therapeutic foods will help you stay well:

Cultured goat's milk dairy products: Consume 8 to 32 ounces of the highest quality cultured dairy products from goat's milk. Try to find yogurt that does not contain the organism *Streptococcus thermophilus*, a bacterial microbe that has been known to make immune system disorders worse.

Grass-fed red meat: Red meat from grass-fed cattle, buffalo, and lamb is very healthy and can be eaten a few times per week. This meat is a great source of protein, minerals, vitamin B_{12}, vitamins A and D, omega-3 fats, and CLA.

Organic, pasture-raised eggs: Consume as many as one to three organic eggs high in omega-3 fatty acids each day. These eggs contain DHA, vitamins E and B_{12}, and antioxidants including lutein.

Extra virgin coconut oil: This oil is perhaps the healthiest of the widely available oils. I recommend cooking almost exclusively with extra virgin coconut oil. Consume as much as two to four tablespoons per day of the oil in cooking, smoothies, or right off the spoon. Coconut oil contains large amounts of lauric acid, a potent antimicrobial and one of the chief fatty acids found in breast milk.

Using extra virgin coconut oil topically can be great for skin problems of any kind. Rub a small amount on the affected area daily. Be sure not to over-apply as the oil may rub off onto clothing or furniture.

Ocean-caught fish: This type of fish is perhaps the healthiest of all protein sources. Salmon, sardines, mackerel, herring, and albacore tuna are high in the omega-3 fatty acids EPA and DHA. Ocean-caught fish can be consumed every day to enhance digestive and immune system health.

Cod liver oil: Take one to three teaspoons of an excellent cod liver oil each day, or caplets. The amount consumed should be based upon the amount of sunlight you receive. People in colder climates generally need to consume larger amounts. Cod liver oil is a fantastic source of the omega-3 fats DHA and EPA, as well as fat-soluble vitamins A and D.

Berries: The daily consumption of berries, including blueberries, strawberries, blackberries, and raspberries, can provide the body with antioxidants that can neutralize harmful toxins damaging to the body. Berries supply rich sources of dietary fiber.

Vegetable juice: Consume vegetable juices that are low in carbohydrates, such as celery and green juices mixed with a small amount of higher carbohydrate veggies such as carrot or beet. Mix in some form of healthy fat with each glass of the juice. One to three teaspoons of cultured goat's milk, extra virgin coconut oil, canned or fresh coconut milk and cream, or flaxseed oil enhance absorption of minerals and prevents spikes in blood sugar.

Fermented vegetables: Consume a few tablespoons of fermented vegetables such as sauerkraut with each meal to aid in digestion. Fermented vegetables are an excellent source of naturally occurring probiotics and enzymes.

Stocks: It is a great idea to consume stocks on a regular basis, especially when you have a cold or flu. Stocks made from the bones of chicken, fish, lamb, and beef contain minerals, gelatin, cartilage, collagen, and electrolytes from the vegetables. Stocks are an excellent source of proteins, especially collagen. They help to heal the gut lining and reduce inflammation.

Supplements

Take these health supplements to alleviate symptoms and get well:

A probiotic with SBOs. Start with one caplet per day on an empty stomach, thirty minutes before or one hour after meals. Increase usage by adding one additional caplet per day (i.e., one caplet the first day, two the second day, three the third day, and so on). Once your dosage is up to 12 cap lets per day, stay on that amount for a minimum of three months and then begin to gradually decrease to a maintenance dosage of between three to six caplets per day.

Probiotics with SBOs are best taken first thing in the morning and right before bedtime with eight ounces pure water. Probiotics with SBOs may be taken with other nutritional supplements, but should be taken one hour apart from medications. If you experience symptoms of detoxification (i.e., increased elimination, loose stools, constipation, excess gas, flu-like symptoms, or fever), reduce the dosage and work up slowly to twelve per day.

A green superfood powder. Take two tablespoons twice daily with eight ounces water or fresh vegetable juice. Best taken on an empty stomach away from food.

Digestive enzymes. Take one to three capsules with each meal or snack.

An organic fiber supplement with chia seed. Consume one serving twice per day, morning and evening, with eight or more ounces of purified water. (Consuming a fiber supplement is essential during the first two weeks of the program. Thereafter, consume fiber as needed.)

A protein powder from bone broth. Take one to three servings per day mixed in water, juice, smoothies, yogurt, or can be used in many recipes.

Additional Therapies

For people who have or may have imbalanced intestinal flora or a weak immune system, avoiding contact with chlorinated water is of the utmost importance. That includes bathing water and drinking water. Chlorine kills bacteria, friendly and unfriendly, in the intestines and can be absorbed through the skin. I recommend installing a shower filter to remove chlorine. Avoid swimming in chlorinated water as well.

Sleep Disorders

Overview

America has a sleep deficit and has had one for a long time. There are many mornings that my wife, Nicki, and I count ourselves among the 100 million Americans who get up shortly after dawn without getting proper rest. Our excuse is that we have children underfoot, but that's not much of an excuse because millions of parents are in our boat.

Whether you possess a good excuse or not for not getting enough sleep, the consequences of a sleep deficit are profound upon our culture:

- Sleepy children daydream in the classroom.
- Tired employees cost their companies billions in lost productivity each year.
- Drivers falling asleep behind the wheel cause accidents that kill thousands annually.
- Interpersonal relationships become strained and often fracture when couples are too tired to deal with each other.

The root causes of our national sleep debt are overcrowded schedules, the desire to accomplish one more thing before retiring, and too much stimulation from watching TV in bed, which is a shame. Sleep and relaxation are basic necessities of life—right up there with diet and exercise in my book—but you'd never know it by the way we treat this foundation of good health. "Sleep plays a major role in preparing the body and brain for an alert, productive, psychologically, and physiologically healthy tomorrow," said Dr. James B. Maas, author of *Power Sleep*.

This is as good a place as any to issue a wake-up call about the importance of sleep, a body therapy that is the most important non-nutrient you can incorporate into your healthy lifestyle. A good night's rest revitalizes tired bodies, gives us more energy, and helps us think more clearly throughout the day.

The magic number that sleep experts say we have to shoot for is eight hours. Why eight hours? Because when people can control the amount of time they sleep, such as in a sleep laboratory, they naturally sleep eight hours in a twenty-four-hour period. Yet, medical sleep experts note that individual requirements vary widely, and that no two people's sleep needs are necessarily alike.

The quality of one's sleeping hours is also important. Deep, refreshing sleep is a great restorer of both physical and emotional health, but a lot of people have trouble sleeping.

The causes of chronic insomnia and poor sleep vary widely. Some medical professionals says that insomnia is related to psychiatric problems such as depression, anxiety, or stress. But prescription drugs affect sleep, including appetite suppressants, steroids, blood pressure drugs like reserpine, and thyroid hormones.

Another cause of insomnia includes one's sleep environment. Changes in the temperature or light in the bedroom, environmental noises and smells, and the quality of the mattress and pillows may lead to disruptions of the initiation or maintenance of sleep. Using the bedroom for cooking, eating, studying, or watching television, like in a studio apartment, may cause insomnia in those whose sleep is fragile.

The use of alcohol and illegal drugs can also impair one's sleep quality. Finally, organic causes of poor sleep and insomnia, such as the chronic pain from rheumatoid arthritis, can cause an overall decrease in sleep efficiency.

Finally, advancing age itself also is associated with declining sleep quality. It's a fact that most people sleep less at a single stretch than they did when they were younger.

Many older people believe that because they are more advanced in years they should not need as much sleep as when they were younger, and they cannot understand why they no longer feel rested in the morning. But if they think they can get by with less sleep or a reduced quality of sleep, they are possibly harboring an illusion potentially dangerous to their health.

When I get behind, I compensate by going to bed earlier. I've heard that each hour of sleep *before* midnight is equal to twice the hours of sleep after midnight. The formula makes sense to me. If I go to bed real late, say around 2 a.m., I just don't feel well for a couple of days. When I get to bed before midnight, I perform better the next day. Apparently, the first third of the night is when we experience the deepest part of our sleep.

I urge you to go to bed earlier, even if it's just thirty minutes before you normally go to bed.

Diet

It's interesting to note that sleep disorders are frequently associated with gastrointestinal conditions. Thus, by enhancing your gastrointestinal health, you will also be supporting healthful sleep. Follow the Maker's Diet diligently for three to six months. After symptoms are completely gone for at least three months, you may gradually add foods from the "Average" or "Trouble" categories if desired.

Therapeutic Foods

These therapeutic foods will help you sleep better:

Cultured goat's milk dairy products: Consume 8 to 32 ounces of the highest quality cultured dairy products from goat's milk. Try to find yogurt that does not contain the organism *Streptococcus thermophilus*, a bacterial microbe that has been known to make immune system disorders worse.

Grass-fed red meat: Red meat from grass-fed cattle, buffalo, and lamb is very healthy and can be eaten a few times per week. This meat is a great source of protein, minerals, vitamin B_{12}, vitamins A and D, omega-3 fats, and CLA.

Organic, pasture-raised eggs: Consume as many as two organic eggs high in omega-3 fatty acids each day. These eggs contain DHA, vitamins E and B_{12}, and antioxidants including lutein.

Extra virgin coconut oil: This oil is perhaps the healthiest of the widely available oils. I recommend cooking almost exclusively with extra virgin coconut oil. Consume as much as two to four tablespoons per day of the oil in cooking, smoothies, or right off the spoon. Coconut oil contains large amounts of lauric acid, a potent antimicrobial and one of the chief fatty acids found in breast milk.

Ocean-caught fish: This type of fish is perhaps the healthiest of all protein sources. Salmon, sardines, mackerel, herring, and albacore tuna are high in the omega-3 fatty acids EPA and DHA. Ocean-caught fish can be consumed every day to enhance digestive and immune system health.

Cod liver oil: Take one to three teaspoons of an excellent cod liver oil each day, or caplets. The amount consumed should be based upon the amount of sunlight you receive. People in colder climates generally need to consume larger amounts. Cod liver oil is a fantastic source of the omega-3 fats DHA and EPA, as well as fat-soluble vitamins A and D.

Vegetable juice: Consume vegetable juices that are low in carbohydrates, such as celery and green juices mixed with a small amount of higher carbohydrate veggies such as carrot or beet. Mix in some form of healthy fat with each glass of the juice. One to three teaspoons of cultured goat's milk, extra virgin coconut oil, canned or fresh coconut milk and cream, or flaxseed oil enhance absorption of minerals and prevents spikes in blood sugar.

Fermented vegetables: Consume a few tablespoons of fermented vegetables such as sauerkraut with each meal to aid in digestion. Fermented vegetables are an excellent source of naturally occurring probiotics and enzymes.

Stocks: It is a great idea to consume stocks on a regular basis, especially when you are undergoing treatment. Stocks made from the bones of chicken, fish, lamb, and beef contain minerals, gelatin, cartilage, collagen, and electrolytes from the vegetables. Stocks are an excellent source of proteins, especially collagen. They help to heal the gut lining and reduce inflammation.

Supplements

Take these health supplements to give yourself the best possible chance to sleep well:

A green superfood powder. Take two tablespoons twice daily with eight ounces water or fresh vegetable juice. Best taken on an empty stomach away from food.

Digestive enzymes. Take one to three capsules with each meal or snack.

An organic fiber supplement with chia seed. Consume one serving twice per day, morning and evening, with eight or more ounces of purified water. (Consuming a fiber supplement is essential during the first two weeks of the program. Thereafter, consume fiber as needed.)

A protein powder from bone broth. Take one to three servings per day mixed in water, juice, smoothies, yogurt, or can be used in many recipes.

Additional Therapies

Relaxation therapy can be extraordinarily helpful. Some insomniacs are unable to recognize that they are insensitive to the internal state of their bodies. They are unable to realize they are tense, even though their fingers may be drumming the table and their feet may be tapping nervously.

Techniques used to teach relaxation skills include abdominal breathing and progressive muscle relaxation (tensing and then relaxing individual muscle groups). Learning relaxation skills helps most patients with insomnia to sleep better.

Other ways to induce sleep include exercise in the late afternoon or early evening or eating a light bedtime snack consisting of a food high in the amino acid tryptophan and calcium. Examples would be goat's milk yogurt, cream, or soft cheese.

Restoring the health of the gut and immune system has an amazing balancing effect on the body, which promotes good sleep. This restored level of balance usually brings about improved sleeping patterns, even in those with insomnia. There is little or no evidence that people eating a more primitive diet suffered from sleeping disorders. Therefore, adopting the age-old principles of primitive health can go a long way toward reversing sleeping disorders.

Sports Injuries…see Inflammatory Conditions

Stress

Overview

Stress can be a killer, which is a medical fact. Neuropsychologist Kenneth R. Pelletier, a Clinical Professor of Medicine at the University of California School of Medicine San Francisco, notes that stress-related psychological and physiological disorders have become the number-one social and health problem in America in the last twenty years. He goes on to point out that stress-induced disorders have long since replaced epidemics of infectious disease as the major medical problem of the modern era.

Look at your friends. Look at yourself. The stressed ones—the ones who are always rushed and under the gun—are the ones who always seem to be at greater risk for high blood pressure, insomnia, migraines, impotency, asthma, hay fever, arthritis, ulcers, alcoholism, and drug addiction.

Stress is a killer. The belief that stress, depression, and hopelessness contribute to susceptibility to disease dates to 200 A.D. when Galen, the Greek physician, commented that cancer seems to afflict sad and pensive women more frequently than the happy. Yet, for most people, these influences on cancer susceptibility are generally unappreciated.

Heart disease, a major killer of men and women, has been shown to have a strong link to stress and depression. Landmark studies conducted by Psychologist John Barefoot of the Duke University Medical Center conclusively proved that depression plays a role in the development of heart disease. In the Barefoot study, which began in 1964, those people with the highest scores for despair, low self-esteem, difficulties concentrating, and low motivation had a 70 percent higher risk of suffering a heart attack and 60 percent higher risk of death overall compared to men and women with low scores.

Feeling stressed has real implications for health, causing increased heart rate, constricted blood vessels, and high blood pressure. Ominously, those who took part in the Barefoot study were, for the most part, suffering from what is known as subclinical depression, which is often precipitated by prolonged chronic, low-level stress that at first seems acceptable but over time becomes cumulatively devastating to health.

This is the type of stress that most of us go through. Unfortunately, prolonged stress, when we feel helpless to change, turns into depression and also anger. In other words, stress brews all of the dark, dangerous emotions, attitudes, and feelings of hopelessness. This dangerous matrix of emotions with outside triggers becomes a trap due to *conditioning* when we are unable to break dangerous behavioral and thought patterns.

These signals of desperation are not taken seriously by patients themselves or their doctors, and they are usually not treated comprehensively with a program for turning on the body's own healing powers. The irony is that this type of "subclinical" stress is the kind we all need to beat, and the kind that outsmarts too many people. Further exacerbating the situation is that many patients with stress are treated with tranquilizing and other symptom-masking drugs. This doesn't promote healing or insight into the condition.

Steps for Stress

While there may be many reasons for feeling helpless, trying to avoid constant suppression of aggression is important. Dealing with problems directly by voicing concerns and taking constructive action is essential to dealing effectively with stress. Feeling free to ask questions, voice concerns, and question authority are examples of active responses.

Being able to see the larger picture and the orderly beauty of Nature is calming and relaxing. Everyone needs a way to work out his or her problems while being alone and yet not lonely. This can come from walks in Nature or a regular program of exercise. By getting your mind off your problems on a conscious level, you give yourself a chance to go to work on those problems unconsciously and get the answers you need, but you must be willing to *let go* to accomplish this.

The Role of Exercise

It's important to exercise daily. Not only is exercise a great stress reliever, but being active helps people to lose weight by readjusting their metabolism naturally. Studies have shown that people who exercise tend to eat healthier. Their bodies don't seem to crave the same amount of sugar as those who are sedentary. They end up eating fruits, vegetables, high-quality proteins, fats, and high-fiber foods with copious amounts of water because that is what their bodies crave.

Exercise, the best defense against stress, seems to tune up all aspects of healthy function and even makes the body more resistant to environmental carcinogens and other toxins. Exercise may be as organized as attending a fitness class at a local gym or as spontaneous as walking a country road or pulling weeds in the garden.

When you're taking time to exercise, be sure to discard any sense of time urgency that can turn exercise into a stressful event. When you're not operating with time urgency, you get to know what you really need deep within, which is to chill out.

A New Spirit

Think about developing a warrior or fighting spirit. A warrior or fighting spirit is based on confidence that positive steps can be taken in response to any stressful situation. A fighting spirit is also based on a sense of hope for the future and is the opposite of helplessness and hopelessness.

All sorts of self-enhancing projects can help people to fight off stress. If you love gardening, set aside time each day to get your hands dirty or rake up some leaves. If you love playing guitar, strum the chords to your favorite songs every day. If you love playing with your children or grandchildren, play with them. Take up a new hobby that you always wanted to try. Everyone has *something* that they love doing. Maybe it's riding horses or cycling with a local bike group.

Whatever floats your boat, get out there and do something you've wanted to do or try for a long time!

Stress Triggers

To deal effectively with stress, conduct a personal appraisal of your own stress triggers. It's also important to recognize that stress triggers are often overlapping, fueling each other. For instance, financial difficulties can create relationship difficulties. Illness can become financially devastating and test any relationship. Here are five areas that experts say seem to produce the greatest stress:

Physical: Air, noise, and light pollution can create extreme stress, turning homes and workplaces into pressure chambers. Overcrowding in urban living situations also creates stress. Loss of health is a catalyst for many other stresses, particularly financial, relationship, and work.

Job-related: Deadline pressures on the job, the constant sense of competition in work, an individual's poor relationship with a difficult boss, and not working at a meaningful or enjoyable job are all major stresses. Major stresses occur for those laid off. University of Michigan researcher Sidney Cobb studied one hundred auto paint factory workers, starting from six weeks before their jobs were to be terminated, following them for two years. Incidence of hypertension, peptic ulcers, arthritis, and psychosomatic disorders all increased. Moreover, three wives were hospitalized with rare peptic ulcers.

Financial: Money difficulties are a prime cause of divorce, domestic violence, and worry.

Relationship: A difficult time with a relative, mate, child, or friend can create unyielding stress. A death in the family or loss of a relationship can also be stressful.

Social change: Marriage, pregnancy, job changes, or moving can also become excessively stressful if focused into too short of a period. One of the first modern scientists to document the stress of social change was Adolph Meyer, a professor of psychiatry at Johns Hopkins University. By keeping "life charts," he found that illnesses tended to occur at times when clusters of major events occurred in people's lives within a fairly short period of time.

Diet

To avoid and reverse the damaging effects of stress on the body, it's best to consume a diet of foods in the "Extraordinary" category.

Therapeutic Foods

These therapeutic foods will help you keep the stress levels down:

Cultured goat's milk dairy products: Consume 8 to 32 ounces of the highest quality cultured dairy products from goat's milk. Try to find yogurt that does not contain the organism *Streptococcus thermophilus*, a bacterial microbe that has been known to make immune system disorders worse.

Grass-fed red meat: Red meat from grass-fed cattle, buffalo, and lamb is very healthy and can be eaten a few times per week. This meat is a great source of protein, minerals, vitamin B_{12}, vitamins A and D, omega-3 fats, and CLA.

Organic, pasture-raised eggs: Consume as many as two organic eggs high in omega-3 fatty acids each day. These eggs contain DHA, vitamins E and B_{12}, and antioxidants including lutein.

Extra virgin coconut oil: This oil is perhaps the healthiest of the widely available oils. I recommend cooking almost exclusively with extra virgin coconut oil. Consume as much as two to four tablespoons per day of the oil in cooking, smoothies, or right off the spoon. Coconut oil contains large amounts of lauric acid, a potent antimicrobial and one of the chief fatty acids found in breast milk.

Ocean-caught fish: This type of fish is perhaps the healthiest of all protein sources. Salmon, sardines, mackerel, herring, and albacore tuna are high in the omega-3 fatty acids EPA and DHA. Ocean-caught fish can be consumed every day to enhance digestive and immune system health.

Cod liver oil: Take one to three teaspoons of an excellent cod liver oil each day, or caplets. The amount consumed should be based upon the amount of sunlight you receive. People in colder climates generally need to consume larger amounts. Cod liver oil is a fantastic source of the omega-3 fats DHA and EPA, as well as fat-soluble vitamins A and D.

Vegetable juice: Consume vegetable juices that are low in carbohydrates, such as celery and green juices mixed with a small amount of higher carbohydrate veggies such as carrot or beet. Mix in some form of healthy fat with each glass of the juice. One to three teaspoons of cultured goat's milk, extra virgin coconut oil, canned or fresh coconut milk and cream, or flaxseed oil enhance absorption of minerals and prevents spikes in blood sugar.

Fermented vegetables: Consume a few tablespoons of fermented vegetables such as sauerkraut with each meal to aid in digestion. Fermented vegetables are an excellent source of naturally occurring probiotics and enzymes.

Stocks: It is a great idea to consume stocks on a regular basis, especially when you are feeling under the weather. Stocks made from the bones of chicken, fish, lamb, and beef contain minerals, gelatin, cartilage, collagen, and electrolytes from the vegetables. Stocks are an excellent source of proteins, especially collagen. They help to heal the gut lining and reduce inflammation.

Supplements

Take these health supplements to alleviate symptoms of stress:

A probiotic with SBOs. Start with one caplet per day on an empty stomach, thirty minutes before or one hour after meals. Increase usage by adding one additional caplet per day (i.e., one caplet the first day, two the second day, three the third day, and so on). Once your dosage is up to twelve caplets per day, stay on that amount for a minimum of three months and then begin to gradually decrease to a maintenance dosage of between three to six caplets per day.

Probiotics with SBOs are best taken first thing in the morning and right before bedtime with eight ounces pure water. Probiotics with SBOs may be taken with other nutritional supplements, but should be taken one hour apart from medications. If you experience symptoms of detoxification (i.e., increased elimination, loose stools, constipation, excess gas, flu-like symptoms, or fever), reduce the dosage and work up slowly to twelve per day.

A green superfood powder. Take two tablespoons twice daily with eight ounces water or fresh vegetable juice. Best taken on an empty stomach away from food.

Digestive enzymes. Take one to three capsules with each meal or snack.

An organic fiber supplement with chia seed. Consume one serving twice per day, morning and evening, with eight or more ounces of purified water. (Consuming a fiber supplement is essential during the first two weeks of the program. Thereafter, consume fiber as needed.)

A protein powder from bone broth. Take one to three servings per day mixed in water, juice, smoothies, yogurt, or can be used in many recipes.

Additional Therapies

Stress levels will benefit from healthy intestinal flora. For those who have or may have imbalanced intestinal flora, avoiding contact with chlorinated water is of the utmost importance. That includes bathing water and drinking water. Chlorine kills bacteria, friendly and unfriendly, in the intestines and can be absorbed through the skin. I recommend installing a shower filter to remove chlorine. Avoid swimming in chlorinated water as well.

Syndrome X…see Blood Sugar Imbalances

Triglycerides (Elevated)…see Cardiovascular Health

Ulcerative Colitis…see Chronic Digestive Disease

Upper Respiratory Health

- Asthma
- Seasonal Allergies
- Sinusitis

Overview

Asthma

Asthma, the leading chronic illness of childhood, is responsible for substantial infant morbidity and has a significant impact on use of our finite health resources, say researchers from the Department of Pediatrics, University of Washington, and the Center for Health Studies, Group Health Cooperative, Seattle.

Other researchers note that asthma prevalence in children doubled from 1980 to 1995 but increased more slowly from 2001 to 2010. Interestingly, the burden of the disease is most acute in urban areas and among racial and ethnic minority populations; hospitalization and morbidity rates for nonwhites were more than twice those for whites.

Although studies illustrating causal effects between outdoor air pollution and asthma prevalence are scant, air pollution appears to significantly worsen symptoms among children already with the disease. Decreased lung function, bronchial inflammation, and other asthma symptoms such as recurrent wheezing, breathlessness, chest tightness, and coughing have been associated with exposure to particulates, ozone, smoke, sulfur dioxide, and nitric oxide.

Research in the past twenty years has revealed the importance of inflammation of the airways in asthma and successful clinical therapies aimed at reducing chronic inflammation. Asthma is associated with the body's production of pro-inflammatory fatty compounds called leukotrienes, secreted by the immune system's white blood cells (leukocytes) as a reaction to common environmental allergens and pollutants including house dust mites, animal dander, cockroaches, fungal spores, pollens, and industrial airborne contaminants.

Ordinarily, white blood cells defend the body against infecting organisms and foreign agents, both in the tissues and in the bloodstream itself.

But in persons with asthma, the white blood cells tend to produce excess amounts of pro-inflammatory leukotrienes.

One way to counter the body's excess production of leukotrienes is to enhance intake of omega-3 fatty acids. The omega-3 fatty acids cause the body to produce more of the less-inflammatory 5-series leukotrienes. This shift is directly related to relief from asthma symptoms.

Seafood, a rich source of omega-3 fatty acids, has been shown to help children. Youngsters who eat fish more than once a week have only one-third the risk of asthma compared with children who do not eat fish regularly. It's sometimes difficult, however, to convince children to consume those seafood dishes highest in omega-3 fatty acids, such as salmon, tuna, and mackerel. What can help is blending flaxseed oil, also a rich source of omega-3 fatty acids, into tasty smoothies, yogurt, or veggie juice.

Please keep in mind that children also need to get "dirty." When they're outside, messing with dirt, they're more likely to be exposed to germs and microbes naturally present in the soil. Any incidental exposures educate the immune system and enable it to mature so that it doesn't overreact to every little antigen or allergen present in the environment.

Remember: your children will not benefit from being kept in an overly sterile environment. Such seclusion could well lead to imbalances in their immune systems.

Allergies (Seasonal)

The same principles detailed above for asthma apply to seasonal allergies.

Sinusitis

Closely related in occurrence to bronchitis, chronic tracheobronchial inflammations are often found concomitantly with chronic sinusitis. Sinusitis usually develops by continuous spreading of rhinitis, but may also arise following injury.

Increasing exposure to environmental pollutants is thought to be responsible for the growing incidence of chronic inflammations of the nasal sinuses.

Chronic sinusitis is difficult to treat. Today, operative therapy with curettage of the mucosa is often considered inadequate because it's generally limited to correction of the airway blockage. Medical therapy includes the prescription of locally applied decongestants. Furthermore, a number of antibiotics are available, although they rarely attain effective concentrations in the mucosa or bone of the nasal sinuses.

Healing of the chronic inflammation is seldom possible with the usual conservative measures. Surgical irritation with instillation of antibiotics and corticosteroids entails the risk of sensitization of the mucous membranes. Corticosteroids additionally interfere with the defensive mechanisms that are already somewhat impaired.

The goal, once again, is to support the normal inflammatory process and the natural eliminative functions while stimulating the immune system. With this in mind, natural strategies to moderate inflammatory reactions within the body are quite helpful.

Diet

Follow the Maker's Diet diligently for six to twelve months. After symptoms are completely gone for at least three months, you may gradually add foods from the "Average" or "Trouble" categories if desired.

Because people suffering from upper respiratory disorders appear to have a predisposed weakness in their intestinal tracts, I strongly recommend that they adhere to a diet of foods in the "Extraordinary" category for the rest of their lives.

Therapeutic Foods

These therapeutic foods will help you stay well:

Cultured goat's milk dairy products: Consume 8 to 32 ounces of the highest quality cultured dairy products from goat's milk. Try to find yogurt that does not contain the organism *Streptococcus thermophilus*, a bacterial microbe that has been known to make immune system disorders worse.

Grass-fed red meat: Red meat from grass-fed cattle, buffalo, and lamb is very healthy and can be eaten a few times per week. This meat is a great source of protein, minerals, vitamin B_{12}, vitamins A and D, omega-3 fats, and CLA.

Organic, pasture-raised eggs: Consume as many as one to three organic eggs high in omega-3 fatty acids each day. These eggs contain DHA, vitamins E and B_{12}, and antioxidants including lutein.

Extra virgin coconut oil: This oil is perhaps the healthiest of the widely available oils. I recommend cooking almost exclusively with extra virgin coconut oil. Consume as much as two to four tablespoons per day of the oil in cooking, smoothies, or right off the spoon. Coconut oil contains large amounts of lauric acid, a potent antimicrobial and one of the chief fatty acids found in breast milk.

Ocean-caught fish: This type of fish is perhaps the healthiest of all protein sources. Salmon, sardines, mackerel, herring, and albacore tuna are high in the omega-3 fatty acids EPA and DHA. Ocean-caught fish can be consumed every day to enhance digestive and immune system health.

Cod liver oil: Take one to three teaspoons of an excellent cod liver oil each day, or caplets. The amount consumed should be based upon the amount of sunlight you receive. People in colder climates generally need to consume larger amounts. Cod liver oil is a fantastic source of the omega-3 fats DHA and EPA, as well as fat-soluble vitamins A and D.

Vegetable juice: Consume vegetable juices that are low in carbohydrates, such as celery and green juices mixed with a small amount of higher carbohydrate veggies such as carrot or beet. Mix in some form of healthy fat with each glass of the juice. One to three teaspoons of cultured goat's milk, extra virgin coconut oil, canned or fresh coconut milk and cream, or flaxseed oil enhance absorption of minerals and prevents spikes in blood sugar.

Fermented vegetables: Consume a few tablespoons of fermented vegetables such as sauerkraut with each meal to aid in digestion. Fermented vegetables are an excellent source of naturally occurring probiotics and enzymes.

Stocks: It is a great idea to consume stocks on a regular basis, especially when you have a cold or flu. Stocks made from the bones of chicken, fish, lamb, and beef contain minerals, gelatin, cartilage, collagen, and electrolytes from the vegetables. Stocks are an excellent source of proteins, especially collagen. They help to heal the gut lining and reduce inflammation.

Supplements

Take these health supplements to alleviate symptoms and get well:

A probiotic, enzyme, and herbs formulation designed to support upper respiratory health.

A probiotic with SBOs. Start with one caplet per day on an empty stomach, thirty minutes before or one hour after meals. Increase usage by adding one additional caplet per day (i.e., one caplet the first day, two the second day, three the third day, and so on). Once your dosage is up to twelve caplets per day, stay on that amount for a minimum of three months and then begin to gradually decrease to a maintenance dosage of between three to six caplets per day.

Probiotics with SBOs are best taken first thing in the morning and right before bedtime with eight ounces pure water. Probiotics with SBOs may be taken with other nutritional supplements, but should be taken one hour apart from medications. If you experience symptoms of detoxification (i.e., increased elimination, loose stools, constipation, excess gas, flu-like symptoms, or fever), reduce the dosage and work up slowly to twelve per day.

A green superfood powder. Take two tablespoons twice daily with eight ounces water or fresh vegetable juice. Best taken on an empty stomach away from food.

Digestive enzymes. Take one to three capsules with each meal or snack.

An organic fiber supplement with chia seed. Consume one serving twice per day, morning and evening, with eight or more ounces of purified water. (Consuming a fiber supplement is essential during the first two weeks of the program. Thereafter, consume fiber as needed.)

A protein powder from bone broth. Take one to three servings per day mixed in water, juice, smoothies, yogurt, or can be used in many recipes.

Additional Therapies

For people who have or may have imbalanced intestinal flora or a weak immune system, avoiding contact with chlorinated water is of the utmost importance. That includes bathing water and drinking water. Chlorine kills bacteria, friendly and unfriendly, in the intestines and can be absorbed through the skin. I recommend installing a shower filter to remove chlorine. Avoid swimming in chlorinated water as well.

Urinary Tract Infections

Overview

A urinary tract infection (UTI) is an infection anywhere in the urinary tract. Your urinary tract includes the organs that collect and store urine and release it from your body. Taken together, they are the kidneys, ureters, bladder, and urethra.

Usually, a UTI (also known as cystitis) is caused by bacteria that can also live in the digestive tract, in the vagina, or in and around the urethra, which is at the entrance to the urinary tract. Most often these bacteria enter the urethra and travel to the bladder and kidneys.

Most of the time, your body effectively removes the bacteria, and you have no symptoms. However, some people seem to be prone to infection, including women and older people. People with UTIs as well as cystitis have improved greatly by following the diet, supplement, and lifestyle program outlined in this book.

Diet

Follow the Maker's Diet diligently for six to twelve months. After symptoms are completely gone for at least three months, you may gradually add foods from the "Average" or "Trouble" categories if desired.

Because people with recurrent bladder infections appear to have a predisposed weakness in their urinary tracts, I strongly recommend that you adhere to a diet of foods in the "Extraordinary" category for the rest of your life. Please note that maintaining a healthy gastrointestinal flora is critical to reducing your risk of getting a UTI and their recurrence.

Therapeutic Foods

These therapeutic foods will help you get well:

Cultured goat's milk dairy products: Consume 8 to 32 ounces of the highest quality cultured dairy products from goat's milk. Try to find yogurt that does not contain the organism *Streptococcus thermophilus*, a bacterial microbe that has been known to make immune system disorders worse.

Grass-fed red meat: Red meat from grass-fed cattle, buffalo, and lamb is very healthy and can be eaten a few times per week. This meat is a great source of protein, minerals, vitamin B_{12}, vitamins A and D, omega-3 fats, and CLA.

Organic, pasture-raised eggs: Consume as many as two organic eggs high in omega-3 fatty acids each day. These eggs contain DHA, vitamins E and B_{12}, and antioxidants including lutein.

Extra virgin coconut oil: This oil is perhaps the healthiest of the widely available oils. I recommend cooking almost exclusively with extra virgin coconut oil. Consume as much as two to four tablespoons per day of the oil in cooking, smoothies, or right off the spoon. Coconut oil contains large amounts of lauric acid, a potent antimicrobial and one of the chief fatty acids found in breast milk.

Ocean-caught fish: This type of fish is perhaps the healthiest of all protein sources. Salmon, sardines, mackerel, herring, and albacore tuna are high in the omega-3 fatty acids EPA and DHA. Ocean-caught fish can be consumed every day to enhance digestive and immune system health.

Cod liver oil: Take one to three teaspoons of an excellent cod liver oil each day, or caplets. The amount consumed should be based upon the amount of sunlight you receive. People in colder climates generally need to consume larger amounts. Cod liver oil is a fantastic source of the omega-3 fats DHA and EPA, as well as fat-soluble vitamins A and D.

Vegetable juice: Consume vegetable juices that are low in carbohydrates, such as celery and green juices mixed with a small amount of higher carbohydrate veggies such as carrot or beet. Mix in some form of healthy fat with each glass of the juice. One to three teaspoons of cultured goat's milk, extra virgin coconut oil, canned or fresh coconut milk and cream, or flaxseed oil enhance absorption of minerals and prevents spikes in blood sugar.

Fermented vegetables: Consume a few tablespoons of fermented vegetables such as sauerkraut with each meal to aid in digestion. Fermented vegetables are an excellent source of naturally occurring probiotics and enzymes.

Berries: Blueberries and cranberries are extremely important for those suffering from recurrent bladder infections as they are able to inhibit bacteria from sticking to the wall of the bladder. These berries are some of the best sources of antioxidants found in any foods. Berries also supply rich sources of dietary fiber.

Stocks: It is a great idea to consume stocks on a regular basis, especially when you are undergoing treatment for a UTI. Stocks made from the bones of chicken, fish, lamb, and beef contain minerals, gelatin, cartilage, collagen, and electrolytes from the vegetables. Stocks are an excellent source of proteins, especially collagen. They help to heal the gut lining and reduce inflammation.

Supplements

Take these health supplements to give yourself the best possible chance to get well:

A probiotic with SBOs. Start with one caplet per day on an empty stomach, thirty minutes before or one hour after meals. Increase usage by adding one additional caplet per day (i.e., one caplet the first day, two the second day, three the third day, and so on). Once your dosage is up to twelve caplets per day, stay on that amount for a minimum of three months and then begin to gradually decrease to a maintenance dosage of between three to six caplets per day.

Probiotics with SBOs are best taken first thing in the morning and right before bedtime with eight ounces pure water. Probiotics with SBOs may be taken with other nutritional supplements, but should be taken one hour apart from medications. If you experience symptoms of detoxification (i.e., increased elimination, loose stools, constipation, excess gas, flu-like symptoms, or fever), reduce the dosage and work up slowly to twelve per day.

A green superfood powder. Take two tablespoons twice daily with eight ounces water or fresh vegetable juice. Best taken on an empty stomach away from food.

Digestive enzymes. Take one to three capsules with each meal or snack.

An organic fiber supplement with chia seed. Consume one serving twice per day, morning and evening, with eight or more ounces of purified water. (Consuming a fiber supplement is essential during the first two weeks of the program. Thereafter, consume fiber as needed.)

A protein powder from bone broth. Take one to three servings per day mixed in water, juice, smoothies, yogurt, or can be used in many recipes.

Additional Therapies

Changing some of your daily habits may help you avoid UTIs. Here are some ideas:

- Drink lots of fluid to flush the bacteria from your system. Water is best. Try for six to eight glasses a day.
- Urinate frequently and go when you first feel the urge. Bacteria can grow when urine stays too long in the bladder.
- Urinate shortly after sex. This can flush away bacteria that might have entered your urethra during sexual contact.
- After using the toilet, always wipe from front to back, especially after a bowel movement.
- Wear cotton underwear and loose-fitting clothes so that air can keep the area dry. Avoid tight-fitting jeans and nylon underwear, which trap moisture and can help bacteria grow.
- For women, using a diaphragm or spermicide for birth control can lead to UTIs by increasing bacteria growth. If you have trouble with UTIs, consider modifying your birth control method. Unlubricated condoms or spermicidal condoms increase irritation and foster bacterial symptoms. Consider switching to lubricated condoms without spermicide, or use a non-spermicidal lubricant.

Finally, avoid contact with chlorinated water. That includes bathing water and drinking water. Chlorine kills bacteria, friendly and unfriendly, in the intestines and can be absorbed through the skin. I recommend installing a shower filter to remove chlorine. Avoid swimming in chlorinated water as well.

Uterine Fibroids…see Female Health

Vaginitis…see Female Health

Violent, Impulsive Behavior…see Mental Disorders

Viral Disease

- Colds
- Epstein–Barr Virus
- Flu
- Hepatitis
- Herpes Simplex
- Shingles

Overview

Viruses, the smallest of parasites, are completely dependent on cells (bacterial, plant, or animal) to reproduce. Viruses are composed of an outer cover of protein and sometimes lipid and contain a nucleic acid core of RNA or DNA. In many cases, this core penetrates susceptible cells and initiates the infection.

Viruses range from 5 to 300 nanometers—too small for light microscopy but visible using electron microscopy. Viruses can be identified by biophysical and biochemical methods. Like most other parasites, viruses stimulate host antibody production.

Several hundred different viruses infect humans every day, or so it seems. Because many have been only recently recognized, their clinical effects are not fully understood. Many viruses infect hosts without producing symptoms; nevertheless, because of their wide and sometimes universal prevalence, they create important medical and public health problems.

Viruses that primarily infect humans are spread mainly via respiratory and enteric excretions. These viruses are found worldwide, but their spread is limited by inborn resistance, prior immunizing infections or vaccines, sanitary and other public health control measures, and prophylactic antiviral drugs.

Zoonotic viruses pursue their biologic cycles chiefly in animals; humans are secondary or accidental hosts. These viruses are limited to areas and environments able to support their nonhuman natural cycles of infection (vertebrates or arthropods or both).

Some viruses have oncogenic properties. Human T-cell lymphotropic virus type 1 (a retrovirus) is associated with human leukemia and lymphoma. Epstein–Barr Virus has been associated with malignancies such as nasopharyngeal carcinoma, Burkitt's lymphoma, Hodgkin's disease, and lymphomas in immunosuppressed organ transplant recipients.

Slow viral diseases are characterized by prolonged incubations and cause some chronic degenerative diseases, including subacute sclerosing panencephalitis (measles virus), progressive rubella panencephalitis (PRP), progressive multifocal leukoencephalopathy (JC virus), and Creutzfeldt–Jakob disease (a rare but fatal brain disease).

Latency—a quiescent infection by a virus—permits recurrent infection despite immune responses and facilitates person-to-person spread. Herpes viruses exhibit latency.

Only a few viral diseases can be diagnosed clinically or epidemiologically (e.g., by well-known viral syndromes). Diagnosis usually requires testing. Serologic examination during acute and convalescent stages is sensitive and specific but slow; more rapid diagnosis can sometimes be made using culture, polymerase chain reaction, or viral antigen tests. Histopathology can sometimes be helpful.

Conventional medicine utilizes vaccines for active immunity against influenza, measles, mumps, poliomyelitis, rabies, rubella, hepatitis A, hepatitis B, varicella, and yellow fever. An effective adenovirus vaccine is available but is used only in high-risk groups, such as military recruits. Immunoglobulins are also available for passive immune prophylaxis.

Exciting research has shown that two microorganisms found in the soil, *Bacillus subtilis* and *Bacillus lichenformis,* produce surfactants that are capable of destroying lipid-enveloped viruses such HHV-6, other members of the herpes family, and many other types of viruses. These SBOs are believed to stimulate the body to produce up to sixteen types of alpha interferon, all of which are capable of reducing the viral load of the body.

Diet

Follow the Maker's Diet diligently for six to twelve months. After symptoms are completely gone for at least three months, you may gradually add foods from the "Average" or "Trouble" categories if desired.

Because people suffering from chronic viral diseases appear to have a predisposed weakness in their immune systems, I strongly recommend that they adhere to a diet of foods in the "Extraordinary" category for the rest of their lives.

Therapeutic Foods

These therapeutic foods will help you stay healthy against viral intruders:

Cultured goat's milk dairy products: Consume 8 to 32 ounces of the highest quality cultured dairy products from goat's milk. Try to find yogurt that does not contain the organism *Streptococcus thermophilus*, a bacterial microbe that has been known to make immune system disorders worse.

Grass-fed red meat: Red meat from grass-fed cattle, buffalo, and lamb is very healthy and can be eaten a few times per week. This meat is a great source of protein, minerals, vitamin B_{12}, vitamins A and D, omega-3 fats, and CLA.

Organic, pasture-raised eggs: Consume as many as two organic eggs high in omega-3 fatty acids each day. These eggs contain DHA, vitamins E and B_{12}, and antioxidants including lutein.

Extra virgin coconut oil: This oil is perhaps the healthiest of the widely available oils. I recommend cooking almost exclusively with extra virgin coconut oil. Consume as much as two to four tablespoons per day of the oil in cooking, smoothies, or right off the spoon. Coconut oil contains large amounts of lauric acid, a potent antimicrobial and one of the chief fatty acids found in breast milk.

Ocean-caught fish: This type of fish is perhaps the healthiest of all protein sources. Salmon, sardines, mackerel, herring, and albacore tuna are high in the omega-3 fatty acids EPA and DHA. Ocean-caught fish can be consumed every day to enhance digestive and immune system health.

Cod liver oil: Take one to three teaspoons of an excellent cod liver oil each day, or caplets. The amount consumed should be based upon the amount of sunlight you receive. People in colder climates generally need to consume larger amounts. Cod liver oil is a fantastic source of the omega-3 fats DHA and EPA, as well as fat-soluble vitamins A and D.

Vegetable juice: Consume vegetable juices that are low in carbohydrates, such as celery and green juices mixed with a small amount of higher carbohydrate veggies such as carrot or beet. Mix in some form of healthy fat with each glass of the juice. One to three teaspoons of cultured goat's milk, extra virgin coconut oil, canned or fresh coconut milk and cream, or flaxseed oil enhance absorption of minerals and prevents spikes in blood sugar.

Fermented vegetables: Consume a few tablespoons of fermented vegetables such as sauerkraut with each meal to aid in digestion. Fermented vegetables are an excellent source of naturally occurring probiotics and enzymes.

Stocks: It is a great idea to consume stocks on a regular basis, especially when you are feeling under the weather. Stocks made from the bones of chicken, fish, lamb, and beef contain minerals, gelatin, cartilage, collagen, and electrolytes from the vegetables. Stocks are an excellent source of proteins, especially collagen. They help to heal the gut lining and reduce inflammation.

Supplements

Take these health supplements to alleviate symptoms and get well:

A probiotic, enzyme, and herbs formulation designed to support viral health.

A probiotic with SBOs. Start with one caplet per day on an empty stomach, thirty minutes before or one hour after meals. Increase usage by adding one additional caplet per day (i.e., one caplet the first day, two the second day, three the third day, and so on). Once your dosage is up to twelve caplets per day, stay on that amount for a minimum of three months and then begin to gradually decrease to a maintenance dosage of between three to six caplets per day.

Probiotics with SBOs are best taken first thing in the morning and right before bedtime with eight ounces pure water. Probiotics with SBOs may be taken with other nutritional supplements, but should be taken one hour apart from medications. If you experience symptoms of detoxification (i.e., increased elimination, loose stools, constipation, excess gas, flu-like symptoms, or fever), reduce the dosage and work up slowly to twelve per day.

A green superfood powder. Take two tablespoons twice daily with eight ounces water or fresh vegetable juice. Best taken on an empty stomach away from food.

Digestive enzymes. Take one to three capsules with each meal or snack.

An organic fiber supplement with chia seed. Consume one serving twice per day, morning and evening, with eight or more ounces of purified water. (Consuming a fiber supplement is essential during the first two weeks of the program. Thereafter, consume fiber as needed.)

A protein powder from bone broth. Take one to three servings per day mixed in water, juice, smoothies, yogurt, or can be used in many recipes.

Additional Therapies

For those who have or may have imbalanced immune system, avoiding contact with chlorinated water is of the utmost importance. That includes bathing water and drinking water. Chlorine kills bacteria, friendly and unfriendly, in the intestines and can be absorbed through the skin. I recommend installing a shower filter to remove chlorine. Avoid swimming in chlorinated water as well.

Weight Management

Overview

Health professionals define *overweight* as an excess amount of body weight that includes muscle, bone, fat, and water. Obesity specifically refers to an excess amount of body weight greater than 30 percent over one's ideal weight.

Everyone needs a certain amount of body fat for stored energy, heat insulation, shock absorption, and other functions. Some people, such as body-builders or other athletes with a lot of muscle, can be overweight without being obese. But those are the exceptions, not the rule. The fact remains that way too many today are overweight, which has severe health complications.

Health care providers are concerned not only with how much fat a person has, but also where the fat is located on the body. As a rule, women have more body fat than men. Women typically collect fat in their hips and buttocks, giving them a "pear" shape. Men usually build up fat around their bellies, giving them more of an "apple" shape. Of course some men are pear-shaped and some women become apple-shaped, especially after menopause.

If you carry fat mainly around your waist, you are more likely to develop obesity-related health problems. Women with a waist measurement of more than 35 inches or men with a waist measurement of more than 40 inches have a higher health risk because of their fat distribution.

Obesity is more than a cosmetic problem; it is a health hazard. Approximately 300,000 adult deaths in the United States each year are related to obesity. Several serious medical conditions have been linked to obesity, including adult-onset diabetes, heart disease, high blood pressure, and stroke.

Obesity is also linked to higher rates of certain types of cancer. Obese men are more likely than non-obese men to die from cancer of the colon, rectum, or prostate. Obese women are more likely than non-obese women to die from cancer of the gallbladder, breast, uterus, cervix, or ovaries.

Other diseases and health problems linked to obesity include:

- Gallbladder disease and gallstones
- Liver disease
- Osteoarthritis, a disease in which the joints deteriorate. This is possibly the result of excess weight on the joints.
- Gout, another disease affecting the joints
- Pulmonary (breathing) problems, including sleep apnea in which a person can stop breathing for a short time during sleep
- Reproductive problems in women, including menstrual irregularities and infertility.

Health care providers generally agree that the more obese a person is, the more likely he or she is to develop health problems.

Emotional suffering may be one of the most painful parts of obesity. American society emphasizes physical appearance and often equates attractiveness with slimness, especially for women. Such messages make overweight people feel unattractive.

By following the diet, lifestyle, and supplement programs outlined in this book, people who are overweight and even obese can greatly improve their health and lose excess body fat without being deprived of essential nutrients or the foods they enjoy.

Diet

Follow the Maker's Diet diligently for six to twelve months. People with weight problems should be careful to avoid or limit high-carbohydrate foods as well as polyunsaturated fats such as corn, soy, and safflower oil. People with metabolic disorders should participate in moderate exercise.

After you have reached your ideal weight, you may gradually add foods from the "Average" or "Trouble" categories if desired. Because people suffering with weight problems appear to have a predisposed weakness in their intestinal tracts, I strongly recommend that they adhere to a diet of foods in the "Extraordinary" category for the rest of their lives.

Therapeutic Foods

These therapeutic foods will help you stay well and lose weight:

Cultured goat's milk dairy products: Consume 8 to 32 ounces of the highest quality cultured dairy products from goat's milk. Try to find yogurt that does not contain the organism *Streptococcus thermophilus*, a bacterial microbe that has been known to make immune system disorders worse.

Grass-fed red meat: Red meat from grass-fed cattle, buffalo, and lamb is very healthy and can be eaten a few times per week. This meat is a great source of protein, minerals, vitamin B$_{12}$, vitamins A and D, omega-3 fats, and CLA.

Organic, pasture-raised eggs: Consume as many as one to three organic eggs high in omega-3 fatty acids each day. These eggs contain DHA, vitamins E and B$_{12}$, and antioxidants including lutein.

Extra virgin coconut oil: This oil is perhaps the healthiest of the widely available oils. I recommend cooking almost exclusively with extra virgin coconut oil. Consume as much as two to four tablespoons per day of the oil in cooking, smoothies, or right off the spoon. Coconut oil contains large amounts of lauric acid, a potent antimicrobial and one of the chief fatty acids found in breast milk.

Ocean-caught fish: This type of fish is perhaps the healthiest of all protein sources. Salmon, sardines, mackerel, herring, and albacore tuna are high in the omega-3 fatty acids EPA and DHA. Ocean-caught fish can be consumed every day to enhance digestive and immune system health.

Cod liver oil: Take one to three teaspoons of an excellent cod liver oil each day, or caplets. The amount consumed should be based upon the amount of sunlight you receive. People in colder climates generally need to consume larger amounts. Cod liver oil is a fantastic source of the omega-3 fats DHA and EPA, as well as fat-soluble vitamins A and D.

Vegetable juice: Consume vegetable juices that are low in carbohydrates, such as celery and green juices mixed with a small amount of higher carbohydrate veggies such as carrot or beet. Mix in some form of healthy fat with each glass of the juice. One to three teaspoons of cultured goat's milk, extra virgin coconut oil, canned or fresh coconut milk and cream, or flaxseed oil enhance absorption of minerals and prevents spikes in blood sugar.

Fermented vegetables: Consume a few tablespoons of fermented vegetables such as sauerkraut with each meal to aid in digestion. Fermented vegetables are an excellent source of naturally occurring probiotics and enzymes.

Stocks: It is a great idea to consume stocks on a regular basis, especially when you have a cold or flu. Stocks made from the bones of chicken, fish, lamb, and beef contain minerals, gelatin, cartilage, collagen, and electrolytes from the vegetables. Stocks are an excellent source of proteins, especially collagen. They help to heal the gut lining and reduce inflammation.

Supplements

Take these health supplements to alleviate symptoms and lose weight:

A probiotic, enzyme, and herbs formulation designed to support good health.

A probiotic with SBOs. Start with one caplet per day on an empty stomach, thirty minutes before or one hour after meals. Increase usage by adding one additional caplet per day (i.e., one caplet the first day, two the second day, three the third day, and so on). Once your dosage is up to twelve caplets per day, stay on that amount for a minimum of three months and then begin to gradually decrease to a maintenance dosage of between three to six caplets per day.

Probiotics with SBOs are best taken first thing in the morning and right before bedtime with eight ounces pure water. Probiotics with SBOs may be taken with other nutritional supplements, but should be taken one hour apart from medications. If you experience symptoms of detoxification (i.e., increased elimination, loose stools, constipation, excess gas,

flu-like symptoms, or fever), reduce the dosage and work up slowly to twelve per day.

A green superfood powder. Take two tablespoons twice daily with eight ounces water or fresh vegetable juice. Best taken on an empty stomach away from food.

Digestive enzymes. Take one to three capsules with each meal or snack.

An organic fiber supplement with chia seed. Consume one serving twice per day, morning and evening, with eight or more ounces of purified water. (Consuming a fiber supplement is essential during the first two weeks of the program. Thereafter, consume fiber as needed.)

A protein powder from bone broth. Take one to three servings per day mixed in water, juice, smoothies, yogurt, or can be used in many recipes.

Additional Therapies

When trying to lose weight, avoiding contact with chlorinated water is of the utmost importance. That includes bathing water and drinking water. Chlorine kills bacteria, friendly and unfriendly, in the intestines and can be absorbed through the skin. I recommend installing a shower filter to remove chlorine. Avoid swimming in chlorinated water as well.

ACKNOWLEDGMENTS

I guess one never realizes how lucky he is to have so many wonderful people in his life until he is asked to thank those who have helped him become who he is today.

I would first like to thank the Lord my God for turning my mourning into gladness and giving me more than I could ever ask for or imagine. You are my Rock and my Salvation.

To my wife of eighteen years, Nicki. Every time I look into your eyes, I *realize* the man I was created to be. Your help and support means more to me than you can ever imagine.

To my mother, who always made me believe that I could accomplish anything I set my mind to. In a dictionary defining the words "a mother's love," there's a display of your picture.

To my father, who laid for me a foundation in natural health that would one day become my life's work. You always knew there was an answer for me. Dad, we found it!

To all of my close friends, if a man ever wonders what kind of person he is, he needs to look no further than the men of valor who surround him. Thank you for sticking with me through thick and thin and agreeing to help me to "never grow old."

SOURCE MATERIAL

Chapter 1

"Since the time of Hippocrates, it has been understood…" is from Van Winkle, E., "The toxic mind: the biology of mental illness and violence." *Medical Hypotheses,* 2000; 55(4): 356–368.

"The article about my recovery generated over two thousand phone calls from doctors…" is from Walker, M., "Medical journalist report of innovative biologics: Homeostatic Soil Organisms support immune system functions from the ground up." *The Townsend Letter for Doctors & Patients,* August/September 1997.

Chapter 3

"Abnormal bacterial populations that lead to dysfunctional gut fermentation have adverse effects on nutrient assimilation and production…" is from Eaton, K.K., et al., "Abnormal gut fermentation: laboratory studies reveal deficiency of B vitamins, zinc, and magnesium." *Journal of Nutritional Biochemistry,* 1993:635-637.

"Digestive, liver, and pancreatic diseases, which often are caused in part by or result in dysbiosis, results in more than 100 million outpatient visits…" can be found at "Costs of Digestive Diseases Has Grown to $141 Billion a Year," by the American Gastroenterological Association, February 10, 2009, and available at https://www.sciencedaily.com/releases/2009/02/090210133922.htm.

"So wide-ranging is the impact of our gut on human health that each of the following conditions may be caused by intestinal toxemia…" is from Anderson, R. "Mucoid plaque." Internet source: www.cleanse.net, accessed October 15, 2002.

"These studies have been accepted for publication in a special supplement of the peer-reviewed *Progress in Nutrition…* " is from Halpem, G.M., et al., "Analysis of the effect of various commercial nutraceutical preparations on the immune system." *Progress in Nutrition,* 2002;4(S1).

Chapter 4

"Antibiotic resistance has become a major public health problems, with more 2 million infections and 23,000 deaths annually…" is from "The hidden societal cost of antibiotic resistance per antibiotic prescribed in the United States." *BMC Infectious Diseases* 2016;16:655, and available at https://www.ncbi.nlm.nih.gov/pmc/articles/PMC5101711/.

"For instance, a medical article published in *Nutrition Reviews*, R. Chang of the Department of Medicine at Memorial Sloan-Kettering Cancer Center…" is from Chang, R., "Functional properties of edible mushrooms." *Nutrition Reviews,* 1996;54(11 Pt 2):S91–93.

Chapter 5

"A lamentable outcome of our modern meat processing techniques…" is excerpted from *Nourishing Traditions: The Cookbook That Challenges Politically Correct Nutrition and the Diet Dictocrats* by Sally Fallon and Mary G. Enig, Ph.D., NewTrends Publishing, 1999.

"An interesting article in the *European Journal of Nutrition* stated that sodium chloride (NaCl)…" is from Frassetto, L., et al., "Diet, evolution and aging—the pathophysiologic effects of the post-agricultural inversion of the potassium to sodium and base to chloride ratios in the human diet." *European Journal of Nutrition,* 2001;40(5):200–213.

"In a Russian-language medical journal, researchers studied changes in joint fluid acid–base balance in sixty-five rheumatoid arthritis patients…" is from Bobkov, V.A., et al., "[Changes in the acid–base status of the synovial fluid in rheumatoid arthritis patients]." *Ter Arkh,* 1999;71(5):20–22.

Chapter 6

"Enzymes are the 'labor force' that builds your body, just like construction workers are the labor force that builds your house…" from *Food Enzymes for Healthy & Longevity* by Dr. Edward Howell, Lotus Press, 1994.

Chapter 7

"In *The Whispering Pond: A Personal Guide to the Emerging Vision of Science,* author Ervin Laszlo gave a version…" is from Gurwitsch, A.G., "Uber Ursachen der Zellteilung." *ArchEntw Mech Org,* 1922;51:383–415.

"Popp, who placed the prefix bio- in front of photons, did so with the intention of suggesting…" is from Popp, FA., et al., "Evidence of non-classical (squeezed) light in biological systems." *Physics Letters A,* 2002;293 (1–2):98–102.

Chapter 8

"I like what popular writer Steve Meyerowitz has to say. He made this observation about grass…" from *Wheat Grass: Nature's Finest Medicine* by S. Meyerowitz, Sproutman Publications, 1999.

"Then in 1939, the *Journal of the American Medical Association Council on Foods* announced that Cerophyl…" is from Cannon, M. & Emerson, G., *Journal of Nutrition,* 1939;18:155.

"In the 1930s and 1940s, America's leading scientists, led by biochemist George Kohler…" is from Kohler, G.O., "The relation of the grass factor to guinea pig nutrition." *Journal of Nutrition,* 1937;15(5):445.

"Authors Sally Fallon and Mary Enig of *Nourishing Traditions* put it this way…" is excerpted from *Nourishing Traditions: The Cookbook That Challenges Politically Correct Nutrition and the Diet Dictocrats* by Sally Fallon and Mary G. Enig, Ph.D., NewTrends Publishing, 1999.

Chapter 9

"Researchers made a survey of cardiovascular disease incidence and related risk factors among 2,300 subsistence horticulturists in the tropical island of Kitava…" is from Lindeberg, S. & Lundh, B., "Apparent absence of stroke and ischaemic heart disease in a traditional Melanesian island: a clinical study in Kitava." *Journal of Internal Medicine,* 1993;233(3):269–275.

"Michael Murray, N.D., a leading natural healing expert, has also written extensively about the absence of modern disease…" from *Encyclopedia of Natural Medicine* by Murray, M. & Pizzomo, J., Prima Publishing, 1998.

"Professor Peter Piper, a professor of molecular biology at Sheffield University…" is from Hickman, M., "Caution: Some soft drinks may seriously harm your health." *The Independent* newspaper, London, England, May 27, 2007.

Chapter 11

"Currently, 9 percent of our population presently has diabetes. That's 30.3 million Americans…" is from "Statistics about Diabetes," American Diabetes Organization, and available at http://www.diabetes.org/diabetes-basics/statistics/.

"Syndrome X, also known as metabolic syndrome, was first coined by a group of researchers at Stanford University…" is from Groop, L.C., "Insulin resistance: the fundamental trigger of type 2 diabetes." *Diabetes Obesity and Metabolism,* 1999;19(suppl.):S1–S7.

"A decline in mental function can have a significant impact on both our physical and emotional health…" is from Barefoot, J.C. & Schroll, M., "Symptoms of depression, acute myocardial infarction, and total mortality in a community sample." *Circulation,* 1996;93:1976–1980.

"Cancer is one of the leading killers in the world today…" is from "Cancer Facts & Figures 2017, American Cancer Society, and available at https://www.cancer.org/research/cancer-facts-statistics/all-cancer-facts-figures/cancer-facts-figures-2017.html.

"More than 800,000 Americans die of cardiovascular disease each year, accounting for one in three deaths..." is from "New Statistics Show One of Every Three U.S. Deaths Caused by Cardiovascular Disease," American Heart Association, available at http://newsroom.heart.org/news/new-statistics-show-one-of-every-three-u-s-deaths-caused-by-cardiovascular-disease.

"What makes the homocysteine theory even more appealing is that Kilmer McCully M.D...." is from "We are living in a graying world..." is from McCully K., "Atherosclerosis, serum cholesterol and the homocysteine theory: a study of 194 consecutive autopsies." *American Journal of Medical Science,* 1990;299:217–221.

"ADHD is implicated in learning disorders and is diagnosed two or three times more frequently in boys than girls, according to Mayo Clinic researchers..." is from "Gender Differences in Children," by Lesley Jamison, Ph.D., and is available at http://cpancf.com/articles_files/art_57attached_file.asp.

"Once considered a rare disorder with an incidence of only one case per 10,000 births thirty years ago..." is from "How Common Is Autism?" from the Autism Science Foundation, and is available at http://autismsciencefoundation.org/what-is-autism/how-common-is-autism/.

"The body converts estradiol, the most potent estrogen, either to "good" estrogen (2-hydroxyestrone)..." is from Davis, D.L. & Bradlow, H.L., "Can environmental estrogens cause breast cancer?" *Scientific American,* October 1, 1995.

"High levels of this bad estrogen are a 'risk marker' or an indication of increased risk of breast cancer..." is from Bradlow, H.L., et al., "Re: estrogen metabolism and excretion in oriental and Caucasian women." *Journal of the National Cancer Institute,* 86(21):1643-1644 and from Taioli, E., et al. "Ethnic differences in estrogen metabolism in healthy women." *Journal of the National Cancer Institute,* 1996;86:617.

"That answer comes to us from a report published in the *European Journal of Clinical Nutrition*..." is from Tarpila, S., et al., "The effect of flaxseed supplementation in processed foods on serum fatty acids and enterolactone." *European Journal of Clinical Nutrition* 2002;56(2):157–165.

"To clinically evaluate whether omega-3 fatty acids protect against breast cancer..." is from Maillard V, et al. "N-3 and N-6 fatty acids in breast adipose tissue and relative risk of breast cancer in a case-control study in Tours, France." *International Journal of Cancer,* 2002;98(l):78–83.

"Irritable bowel syndrome (IBS) and dyspepsia are the most common, notes the International Foundation for Functional Gastrointestinal Disorders…" is from Joint Research Unit for Neurogastroenterology and Nutrition INRA, Universite Toulouse III, Nutrition, Food and Food Safety Department, Toulouse Research Centre.

"Arthritis and related conditions affect more than 50 million Americans…" is from http://www.arthritis.org/about-arthritis/understanding-arthritis/arthritis-statistics-facts.php.

"Ankylosing spondylitis (spinal arthritis) causes immobility of the back and often the shoulders and neck…" is from "Ankylosing Spondylitis," University of Washington Orthopaedics and Sports Medicine, and is available at http://www.orthop.washington.edu/?q=patient-care/articles/arthritis/ankylosing-spondylitis.html.

"Some 30 million Americans suffer from disabling osteoarthritis…" is from "Osteoarthritis," Centers for Disease Control, and is available at https://www.cdc.gov/arthritis/basics/osteoarthritis.htm.

"Rheumatoid arthritis, also known simply as RA, affects about 1.3 million people…" is from "RA and Women's Health," RrheumatoidArthritis.net, and is available at https://rheumatoidarthritis.net/women-health/.

"In terms of gender differentiation, rheumatoid arthritis is most likely to strike women aged thirty to fifty…" is from "How RA Affects Your Body," Healthline.com, and is available at https://www.healthline.com/health/rheumatoid-arthritis-early-signs-and-symptoms#overview1.

"The prostate plays a key role in men's sexuality, providing more than 90 percent of his ejaculate…" is from *The Prostate Report: Prevention and Healing* by J. Whitaker, Phillips Publishing, 1994.

"By age sixty, at least half of all men are suffering from symptoms of an enlarged prostate…" is from "Enlarged Prostrate: A Complex Problem," WebMD.com, and available at https://www.webmd.com/men/prostate-enlargement-bph/features/enlarged-prostate-bph-complex-problem#1.

"Experts believe impotence affects more than 30 million American men…" is from "Impotence Imposes on Relationships," WebMD.com, and is available at https://www.webmd.com/erectile-dysfunction/features/impotence-imposes-on-relationships#1.

"This is buttressed by a Massachusetts Male Aging Study…" is from Feldman, A., et al., "Impotence and its medical and psychological correlate: results of the Massachusetts Male Aging Study." *The Journal of Urology,* 1994;151:54–61.

"An estimated 18 percent of Americans ages eighteen and older—a little less one in five adults—suffer from a diagnosable mental disorder…" is from "Any Mental Illness Among U.S. Adults," National Institutes for Health, and is available at https://www.nimh.nih.gov/health/statistics/prevalence/any-mental-illness-ami-among-us-adults.shtml.

"Anxiety disorders are the most common mental illness in the U.S., affecting 40 million adults in the U.S. eighteen and older…" is from "Understand the Facts," Anxiety and Depression Association of America, and is available at https://adaa.org/understanding-anxiety.

"Approximately 1.8 million American adults ages eighteen and over have agoraphobia with a history of panic disorder…" is from "Agoraphobia Causes, Statistics, Signs, Symptoms & Side Effects," AddictionHope.com, and is available at https://www.addictionhope.com/mood-disorder/agoraphobia/.

"Approximately 16 million American adults, or around 7 percent of the U.S. population age eighteen and older, have a major depressive episode in the last year…" is from "Facts & Statistics," Anxiety and Depression Association of America, and is available at https://adaa.org/about-adaa/press-room/facts-statistics.

"Between 11 percent and 20 percent of new mothers, however, have a greater problem called postpartum depression…" is from "The Statistics," PostpartumProgress.com, and is available at http://postpartumprogress.org/the-facts-about-postpartum-depression/.

"Approximately 2.4 million American adults, or about 1.1 percent of the population age eighteen and older in a given year, have schizophrenia…" is from "Mental Health Facts," National Association for Mental Illness, and is available at https://www.nami.org/NAMI/media/NAMIMedia/Infographics/GeneralMHFacts.pdf.

"Approximately 85 percent of people between the ages of twelve and twenty-four experience at least minor acne…" is from "Acne," American Academy of Dermatology Association, and is available at https://www.aad.org/media/stats/conditions.

"Psoriasis affects around 2 percent of the United States population, or about 7.5 million people…" is from "Everything You Need to Know About Psoriasis," HealthLine.com, and is available at https://www.healthline.com/health/psoriasis.

"Stress can be a killer, which is a medical fact. Neuropsychologist Kenneth R. Pelletier…" is from *Mind as Healer, Mind as Slayer*, by K. Pelletier, Dell Publishing, 1977, p. 6.

"The belief that stress, depression, and hopelessness contribute to susceptibility to disease dates to 200 A.D. when Galen, the Greek physician…" is from Peteet, J.R., "Psychological factors in the causation and course of cancer." *Cancer, Stress, and Death,* [ed. Day, S.B.], Plenum Medical Book Company, 1989: 63–77.

"Landmark studies conducted by psychologist John Barefoot of the Duke University Medical Center conclusively proved that depression plays a role in the development of heart disease…" is from "Conflict with Close Family Can Trigger Unhealthy Levels of Stress and Depression Among Heart Disease Patients," Duke Health, and available at https://corporate.dukehealth.org/news-listing/conflict-close-family-can-trigger-unhealthy-levels-stress-and-depression-among-heart.

"In the Barefoot study, which began in 1964, those people with the highest scores for despair, low self-esteem, difficulties concentrating, and low motivation…" is from "Penetrating the Riddle of Heart Attack," *MIT Technology Review*, and available at https://www.technologyreview.com/s/400087/penetrating-the-riddle-of-heart-attack/.

"Asthma, the leading chronic illness of childhood, is responsible for substantial infant morbidity and has a significant impact on use of our finite health resources…" is from Lozano, P., et al., "The economic burden of asthma in US children: estimates from the National Medical Expenditure Survey," *Journal of Allergy and Clinical Immunology,* 1999;104(5):957–963.

"Other researchers note that asthma prevalence in children doubled from 1980 to 1995 but increased more slowly from 2001 to 2010…" is from "Changing trends in asthma prevalence among children," *Pediatrics* magazine, and available at http://pediatrics.aappublications.org/content/early/2015/12/24/peds.2015-2354.

"Approximately 300,000 adult deaths in the United States each year are related to obesity…" is from "Obesity Kills 300,000 Yearly, StreetDirectory.com, and is available at http://www.streetdirectory.com/travel_guide/48263/lose_weight/obesity_kills_300000_yearly.html.

ABOUT JORDAN RUBIN

Known as America's Biblical Health Coach, Jordan Rubin is a *New York Times* best-selling author of *The Maker's Diet,* TV personality, motivational speaker, organic farmer and founder of Garden of Life, Beyond Organic, and his latest entrepreneurial effort, Ancient Nutrition, which he co-founded with Dr. Josh Axe and which specializes in bone-broth protein products. Jordan has spent nearly twenty years studying naturopathic medicine, nutrition, and permaculture science. Jordan and his wife, Nicki, have six amazing children.

Experience a personal revival!

Spirit-empowered content from today's top Christian authors delivered directly to your inbox.

Join today!
lovetoreadclub.com

Inspiring Articles

Powerful Video Teaching

Resources for Revival

Get all of this and so much more, e-mailed to you twice weekly!

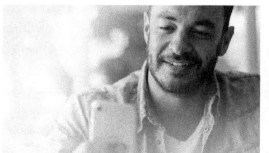

LOVE TO READ CLUB

by **D DESTINY IMAGE**

CPSIA information can be obtained
at www.ICGtesting.com
Printed in the USA
LVHW080422070919
630294LV00004B/12/P